NUTRITION IN EXERCISE AND SPORT

Ira Wolinsky and James Hickson, *Series Editors*

Published Titles

Exercise and Disease, *Ronald Watson and Marianne Eisinger*

Forthcoming Titles

Nutrients as Ergogenic Aids in Sports and Exercise, *Luke Bucci*

Nutrition Applied to Injury Rehabilitation and Sports Medicine, *Luke Bucci*

Nutrition in Exercise and Sport, 2nd Edition, *Ira Wolinsky and James Hickson*

EXERCISE
AND
DISEASE

Ronald R. Watson, Ph.D.
Director
NIAA Specialized Alcohol Research Center
University of Arizona
Tucson, Arizona

Marianne Eisinger, Ph.D.
Department of Family and Community Medicine
University of Arizona
Tucson, Arizona

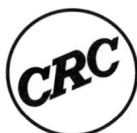

CRC Press
Boca Raton   Ann Arbor   London   Tokyo

Library of Congress Cataloging-in-Publication Data

Exercise and disease / [edited by] Ronald R. Watson and Marianne
Eisinger.
    p. cm. -- (Nutrition in exercise and sport)
    Includes bibliographical references and index.
    ISBN 0-8493-7912-1
    1. Exercise therapy. 2. Exercise--Physiological effect.
  I. Watson, Ronald R. (Ronald Ross) II. Eisinger, Marianne.
  III. Series.
    [DNLM: 1. Exercise--physiology. 2. Preventive Medicine. QT 260
E955]
  RM725.E9 1992
  612'.04--dc20
  DNLM/DLC
  for Library of Congress   92-4003
        CIP

CONTENTS

SERIES PREFACE

The series *Nutrition in Exercise and Sport* is designed to provide the setting for in-depth exploration of the many and varied aspects of nutrition and exercise, including sport. The topic of sports nutrition gained real interest among physiologists in the 1960s, and since then, numerous scientific studies have been performed, many of which have focused on the healthful benefits of good nutrition and exercise. As we enter the present decade (1990s) and move forward, scientists will search ever more for the elusive "optimum" nutritional preparation. As they try to unlock nature's secrets, it will be necessary to remember that there must be a range of diets that will support excellent physical performance. Yet, there will inevitably be attempts by scientists and laymen alike to distill the diets to some common denominator — a formula for success. *Nutrition in Exercise and Sport* is dedicated to providing a stage to explore these issues. Each volume seeks to provide a detailed and scholarly examination of some aspect of the topic. Ultimately, the series will comprise a set of authoritative volumes for consultation by scientists, physicians, and a broad range of health care providers and individuals who participate in exercise and sport, whether for recreation or competition.

We welcome the contribution by Ronald R. Watson and Marianne Eisinger, *Exercise and Disease,* to the series.

James F. Hickson, Jr., Ph.D., R.D.
Ira Wolinsky, Ph.D.
Series Editors

PREFACE

During the last 20 years, physical activity has become a major public health goal of worldwide importance. Economic growth and development are accompanied by a less active lifestyle and diminished physical activity, while mortality rates from chronic diseases are rising. The link between physical exercise and its effect on disease prevention and health promotion seems clear. However, problems in measuring physical activity, the broad spectrum of specific disease, and the various types of physical exercise used, turn scientific efforts to determine cause-effect relationships into a complex task.

It was our intention to provide a summary of the most recent information in this field, as well as a current update. Featured in this volume are the therapeutic and disease-prevention properties of physical exercise. Recently, the growing research in immunology joined the search for an understanding of the effects of exercise on health promotion. It is a fascinating new step towards a discovery of the underlying causes and mechanisms of physical activity and exercise; however, it also enlarges the problem of complexity. This volume contains a detailed resume of the immunologist involvement in the exercise-disease interaction.

As we have tried to reduce overlapping among various chapters, we have found some unavoidable, not only because of its reinforcement value, but also for a different interpretation by the author.

Based upon increasing knowledge through scientific progress, the policies and programs for public health should finally lead to postponed mortality and a better quality of life.

THE EDITORS

Ronald R. Watson, Ph.D. initiated and directs the Specialized Alcohol Research Center at The University of Arizona College of Medicine. The main theme of this NIAAA center grant is to understand the role of ethanol-induced immunosuppression on disease and disease resistance in animals. He has edited 24 books.

Dr. Watson attended the University of Idaho and graduated from Brigham Young University in Provo, Utah with a degree in Chemistry in 1966. He completed his Ph.D. degree in 1971 in Biochemistry from Michigan State University. His postdoctoral schooling was completed at the Harvard School of Public Health in Nutrition and Microbiology, including a two-year post-doctoral research experience in Immunology. He was an Assistant Professor of Immunology and did research at the University of Mississippi Medical Center in Jackson from 1973 to 1974. He was an Assistant Professor of Microbiology and Immunology at the Indiana University Medical School from 1974 to 1978. He was an Associate Professor at Purdue University in the Department of Food and Nutrition from 1978 to 1982. In 1982, he joined the faculty at The University of Arizona in the Department of Family and Community Medicine, Nutrition Section, and is a Research Professor. He has published 225 research papers and review chapters.

Dr. Watson is a member of several national and international nutrition, immunology, and cancer societies, as well as research societies on alcoholism.

Marianne Eisinger, Ph.D. received her Master's degree in Human Nutrition and Home Economics from the Justus Liebig University, Giessen, Germany, in 1983. From 1983 to 1985, she worked in public health education focusing on nutrition related disorders. She has published numerous papers in that field.

From 1985 to 1987, she worked at a cancer clinic as a research associate and nutrition counselor before becoming a research associate in Human Nutrition and Sports Medicine at the Institute of Nutrition, Justus Liebig University, Giessen, and Johannes Gutenberg University, Mainz, Germany, where she received a Ph.D. in Human Nutrition. Her current major research interests comprise policies and programs in public health education.

CONTRIBUTORS

Louis C. Almekinders, M.D.
Assistant Professor, Attending
 Physician
Department of Orthopaedic
 Surgery
University of North Carolina
Chapel Hill, North Carolina

Sally V. Almekinders, M.Ed.
Assistant Professor
Department of Physical Education
North Carolina State University
Raleigh, North Carolina

Manfred Baumstark, Ph.D.
Department of Physical
 Performance Medicine
Center of Internal Medicine
Freiburg University Hospital
Freiburg, Germany

Aloys Berg, M.D.
Professor
Department of Physical
 Performance Medicine
Center of Internal Medicine
Freiburg University Hospital
Freiburg, Germany

**Patricia A. Brill, M.Ed.,
 M.S.S., Ph.D.**
Research Associate
Exercise Physiology
The Cooper Institute for Aerobics
 Research
Dallas, Texas

Rod K. Dishman, Ph.D.
Professor and Director, Exercise
 Psychology Lab
Department of Exercise Science
The University of Georgia
Athens, Georgia

Ingrid Frey, Ph.D.
Department of Physical
 Performance Medicine
Center of Internal Medicine
Freiburg University Hospital
Freiburg, Germany

Michael I. Goran, Ph.D.
Research Assistant Professor
Department of Medicine, Division
 of Endocrinology, Metabolism
 and Nutrition
University of Vermont
Burlington, Vermont

**Neil F. Gordon, M.D., Ph.D.,
 M.P.H.**
Director
Exercise Physiology
The Cooper Institute for Aerobics
 Research
Dallas, Texas

Martin Halle, M.D.
Department of Physical
 Performance Medicine
Center of Internal Medicine
Freiburg University Hospital
Freiburg, Germany

Laurie Hoffman-Goetz, Ph.D.
Professor
Department of Health Studies
Faculty of Applied Health
 Sciences
University of Waterloo
Waterloo, Ontario, Canada

David Keast, Ph.D.
Associate Professor
Department of Microbiology
University of Western Australia
Nedlands, Australia

Joseph Keul, M.D.
Professor and Director
Department of Physical
  Performance Medicine
Center of Internal Medicine
Freiburg University Hospital
Freiburg, Germany

Brian MacNeil, B.Sc.
Doctoral Candidate
Department of Kinesiology
Faculty of Applied Health
  Sciences
University of Waterloo
Waterloo, Ontario, Canada

Robert S. Mazzeo, Ph.D.
Assistant Professor
Department of Kinesiology
University of Colorado
Boulder, Colorado

Alan R. Morton, Ed.D.
Associate Professor
Department of Human Movement
  Studies
University of Western Australia
Nedlands, Australia

Imran Nasrullah, M.S.
Research Associate
Department of Neuroendocrine
  Immunology
Joslin Diabetes Center
Boston, Massachusetts

Sandra L. Nehlsen-Cannarella,
  Ph.D.
Director
Surgery and Pathology Department
Immunology Center
Loma Linda University
Loma Linda, California

David C. Nieman, D.H.Sc.,
  M.P.H.
Associate Professor
Department of Health, Leisure,
  and Exercise Science
Appalachian State University
Boone, North Carolina

Eric T. Poehlman, Ph.D.
Assistant Professor
Department of Medicine and
  Nutritional Sciences
University of Vermont
Burlington, Vermont

Christopher B. Scott, M.S.,
  M.S.S.
Research Associate
Exercise Physiology
The Cooper Institute for Aerobics
  Research
Dallas, Texas

Tony J. Verde, Ph.D.
Physiologist
Human Performance Division
The Graduate Hospital Human
  Performance and Sports Medicine
  Center
Wayne, Pennsylvania

Maryl L. Winningham, RN,
  Ph.D., FACSM
Assistant Professor
College of Nursing
The University of Utah
Salt Lake City, Utah

Chapter 1

THE ROLE OF PHYSICAL ACTIVITY IN THE DEVELOPMENT OF CHILDHOOD OBESITY*

Michael I. Goran and Eric T. Poehlman

TABLE OF CONTENTS

* Supported by grants from the American Diabetes Association (MIG), NIA AG-07857 (ETP),
  and the Andrus Foundation for the American Association of Retired Persons (ETP).

I. INTRODUCTION

Obesity, or excess body fat stores, currently affects 25% of children and is one of the main causes of pediatric hypertension. Obesity also leads to other secondary medical complications, including those of psychosocial and orthopedic origin. In addition, childhood obesity remains a high risk factor for non-insulin-dependent diabetes, coronary heart disease, and early death when it persists into adulthood. Paradoxically, the incidence of obesity in children is rapidly increasing despite a general rise in the awareness of health and fitness in our society. The underlying causes of childhood obesity are poorly understood, especially with regard to the role of energy intake and energy expenditure in regulating body energy stores. Needless to say, the development of obesity is more complicated than simply the result of over-eating. The purpose of this chapter is to specifically examine and review the role of energy expenditure associated with physical activity in the pathogenesis of childhood obesity.

II. BACKGROUND

Obesity is defined as an accumulation of excess body fat and has been estimated to occur in 25% of children.[1] This condition is the main cause of hypertension in children and accounts for 25% of all cases of non-insulin-dependent diabetes.[1] In addition, childhood obesity is the underlying cause of other medical problems of psychosocial and orthopedic origins. Moreover, when obesity persists into adulthood, it remains a high risk factor for coronary heart disease and early death. Although our society is tending to become more health and fitness conscious, the problem of obesity in young children is worsening. In children aged 6 to 11 years, the incidence rates of obesity (defined as a triceps skinfold greater than the 85th percentile) and superobesity (defined as a triceps skinfold greater than the 95th percentile) have increased by 54 and 98%, respectively, over the last 15 years.[2,3]

Although there is much indirect evidence for the persistence of obesity into adulthood, the lack of long term longitudinal data casts doubt over the exact risk factor linking childhood obesity to adulthood obesity.[4] However, the familial trend of obesity has been clearly established.[5,6] The chance of a child becoming obese is 80% if both parents are obese, 40% if one parent is obese, and 7% if neither is obese.[5,7] There is little information on whether the familial clustering of obesity is different in the various forms of obesity. The physiological basis of this heritability is unclear, but is undoubtedly the result of "an interaction of a susceptible host with an environment that promotes disease."[2]

Although the pathogenesis of obesity remains elusive, the condition must be the end result of an imbalance between energy intake and energy expenditure. Energy intake is the caloric content of food that is consumed and absorbed into the body. When there is no change in body energy stores, total daily energy intake is equivalent to total daily energy expenditure. Total daily energy expenditure is composed of three components: resting metabolic rate, thermic effect of food, and energy expenditure associated with physical activity. The resting metabolic rate constitutes about 60% of daily energy expenditure, and is the caloric cost of metabolic processes required to sustain physiological function. The resting metabolic rate is primarily body-size dependent, and is most significantly correlated with lean body mass.[8] The thermic effect of food is the caloric cost of digestion and mobilization of food, comprising about 10% of daily energy expenditure.[9] The energy expenditure associated with physical activity is the most variable component, and has been shown to range from between 30 and 80% of daily energy expenditure in sedentary women[10] and Tour de France cyclists,[11] respectively, and from between 10 and 43% of total energy expenditure in a group of healthy, free-living elderly persons.[12] In children, the energy expenditure required for growth is significant only during early infancy and adolescence, and in young growing children only accounts for about 2% of daily energy expenditure.[13]

Energy expenditure can be measured by a variety of techniques. Direct calorimetry measures heat produced by the body, and indirect calorimetry measures energy expenditure via respiratory gas analysis. Although these methods are both accurate and precise, the main drawback is that energy expenditure can only be measured under sedentary conditions for small periods of time (hours) or longer (days) if whole body chambers are available. The doubly labeled water method is a relatively new research tool that allows accurate[14] and precise[15] measurement of energy expenditure over extended time periods (days to weeks) in subjects who are truly free-living (i.e., living in their normal environment and performing their regular activities). This method is an isotopic approach to indirect calorimetry that directly measures carbon dioxide production. With knowledge of an estimated 24-h food quotient from the composition of the diet, energy expenditure can be calculated. As reviewed elsewhere, the availability of the doubly labeled water technique is beginning to revolutionize our general understanding of the role of energy expenditure in regulating energy balance and energy requirements.[16,17] The resurgence of information is based on the fact that energy expenditure can now be measured by a noninvasive, isotopic approach in which subjects can go about their normal habitual daily activities without constraints on their daily activities.

The doubly labeled water method can also be used to indirectly derive the daily energy expenditure associated with physical activity. This can be achieved by measuring total energy expenditure using doubly labeled water and measuring resting energy expenditure by respiratory gas analysis. With this approach, the energy expenditure of physical activity is equivalent to total energy expenditure minus resting energy expenditure and the energy expenditure of the thermic effect feeding, which is estimated to be 10% of total energy expenditure.[9]

III. OBESITY AND ENERGY EXPENDITURE

The dramatic rise in the incidence of childhood obesity over recent years[2,3] could be reflecting a general increase in sedentary activities in children (e.g., watching more television) with an inappropriately excessive level of energy intake. This concept is supported by data reviewed by Dietz and Gortmaker, showing that the number of hours spent watching television at age 6 to 11 is a powerful predictor for the development of obesity by age 12 to 17 years.[3] Dietz and Strasburger have provided a comprehensive review on the health consequences of television viewing in children.[18] The most extensive data on television viewing in children were collected in a survey designed to help corporate companies select effective commercial time. The data show that 2 to 5 year olds and 6 to 11 year olds watch television for approximately 28 and 24 h per week, respectively. Therefore, as pointed out by Dietz and Strasburger, young children appear to be spending more time in front of the television than in school when the data are considered on an annual basis.[18] There are, however, some limitations to these data. The first concern is selection bias, since data were only collected from surveyed households willing to participate. In addition, the data were based on whether the households concerned had the television set turned on and, in this particular study, the households were asked to electronically "key in" the information on which family members were viewing. Thus, it is possible that children "keyed in" as watching television might actually be performing other activities at the same time or, alternatively, that the television was on, but not being watched.

Given these limitations, there is a general belief, however, that young children are watching too much television. Increased television viewing is a risk factor for obesity for a number of reasons. First, it promotes general inactivity and takes time away from other physical activities, although it is recognized that television viewing is not always a totally passive activity.[18] Furthermore, because of commercials, television viewing influences food intake behavior (for example, the promotion of snack foods) and, moreover, television viewing promotes increased snacking.[19]

The data concerning increased television viewing as a risk factor for obesity could be considered as a behavioral or a social risk factor. There is, however, evidence from a more physiological standpoint that low rates of energy expenditure may be a risk factor in the development of obesity in children. In 1976, for example, Griffiths and Payne measured energy expenditure in 20 nonobese children aged 4 to 5 years[20] who were categorized as being at either high (at least one obese parent) or low risk (two lean parents) of becoming obese later in life. Energy expenditure was measured using the heart rate method, which involves measuring daily heart rate and converting to energy expenditure by performing individual calibrations between heart rate and oxygen consumption. Energy expenditure was found to be 22% lower in children who had at least one obese parent when compared to children with two lean parents (1174 ± 297 kcal/d vs. 1508 ± 352 kcal/d; $p < 0.01$), even though the two groups of children were matched for weight and lean body mass. The same difference was noted for resting energy expenditure (999 ± 146 kcal/d vs. 1183 ± 184 kcal/d; p < 0.05). A similar trend was noted for the energy expenditure associated with physical activity, derived by subtracting resting energy expenditure from total daily energy expenditure, but this did not reach statistical significance.

The study of Griffiths and Payne[20] was the first to suggest a defect in energy expenditure in pre-obese children. However, the heart rate method used by Griffiths and Payne for measurement of energy expenditure is not ideal. Standard methods for calibrating heart rate with energy expenditure (or oxygen consumption) are not reliable.[21] When heart rate monitoring was compared with the doubly labeled water method, the average energy expenditures using either technique compared well, but the discrepancy between the two techniques ranged from −22.2 to +52.1%.[22] In addition, subjects wearing heart rate monitors are aware that activity is being monitored and behavior may be modified. A further concern of the study of Griffiths and Payne is that it is not known whether the children with lower energy expenditure actually became obese in later years.

In a similar study, Payne et al. later reported findings on energy intake in a group of younger pre-obese children, aged 3 to 5 years.[23] Energy intake in children with one obese parent was 16% lower than in children matched in age and weight with no obese parent (1103 ± 196 kcal/d vs. 1314 ± 257 kcal/d; p < 0.02). A recent study reported observations on the same children 12 years later.[24] In this follow up study, gender differences were observed. Parental obesity failed to predict the development of adiposity in boys, but did predict an earlier decline in the resting energy expenditure, a known risk factor for body weight gain.[25] In addition, energy intake in young boys did not predict development of obesity. In contrast, energy intake of young girls did predict adiposity later in life. Although these studies supply useful longitudinal information, the conclusions are based on reported values of food intake which are known to be underestimated, particularly in obese individuals,[26,27] and this general effect is more pronounced in females than in males.[12]

In 1986, Avons and James measured daily energy expenditure by direct calorimetry in young men aged 17 to 27 years who had either one parent with a history of severe obesity (>30% above ideal body weight at some time during their adult life), or both parents with no weight problem.[28] In contrast to the findings of Griffiths and Payne,[20] both groups had similar energy expenditure during the standardized protocol in the calorimeter, even when results were expressed per kilogram fat-free mass. However, as the authors point out, the young men with one obese parent tended to be fatter (19.8 ± 2.1% body fat) than the young men with lean parents (13.7 ± 1.1% body fat). Close inspection of the group of young men with one obese parent revealed that three were lean (body fat 15.2 ± 2.8%) and four were obese (23.2 ± 1.5% body fat). In the three who were lean, daily energy expenditure tended to be lower than the lean men with two lean parents (3569 ± 155 kcal/d vs. 3735 ± 74 kcal/d). This study highlights the importance of studying children before they express obese tendencies. In addition, standardized activity schedules in a confining calorimeter do not represent real life situations and may mask true physiological differences related to differences in habitual lifestyle.

The first study to use the newly available doubly labeled water technique to examine the issue of energy expenditure during the development of obesity was reported by Roberts et al.[29] In this study, energy expenditure was examined in infants (age 3 months) born to either lean or overweight mothers. The conclusion of this study supports the data of Griffiths and Payne,[20] in that daily energy expenditure was 20% lower in the infants born to overweight mothers compared to infants born to lean methods (61.2 ± 6.5 kcal/kg/d vs. 77.2 ± 3.4 kcal/kg/d; $p < 0.05$). Moreover, the infants with lower energy expenditure at 3 months gained more weight during the first year of life.

A number of studies using the Pima Indian model of obesity also suggest that low rates of energy expenditure are involved in the familial aggregation of obesity.[30] These studies demonstrate a familial dependence of resting energy expenditure, independent of the other factors known to contribute to variations in energy expenditure.[31] Another study confirmed that a reduced rate of energy expenditure is a marker for weight gain, since subsequent weight gain was greater in individuals who had a lower rate of resting and 24-h energy expenditure.[25]

There have also been a number of studies in which total energy expenditure has been measured in free living, obese individuals using the doubly labeled water technique. The results from those studies do not provide evidence for a role of energy expenditure (even after adjustment for differences in body mass and lean body mass) in obese adolescents (12 to 18 years old) when compared to non-obese controls.[32] In addition, studies on obese women using the doubly labeled water technique to measure daily energy expenditure conclude that energy expenditure is elevated, but that the difference is entirely explained by the larger body mass of the obese.[33] The conflicting findings of the studies in the pre-obese state compared to the obese state emphasizes that energy expenditure is important in the development, but not necessarily the maintenance, of obesity.

IV. OTHER FACTORS INVOLVED IN THE DEVELOPMENT OF OBESITY

The overall regulation of energy balance via changes in energy intake and energy expenditure is influenced by other factors, including those of environmental and genetic origin. The belief that obese families tend to have obese pets suggests a strong environmental factor to obesity. However, it is not known whether the pets in question become obese because of the environmental factors associated with overfeeding, underexercising, or a combination of both. Although environmental factors relating to food intake and energy expenditure are clearly involved, there is firm evidence supporting the concept that susceptibility to becoming obese is, at least in part, genotype dependent. For example, Bouchard et al. overfed identical twins by 1000 kcal/d for 100 d and showed that the ability to adapt to this overfeeding was genotype dependent.[34,35] In these studies, body weight gain in response to the overfeeding was variable between sets of twins but consistent within, and this was related to metabolic adaptations in resting energy expenditure.[34,35] Interindividual variation in the adaptability of resting energy expenditure during periods of overfeeding may, therefore, explain the widespread variation between individuals in body fat content. Thus, for example, we could speculate that lean children of obese parents would gain more weight than lean children of lean parents when challenged with the same degree of excess caloric intake because of genetic differences in the ability to adapt to overfeeding. However, the biological mechanisms that would tend to promote increased fat deposition remain to be determined.

The aforementioned studies suffer from the limitation that the genetic component is not discernable from the environmental component. It is, therefore, of interest to examine the data of Stunkard et al.[36,37] who studied body mass index as a marker of body fatness in twins who were either reared apart, or in children who were adopted. In studying adoptees, they found significant associations between fatness of the adoptees and fatness in their genetic parents, but no association with fatness in their adopted parents, thus diminishing the role of environmental influences on body fatness. Further studies in twins reared apart also suggested that the environment during childhood development had a limited effect on body fatness later in life.[36]

V. CAN PHYSICAL ACTIVITY BE USED TO PREVENT THE DEVELOPMENT OF OBESITY?

Like adult obesity, childhood obesity has proven difficult to cure. Dietz has reviewed data from seven intervention studies designed to cure obesity in a total of 162 children and adolescents,[38] and the message is a pessimistic one. The key to controlling the worsening health problem of obesity may, therefore, be in prevention rather than cure. Since inactivity and low rates of energy expenditure would seem to be an important risk factor for obesity, it is clear that increased daily energy expenditure via physical activity will play a crucial role in the prevention of obesity. The goal of this approach is to use physical activity to increase total energy expenditure in children at risk of becoming obese, and to longitudinally examine its impact on the regulation of body energy stores and the subsequent development of obesity. However, this is not as straightforward as it would appear, since it is not yet known how increasing the level of physical activity impacts on energy intake and the other components of energy expenditure (resting energy expenditure, thermic effect of a meal, etc.) in children, and whether the response is different among children varying in their susceptibility to becoming obese. It is not an unlikely scenario that extreme levels of physical activity in some children may actually decrease energy expenditure during nonexercising time, thus diminishing the energy enhancing benefits of physical activity on total daily energy expenditure.

Putting the scientific issues aside, the practical matter is that children are unlikely to participate in regimented exercise programs. Childhood is a time for "free play" and the regimentation of physical activity patterns seems impractical and counterproductive to instilling an appreciation for physical activity later in the adult years. An alternative approach would be to have parents provide an atmosphere that encourages a physically active existence in combination with sound nutritional practices. This atmosphere can be achieved by having parents serve as role models themselves by participating regularly in physical activity and by providing ample opportunity for "active free play" instead of encouraging sedentary activities (i.e., watching television).

The educational system should also take an active role in promoting and teaching physical activity. First, physical education (or physical activity) classes should be provided to all students on a regular basis. The curriculum should focus on teaching the physiological basis of physical fitness and how students can effectively plan for their own personal fitness needs later in the adult years. It is discouraging to see how many adults are unaware of such basic information regarding the frequency, intensity, and duration that is required to improve cardiovascular fitness. Physical education programs should de-emphasize the teaching of team sports, as many of these activities have limited fitness and life-time participation values and probably promote a "spectator mentality" later on in the adult years.

VI. CONCLUSION

Childhood obesity is a worsening health problem that affects the general health status of our society. Since there does not appear to be any effective cures for obesity, the key to controlling this worsening health problem may be via far-sighted prevention programs. Unfortunately, effective preventive programs will remain elusive until the sequence of events leading to obesity, with regard to the balance between energy intake and energy expenditure, are fully understood. However, there is substantial evidence indicating that low activity levels and low rates of resting energy expenditure are important risk factors for the development of childhood obesity. Therefore, education of the importance of physical activity is a crucial line of defense for the prevention of childhood obesity.

REFERENCES

1. **Dietz, W.H.,** Childhood obesity: susceptibility, cause, and management, *J. Pediatr.,* 103, 676, 1983.
2. **Dietz, W.H., Bandini, L.G., and Gortmaker, S.,** Epidemiologic and metabolic risk factors for childhood obesity, *Klin. Paediatr.,* 202, 69, 1990.
3. **Dietz, W.H. and Gortmaker, S.L.,** Do we fatten our children at the television set? Obesity and television viewing in children and adolescents, *Pediatrics,* 75, 807, 1985.
4. **Johnston, F.E.,** Health implications of childhood obesity, *Ann. Intern. Med.,* 103, 1068, 1985.
5. **Garn, S.M. and Clark, D.C.,** Trends in fatness and the origins of obesity, *Pediatrics,* 57, 443, 1976.
6. **Garn, S.M.,** *Curr. Probs. Peds.,* 15, 1, 1985.
7. **Paige, D.M.,** Obesity in childhood and adolescence: special problems in diagnosis and treatment, *Postgrad. Med.,* 79, 233, 1986.
8. **Ravussin, E., Lillioja, S., Anderson, T.E., Christin, L., and Bogardus, C.,** Determinants of 24-hour energy expenditure in man. Methods and results using a respiratory chamber, *J. Clin. Invest.,* 78, 1568, 1986.
9. **Poehlman, E.T., Melby, C.L., and Badylack, S.F.,** Relation of age and physical exercise status on metabolic rate in younger and older healthy men, *J. Gerontol.,* 46, B54, 1991.
10. **Prentice, A.M., Davies, H.L., Black, A.E., Ashford, J., Coward, W.A., Murgatroyd, P.R., Goldberg, G.R., and Sawyer, M.,** Unexpectedly low levels of energy expenditure in healthy women, *Lancet,* p. 1419, 1985.
11. **Westerterp, K.R., Saris, W.H., van Es, M., and ten Hoor, F.,** Use of the doubly labeled water technique in humans during heavy sustained exercise, *J. Appl. Physiol.,* 61, 2162, 1986.
12. **Goran, M.I. and Poehlman, E.T.,** Total energy expenditure and energy requirements in healthy elderly persons, *Metabolism,* in press, 1992.
13. WHO, Energy and Protein Requirements, World Health Organization, Technical Report Series, No. 724, World Health Organization, Geneva, 1985.
14. **Schoeller, D.A., Ravussin, E., Schutz, Y., Acheson, K.J., Baertschi, P., and Jequier, E.,** Energy expenditure by doubly labeled water: validation in humans and proposed calculation, *Am. J. Physiol. Regul. Integr. Comp. Physiol.,* 250, R823, 1986.
15. **Goran, M.I., Beer, W.H., Wolfe, R.R., Poehlman, E. T., and Young, V.R.,** Variation in total energy expenditure in healthy free-living subjects, unpublished, 1992.
16. **Schoeller, D.A.,** Measurement of energy expenditure in free-living humans by using doubly labeled water, *J. Nutr.,* 118, 1278, 1988.
17. **Roberts, S.B.,** Use of the doubly labeled water method for measurement of energy expenditure, total body water, water intake, and metabolizable energy intake in humans and small animals, *Can. J. Physiol. Pharmacol.,* 67, 1190, 1989.
18. **Dietz, W.H. and Strasburger, V.C.,** Children, adolescents, and television, *Curr. Probs. Peds.,* 1, 8, 1991.
19. **Taras, H.L., Sallis, J.F., Patterson, T.L., Nader, P.R., and Nelson, J.A.,** Television's influence on children's diet and physical activity, *J. Dev. Behav. Pediatr.,* 10, 176, 1989.
20. **Griffiths, M. and Payne, P.R.,** Energy expenditure in small children of obese and nonobese parents, *Nature (London),* 260, 698, 1976.
21. **Dauncey, M.J. and James, W.P.T.,** Assessment of the heart-rate method for determining energy expenditure in man, using a whole-body calorimeter, *Br. J. Nutr.,* 42, 1, 1979.
22. **Livingstone, M.B.E., Prentice, A.M., Coward, W.A., Ceesay, S.M., Strain, J.J., McKenna, P.G., Nevin, G.B., Barker, M.E., and Hickey, R.J.,** Simultaneous measurement of free-living energy expenditure by the doubly labeled water method and heart-rate monitoring, *Am. J. Clin. Nutr.,* 52, 59, 1990.

23. **Griffiths, M., Rivers, J.P.W., and Payne, P.R.,** Energy intake in children at high risk of obesity, *Hum. Nutr. Clin. Nutr.,* 41C, 425, 1987.

24. **Griffiths, M., Payne, P.R., Stunkard, A.J., Rivers, J.P.W., and Cox, M.,** Metabolic rate and physical development in children at risk of obesity, *Lancet,* 336, 76, 1990.

25. **Ravussin, E., Lillioja, S., Knowler, W.C., Christin, L., Freymond, D., Abbott, W.G.H., Boyce, V., Howard, B.V., and Bogardus, C.,** Reduced rate of energy expenditure as a risk factor for body-weight gain, *N. Engl. J. Med.,* 318, 467, 1988.

26. **Schoeller, D.A., Bandini, L.G., and Dietz, W.H.,** Inaccuracies in self-reported intake identified by comparison with the doubly labeled water method, *Can. J. Physiol. Pharmacol.,* 68, 941, 1990.

27. **Schoeller, D.A.,** How accurate is self-reported dietary energy intake? *Nutr. Rev.,* 48, 373, 1990.

28. **Avons, P. and James, P.T.,** Energy expenditure of young men from obese and non-obese families, *Hum. Nutr. Clin. Nutr.,* 40C, 259, 1986.

29. **Roberts, S.B., Savage, J., Coward, W.A., Chew, B., and Lucas, A.,** Energy expenditure and intake in infants born to lean and overweight mothers, *N. Engl. J. Med.,* 318, 461, 1988.

30. **Bogardus, C., Lillioja, S., and Ravussin, E.,** The pathogenesis of obesity in man: results of studies of Pima Indians, *Int. J. Obesity,* 14 (Suppl. 1), 5, 1990.

31. **Bogardus, C., Lilloja, S., Ravussin, E., Abbott, W., Zawadzki, J.K., Young, A., Knowler, W.C., Jacobowitz, R., and Moll, P.P.,** Familial dependence of the resting metabolic rate, *N. Engl. J. Med.,* 315, 96, 1986.

32. **Bandini, L.G., Schoeller, D.A., and Dietz, W.H.,** Energy expenditure in lean and obese adolescents, *Pediatr. Res.,* 27, 198, 1990.

33. **Prentice, A.M., Black, A.E., Coward, W.A., Davies, H.L., Goldberg, R.R., Murgatroyd, P.R., Ashford, J., Sawer, M., and Whitehead, R.G.,** High levels of energy expenditure in obese women, *Br. Med. J.,* 292, 983, 1986.

34. **Bouchard, C., Tremblay, A., Despres, J.P., Nadeau, A., Lupien, P.J., Theriault, G., Dussault, J., Moorjani, S., Pinault, S., and Fournier, G.,** The response to long-term overfeeding in identical twins, *N. Engl. J. Med.,* 322, 1477, 1990.

35. **Bouchard, C. and Tremblay, A.,** Genetic effects in human energy expenditure components, *Int. J. Obesity,* 14 (Suppl. 1), 49, 1990.

36. **Stunkard, A.J., Harris, J.R., Pedersen, N.L., and McClearn, G.E.,** The body-mass index of twins who have been reared apart, *N. Engl. J. Med.,* 322, 1483, 1990.

37. **Stunkard, A.J., Sorensen, T.I.A., Hanis, C., Teasdale, T.W., Chakraborty, R., Schull, W.J., and Schulsinger, F.,** An adoption study of human obesity, *N. Engl. J. Med.,* 314, 193, 1986.

38. **Dietz, W.H.,** Prevention of childhood obesity, *Pediatr. Clin. North Am.,* 33, 19203, 1986.

Chapter 2

EXERCISE AND CARDIOVASCULAR DISEASE: A GENDER DIFFERENCE

Patricia A. Brill, Christopher B. Scott, and Neil F. Gordon

TABLE OF CONTENTS

I. INTRODUCTION

Life expectancy for a woman today is 78 years, whereas life expectancy for a man is 72 years in the U.S.[1] The wide gap in the life expectancy of men and women reflects an apparent sex difference in mortality rates, with women having the distinct advantage.[2,3] The most important contributor to the difference in mortality rates between men and women in this country is coronary heart disease (CHD). However, although women have been considered to be protected from this disease, it is also the leading cause of death in women aged 50 years and older, and accounts for approximately 250,000 deaths per year in women aged 35 to 74 years.

The CHD mortality rate for male Americans is 298.3 per 1000 persons, whereas the CHD mortality rate for female Americans is 265.2 per 1000 persons.[4] The lower incidence of CHD mortality and morbidity in women is believed to be due largely to four factors.[5] First, there is a lower prevalence of CHD risk factors in women.[6] These risk factors include cigarette smoking, systolic blood pressure, serum lipids and lipoproteins, glucose tolerance, body weight, and physical inactivity. Second, women have a better tolerance for CHD risk factors.[5] This is evidenced by the fact that men develop atherosclerosis at a faster rate than women with a similar risk factor profile. Third, differences in hormonal and consequent metabolic factors apparently provide women with a protective edge. Estrogen seems to provide a protective factor while androgens seem to increase the risk of CHD.[7,8] Finally, there exists a difference in clinical presentation of the disease. Angina is more likely to be the initial presentation of CHD in women, as opposed to myocardial infarction or sudden death in men. The prevalence of angina is similar in men and women, but the prevalence of myocardial infarction and sudden death is greater in men.[9,10]

In recent years, many studies have focused on the role of physical activity, exercise training, and physical fitness (see definitions in Table 1) in CHD prevention, but most of this research has been conducted on men. In view of the gender differences in the development of CHD, we believe that it is timely to discuss the different effects of physical activity in men and women. Therefore, in this chapter, we briefly outline the differential effects of physical activity, exercise training, and physical fitness on CHD risk in men and women, and the possible mechanisms mediating such differences. Finally, we provide basic guidelines for physical activity and exercise training prescriptions for the purpose of reducing CHD risk.

II. PHYSICAL INACTIVITY, LACK OF FITNESS, AND CORONARY HEART DISEASE MORBIDITY AND MORTALITY

Physical inactivity has been strongly associated with accentuated all-cause mortality, CHD mortality, and CHD morbidity in men. In particular, the

TABLE 1
Definitions for Physical Activity, Exercise Training, and Physical Fitness

Physical Activity — ''Any bodily movement produced by skeletal muscles that results in energy expenditure.''[68]

Exercise Training — ''Physical activity that is planned, structured, repetitive and purposive in the sense that improvement or maintenance of one or more components of physical fitness is an objective.''[68]

Physical Fitness — ''A set of attributes that people have or achieve that relates to the ability to perform physical activity.''[68]

Harvard Alumni Study[11] and the Multiple Risk Factor Intervention Trial[12] report lower all-cause and CHD mortality rates, while the British Civil Servants Study[13] reports a reduced incidence of CHD in men who are physically active. Moreover, recent reviews of existing studies have shown the incidence of CHD to be almost twice as high among sedentary men than among those who regularly participate in various physical activities.[14,15]

Blair et al. have indicated further that higher levels of physical fitness appear to delay all-cause mortality in men, primarily due to lowered rates of cardiovascular disease.[16] They have demonstrated that all-cause mortality rates decrease across physical fitness quintiles. In their study, 64, 26, 27, 21, and 19 deaths per 10,000 person-years were seen in the least fit to the most fit groups of men, respectively. These trends remained after statistical adjustment for traditional CHD risk factors. Similarly, lower rates were also observed for cardiovascular disease mortality in the higher fitness groups (Figure 1). Thus, the most fit men were at an eightfold lower risk for mortality from cardiovascular disease than the least fit men in their study. Likewise, a number of additional studies report the relative risk of fatal and nonfatal CHD in unfit men to be approximately 2.0 (range 1.4 to 5.0) compared to fit men, and these results are consistent after adjustment for various confounding variables.[17-21]

The relationship between physical activity, exercise training, physical fitness, and CHD risk in women has not been extensively investigated. The existing studies on physical activity and CHD risk are conflicting, with approximately 50% showing no substantial advantage in the physically active group.[15] However, Blair et al.[16] have investigated all-cause mortality rates in women and documented 40, 21, 12, 7, and 9 deaths per 10,000 person-years in the least fit through the most fit quintiles of women. Indeed, in their study, the least fit women were nine times more likely to die than the most fit women. After statistical adjustment, the observed fitness-mortality relation could not be attributed to differences between groups in cholesterol, blood pressure, smoking, body fat, and, importantly, exercise habits. Lower rates were also observed for cardiovascular disease mortality in the higher fitness groups (Figure 1).

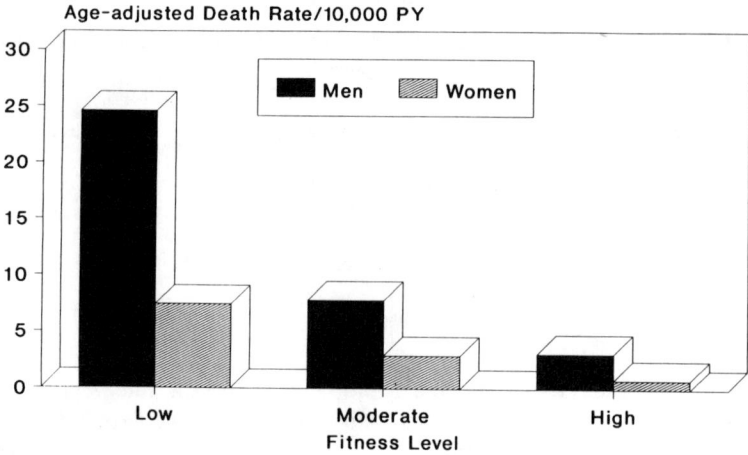

FIGURE 1.   Age-adjusted cardiovascular disease death rates per 10,000 person-years of follow-up in low, moderate, and high fitness categories: Cooper Clinic men and women. (Adapted from Blair, S.N., Kohl, H.W., and Paffenbarger, R.S., et al., *JAMA*, 262, 2397, 1989.)

Although further research is needed to clarify the situation, the seemingly discrepant effects of physical activity, exercise training, and physical fitness on mortality in females may be related to the impreciseness with which physical activity status has been measured in existing studies. The methods of physical activity assessment utilized in such studies were originally designed for use in men. Thus, while being valid in males, these methods may be unacceptable for use in females. This issue should be addressed in future studies.

III. POSSIBLE MECHANISMS OF CHD RISK REDUCTION WITH PHYSICAL ACTIVITY PARTICIPATION OR EXERCISING TRAINING

The precise mechanisms by which regular physical activity or exercise training aid in attenuating the risk of developing or dying from CHD have been the topic of much speculation. Several highly plausible mechanisms have been proposed. Postulated mechanisms are essentially the same in men and women, and are as follows.

A. CIGARETTE SMOKING
A relationship between cigarette smoking and fatal myocardial infarction is seen in men and women.[22,23,24] The Framingham Study showed smoking to be a more prominent risk factor in men than in women,[24,25] the gender difference being attributed to the greater exposure to cigarettes in men. However, since 1980, women aged 20 to 24 have tended to increase their cigarette

consumption, both in terms of the number of women who smoke and the number of cigarettes smoked.[26]

Cigarette smoking is associated with decreased levels of high density lipoprotein cholesterol, increased platelet aggregability, elevated plasma fibrogen levels, increased myocardial oxygen requirements, and greater susceptibility to ventricular arrhythmias.[27] Cigarette smoking also elicits an anti-estrogenic effect,[28] causing women to experience menopause at an earlier age and, thus, presumably increasing their risk for CHD.[23] Individuals who exercise or start an exercise program may be less likely to smoke, and more likely to give up smoking.[29] However, lower mortality rates are seen even in exercisers who continue to smoke. Thus, it is possible that regular exercise might help offset some of the deleterious effects of cigarette smoking on the cardiovascular system.[16]

B. HYPERTENSION

Hypertension, a major risk factor for CHD, occurs in both men and women.[30] The prevalence of hypertension is higher among men than women prior to age 50. Thereafter, the prevalence of hypertension is higher among women.[31]

Though the data sample is greater for men than for women, a recent meta-analysis of 25 longitudinal studies suggests that women may experience a greater blood pressure reduction than men with exercise training.[32] In these studies, the average sample-size-weighted reduction in blood pressure was 7/5 mmHg for men vs. 19/14 mmHg for women. Further studies are needed to clarify this issue and to determine whether the observed reductions in blood pressure with exercise training result from a reduction in cardiac output, peripheral resistance, or both.

C. DIABETES

Persons with diabetes are more likely to develop cardiovascular disease than those without diabetes. Diabetic individuals have a twofold increase in CHD risk and are two to four times more likely to die from CHD than nondiabetic individuals.[33] The prevalence and incidence of diabetes are similar in men and women. However, diabetes increases the risk of CHD threefold in women, placing them at a similar risk to nondiabetic men of the same age.[34]

Acutely, a single bout of submaximal exercise enhances insulin sensitivity in skeletal muscle and other tissues. It, therefore, often causes a decline in the blood glucose levels of patients with insulin-dependent or noninsulin-dependent diabetes mellitus.[35] Such exercise-related improvements in glucose metabolism may persist from hours to days and are postulated to result from an increase in the cell membrane glucose transporter number and intrinsic activity.[36] With chronic exercise training, glycemic control likewise has been observed to improve in persons with noninsulin-dependent and, to a lesser degree, insulin-dependent diabetes.[35] However, it is unclear whether such improvements are largely due to the cumulative effects of the individual acute bouts of exercise rather than a training-related change in fitness per se. Though women may have a greater relative risk of CHD with diabetes than men, it is also currently unknown whether exercise induces a differential gender effect in terms of glycemic control.

D. SERUM LIPIDS

The Framingham Study found total plasma cholesterol levels to be a major predictor of CHD risk in men and women.[37] For every 1% increase in cholesterol levels, a 2% increase in incidence of CHD was observed in both younger and older women.[38] Serum total and low density lipoprotein cholesterol levels increase with age in women, but still remain lower than in men until 50 years of age, at which time the levels begin to approach those of men.[39] High density lipoprotein (HDL) cholesterol is the strongest lipid predictor of CHD in both men and women.[40] HDL cholesterol levels tend to be higher in women of all ages, although they do begin to approach levels found in men after 50 years of age.

Exercise training studies in men indicate that aerobic exercise has positive effects on lipoprotein profiles primarily by increasing HDL cholesterol levels. On the other hand, research involving women has generally not shown as great an increase in HDL cholesterol levels as in men, possibly due to the higher baseline HDL cholesterol levels in women. Alternatively, the volume of activity required to achieve consistent increases in HDL cholesterol levels in women may be greater than that for men.[41,42] In this regard, most studies have examined changes in lipoprotein levels after short-term exercise training, which may not have allowed enough time for significant lipoprotein changes to occur. Recently, we have shown that in young healthy women, a six-month program of either low or high intensity walking can bring about clinically relevant increases in HDL cholesterol levels.[43]

E. OBESITY

Twenty-four percent of all adult women in the U.S. are obese compared to 14% of all adult men.[44] Obesity and being overweight have been recognized to influence other CHD risk factors, such as diabetes and HDL cholesterol levels, which can confound interpreting relationships between obesity and CHD risk.[45,46] Nonetheless, the degree of obesity does seem to be an independent predictor of CHD risk in both men and women.[47]

Caloric restriction through dieting, in combination with caloric expenditure through regular exercise, is the most effective means of preventing obesity and maintaining ideal body weight. Such an approach, compared to dieting alone, better preserves lean body mass and possibly may evoke favorable long-term changes in resting metabolic rate. However, women may be less likely to respond to an exercise training program with a significant loss of weight and fat than men.[42]

Recent studies have indicated that many of the adverse consequences of obesity may be more closely coupled to the distribution of body fat than to the amount of body fat.[48] Individuals with more fat on the trunk (that is, male-pattern fat distribution), especially intra-abdominal fat, are at an increased risk of death when compared to those who are equally fat, but have their fat predominantly located on the extremities (that is, female-pattern obesity). Although additional studies are needed, regular exercise appears capable of evoking favorable changes in body fat distribution.[48] Indeed, preliminary data suggest a preferential mobilization of trunk subcutaneous fat as compared to peripheral subcutaneous fat in response to exercise training.[49]

F. PSYCHOSOCIAL FACTORS

Psychosocial and behavioral risk factors may influence the development of CHD.[50] The Framingham data were the first to report an association between Type A behavior and CHD incidence in women. Women less than 65 years of age who were classified as having Type A behavior were twice as likely to develop CHD as Type B women.[51]

The effect of exercise training on Type A behavior has yet to be investigated comprehensively. However, there is increasing evidence in both males and females that exercise training may help reduce stress, anxiety, and stress related emotions, and enhance general well-being.[52]

G. OTHER PROTECTIVE MECHANISMS OF EXERCISE

Other mechanisms by which physical activity may aid in reducing the risk for developing and/or dying from CHD include an improved balance between myocardial oxygen demand and supply, reduced propensity toward lethal ventricular arrhythmias, reduced platelet aggregation, and increased plasma fibrinolytic activity. The effect of gender on these various mechanisms is currently unknown.

IV. ENERGY EXPENDITURE PRESCRIPTION

The adoption of exercising habits by the American public has not been encouraging. The U.S. Surgeon General had listed an objective of 65% of the American population to be involved with a regular exercise program by the year 1990.[53] Casperson et al. have estimated from the National Health Statistics data that only 8.1% of men and 7.0% of women have met this criterion.[54]

Adherence to exercise programs is a well documented problem for beginning exercisers.[55,56,57] This problem is also prevalent for participants in cardiac rehabilitation programs.[58] Upon first glance at the behavioral data concerning exercise participation, one might question the promotion of exercise training as a means of increasing energy expenditure, and perhaps, rightly so. But this concern with exercise may change as new evidence accrues regarding the possibility of increased physical activity, in place of formal exercise training, as being a cardiovascular health promoter. In terms of public participation, integration of physical activity into one's daily routine may be more likely to be adhered to by a population that needs to increase its energy expenditure, than a formal exercise training program. Unfortunately, the arrival of specific cardiovascular health benefits via such physical activity are, at present, difficult to verify. This is largely due to the inaccuracies of current physical activity quantification measures,[59] the improbability of defining one all-encompassing cardiovascular health variable with a measure of activity, and our current lack of knowledge concerning the relationship between low-intensity energy expenditure and health. Nonetheless, it does appear that while low-intensity energy expenditure may be considerably less effective than high-intensity energy expenditure in enhancing cardiorespiratory fitness, it is of cardiovascular health benefit.

We have subjectively reviewed the literature concerning cardiovascular health enhancement and physical activity and tentatively propose that an energy expenditure of between 14 and 20 kcal/kg of body weight per week may be optimal.[60] The amount and the range of this energy expenditure guideline are certainly premature and do not consider gender or health status differences but, nevertheless, provide a reasonable estimate of what may be needed. Almost any activity apparently can be used to obtain this figure, whether it be gardening, dog walking, ice skating, swimming, weight training, or jogging, provided it can be safely adopted by the sedentary individual. That is, individual activity preferences and safety concerns should represent primary considerations of the physical activity prescription. It is of note, however, that large muscle group activities (in particular, those involving the legs) that have been traditionally defined as aerobic (walking, running, biking, swimming, etc.) usually produce the greatest energy expenditure and, therefore, provide an easier means of obtaining the figures mentioned previously. For those individuals whose main goal is physical fitness improvement along with cardiovascular health improvement, it is recommended that in addition to achieving this level of energy expenditure, the exercise intensity should be sufficient to elicit a heart rate response in excess of 60% of the maximal heart rate.[61] Table 2 provides some insight into the wide variations of activity and energy expenditure that are available.

In addition to exercise intensity, frequency and duration are also important. In this respect, it should be noted that the energy expenditures of low-intensity activities, such as golf and gardening, will most certainly accrue at a slower rate than those of higher-intensity activities, such as biking and cross-country skiing. It would, therefore, stand to reason that golf and gardening will need to be performed more frequently and/or for a longer duration than biking and cross-country skiing for any specific health change to occur. However, if performed regularly and for a long enough period of time, there may indeed be substantial cardiovascular health change. When addressing such issues in future studies, it will be of considerable interest to determine whether individual activity bouts performed throughout the day (such as using

TABLE 2
Energy Expenditure Values for Various Physical Activities

Moderate intensity activity 3–4.9 METS/.050–.068 kcal/kg/min	Hard intensity activity 5–6.9 METS/.071–.10 kcal/kg/min	Very hard intensity activity 7 METS/.111 kcal/kg/min
Calisthenic exercise	Aerobic dance	Backpacking hilly country or rough trails with a heavy pack
Carpentry in workshop (non-competitive)	Basketball	Basketball, soccer, singles tennis, or racquetball (competitive)
Golf (not riding a cart)	Carpentry (outside)	Cross-country skiing
Horseback riding	Construction work (doing physical labor)	Mountain climbing
House painting or paper hanging	Digging in the garden	Rope jumping
Mowing lawn (not on a riding mower)	Doubles tennis	Running
Raking lawn	Downhill skiing	Stair climbing (fast pace)
Sailing	Fishing (wading in stream)	Swimming (fast pace)
Snorkeling	Hiking	Very hard physical labor
Softball	Hunting (small game, walking)	
Table tennis (recreational)	Scuba diving	
Vacuuming carpet	Skating, ice or roller	
Volleyball (recreational)	Snow shoveling (dry snow)	
Walking at 3–4 mph (15 to 20 min per mile)	Square, folk, or fast dancing	
Weeding and cultivating in the garden	Stair climbing (moderate pace)	
Weight lifting	Swimming (slow pace)	
	Walking at 4.5–5.5 mph	
	Water skiing	

Note: The caloric range provided is not intended to accurately quantify energy expenditure. Instead, these values are to be used as a reference point to place individuals within physical activity categories.

Modified from Blair, S.N., *Living with Exercise: Improving Your Health Through Moderate Physical Activity*, American Health Publishing, Dallas, 1991, 112.

TABLE 3
Revised (Fourth Edition) ACSM Guidelines for Exercise Testing Prior to Participation in an Exercise Program

	Apparently healthy		Higher risk[a]		
	Younger (men ≤ 40; women ≤ 50)	Older	No symptoms (all ages)	Symptoms (all ages)	With disease[b]
Medical exam and diagnostic exercise test recommended prior to:					
Moderate exercise[c]	No[d]	No	No	Yes	Yes
Vigorous exercise[e]	No	Yes[f]	Yes	Yes	Yes

[a] Persons with two or more major CAD risk factors or symptoms suggestive of cardiac, pulmonary, or metabolic disease.
[b] Persons with known cardiac, pulmonary, or metabolic disease.
[c] Exercise intensity of 40 to 60% maximal oxygen uptake. It should be well within the individual's current capacity, and the individual should be capable of comfortably sustaining it for a prolonged period of time (that is, 60 min). Progression should be slow and the activity should generally be noncompetitive.
[d] "No" responses do not mean that an exercise test should not be done; rather, they mean that it is not necessary.
[e] Exercise intensity exceeding 60% maximal oxygen uptake. It should represent a substantial challenge to the individual and ordinarily result in fatigue within 20 min.
[f] "Yes" responses mean that an exercise test is recommended.

From American College of Sports Medicine, Guidelines for Exercise Testing and Prescription, Lea & Febiger, Philadelphia, 1991.

the stairs at work instead of the elevator), can be of cardiovascular health benefit as has been suggested by some authors.[9,62,63]

Physical activity prescription of a vigorous nature and/or for a risk-prone individual should begin with a physical exam which includes a graded exercise test to determine the physiological guidelines for the individual (Table 3). In addition to information on individual exertion levels, a task specific warm-up and cool-down (including flexibility exercises) is recommended, even with such activities as mowing the lawn and hunting. The proper safety equipment also must be considered for each respective activity, whether one needs proper footwear for walking and running or a helmet and knee and elbow pads for roller skating.

Although the data are currently unclear, some authors report that injury rates may be higher in women than in men[64] while others indicate that this may not be the case.[65,66] It is possible, however, that men may be more exposed to vigorous exercise than women and, therefore, more greatly exposed to injury.[66] In a study by Blair et al., the risk for injury was greater for females when an exercise program was initiated but not in those with running experience.[65] It appears that, at the very least, activity should start out very gradually in men and women.

For pregnant women or women who wish to become pregnant, exercise should be directed in accordance with current guidelines.[67] Persons with underlying heart disease or other chronic disorders should have their physical activity/exercise training program directed by a medical doctor in accordance with contemporary recommendations.[68]

V. SUMMARY

Cardiovascular disease is the leading cause of morbidity and mortality in women and men. It is evident that a regular physical activity/exercise training program can reduce the risk of CHD via an alteration in many of the known factors which contribute to this condition. Though both women and men share the same risks for this disease, each CHD risk factor may present itself differently within each sex resulting in mortality differences. Similarly, the amount of exercise or physical activity needed to effect each independent risk factor also may be related to gender. While physical exertion needs to be accurately quantified in the research situation to determine dose-response relationships, the fact is most people currently do not or will not participate in formal exercise training programs to achieve these recommended levels. For these individuals, integration of physical activity into their daily routines may be more likely to be adhered to than a formal exercise training program.

REFERENCES

1. WHO, Vital Statistics and Causes of Death, World Health Statistics Annual, World Health Organization, Geneva, 1986.
2. **Cassel, J.C.,** Evans County cardiovascular and cerebrovascular epidemiologic study, *Arch. Intern. Med.,* 128, 883, 1971.
3. **Kannel, W.B., Dawber, T.R., Kagon, A., et al.,** Factors of risk in the development of coronary heart disease — six year follow-up experience. The Framingham Study. *Ann. Intern. Med.,* 55, 33, 1961.
4. National Center for Health Statistics, Vital and Health Statistics, Current estimates from the National Health Interview Survey, 1989. DHHS Publication No. (PHS) 90-1504, U.S. 1990, 86.
5. **Oliver, M.F.,** What is the difference between women and men? in *Myocardial Infarction in Women,* Oliver, N.F., Vedin, A., and Whilhelmsson, C., Eds., Churchill Livingstone, Edinburgh, 1986.
6. **Dawber, T.R., Ed.,** *The Framingham Study: The Epidemiology of Atherosclerotic Disease,* Harvard University Press, Cambridge, MA, 1980.
7. **Bush, T.L. and Barrett-Connor, E.,** Noncontraceptive estrogen use and cardiovascular disease, *Epidemiol. Rev.,* 7, 80, 1985.

8. **McGill, Jr., H.C. and Stern, M.P.,** Sex and atherosclerosis, in *Atherosclerosis Reviews,* Paoletti, R. and Gotto, A.M., Eds., Raven Press, New York, 1979.

9. **Kannel, W.B. and Feinleib, M.,** Natural history of angina pectoris. The Framingham Study. Prognosis and survival, *Am. J. Cardiol.,* 29, 154, 1972.

10. **Wilhelmsen, L.,** Epidemiology of coronary heart disease in young women, in *Coronary Heart Disease in Young Women,* Oliver, M.F., Ed., Churchill Livingston, Edinburgh, 1978.

11. **Paffenbarger, R.S., Hyde, R.J., Wing, A.L., et al.,** Physical activity, all-cause mortality, and longevity of college alumni, *N. Engl. J. Med.,* 315, 605, 1985.

12. **Leon, A.S., Connett, J., Jacobs, Jr., D.R., et al.,** Leisure time physical activity levels and risk of coronary heart disease and death — the multiple risk factor intervention trial, *JAMA,* 258, 2388, 1987.

13. **Morris, J.N., Pollard, R., Everitt, M.G., and Chave, S.P.W.,** Vigorous exercise in leisure-time: protection against coronary heart disease, *Lancet,* 8206, 1207, 1989.

14. **Berlin, J.A. and Colditz, G.A.,** A meta-analysis of physical activity in the prevention of coronary heart disease, *Am. J. Epidemiol.,* 132, 612, 1990.

15. **Powell, K.E., Thompson, P.D., Casperson, C.J., et al.,** Physical activity and the incidence of coronary heart disease, *Annu. Rev. Public Health,* 8, 253, 1987.

16. **Blair, S.N., Kohl, H.W., Paffenbarger, R.S., et al.,** Physical fitness and all-cause mortality: a prospective study of healthy men and women, *JAMA,* 262, 2395, 1989.

17. **Bruce, R.A., Hossack, K.F., DeRoven, T.A., et al.,** Enhanced risk assessment for primary coronary heart disease events by maximal exercise testing: 10 years' experience of Seattle Heart Watch, *J. Am. Coll. Cardiol.,* 2, 565, 1983.

18. **Ekeuland, L.G., Haskell, W.L., Johnson, J.L., et al.,** Physical fitness as a predictor of cardiovascular mortality in asymptomatic North American men: The Lipid Clinics mortality follow-up study, *N. Engl. J. Med.,* 319, 1379, 1988.

19. **Erikssen, J.,** Physical fitness and coronary heart disease morbidity and mortality: a prospective study in apparently healthy middle-aged men, *Acta. Med. Scand. Suppl.,* 711, 189, 1986.

20. **Peters, R.K., Cady, Jr., L.D., Bischoff, D.P., et al.,** Physical fitness and subsequent myocardial infarction in healthy workers, *JAMA,* 249, 3052, 1983.

21. **Wilhelmsen, L., Bjure, J., Ekstrom-Jodal, B., et al.,** Nine year's follow-up of a maximal exercise test in a random population sample of middle-aged men, *Cardiology,* 68 (Suppl. 2), 1, 1981.

22. **Willett, W.C., Green, A., Stampfer, M.J., et al.,** Relative and absolute excess risks of coronary heart disease among women who smoke cigarettes, *N. Engl. J. Med.,* 317, 1303, 1987.

23. **Willett, W.C., Stampfer, M.J., Bain, C., et al.,** Cigarette smoking, relative weight, and menopause, *Am. J. Epidemiol.,* 117, 651, 1983.

24. **Kannel, W.B., McGee, D.L., and Castelli, W.P.,** Latest perspectives on cigarette smoking and cardiovascular disease: The Framingham Study, *J. Cardiol. Rehabil.,* 4, 267, 1984.

25. **Stokes, J., Kannel, W.B., Wolf, P.A., et al.,** The relative importance of selected risk factors for various manifestations of cardiovascular diseaes among men and women from 35–64 years: 30 years of follow-up in The Framingham Study, *Circulation,* 75 (Suppl. V), V65, 1987.

26. Smoking and Health, a National Status Report — A report to Congress, publication No. HHS/PHS/CDC 87-8396. Department of Health and Human Services, Rockville, MD, 1987.

27. A report of the Surgeon General: The Health Consequences of Smoking: Cardiovascular Disease, Office on Smoking and Health, Rockville, MD, 1983.

28. **Baron, J.,** Smoking and estrogen related dosage, *Am. J. Epidemiol.,* 119, 9, 1984.

29. **Sedgwick, A.W., Davidson, A.H., Taplin, R.E., et al.,** Effects of physical activity on risk factors for coronary heart disease in previously sedentary women. A five-year longitudinal study, *Aust. N.Z. J. Med.,* 18, 600, 1988.
30. **Kannel, W.B.,** Status of risk factors and their consideration in antihypertensive therapy, *Am. J. Cardiol.,* 59, 80A, 1987.
31. **Shapiro, A.P. and Rutan, G.H.,** Hypertension in women: differences and implications, in *Coronary Heart Disease in Women,* Proceedings of an NIH workshop, Eaker, E.D., Packard, B., and Wenger, N.H., et al., Eds., Haymarket Doyma, New York, 1987, 172.
32. **Hagberg, J.M.,** Exercise, fitness, and hypertension, in *Exercise, Fitness and Health,* Bouchard, C., Shepard, R.J., Stephens, T., et al., Eds., Human Kinetics Publishers, Champaign, IL, 1990.
33. Diabetes 1991 Vital Statistics. American Diabetes Association, 1991.
34. **Kannel, W.B. and McGee, D.L.,** Diabetes and cardiovascular disease — The Framingham Study, *JAMA,* 241, 2035, 1979.
35. **Vranic, M. and Wasserman, D.,** Exercise fitness and diabetes, in *Exercise Fitness and Health: A Consensus of Current Knowledge,* Bouchard, C., Shephard, R., Stephens, T., et al., Eds., Human Kinetics Publishers, Champaign, IL, 1990.
36. **King, P., Hirshman, M., Horton, E., et al.,** Glucose transport in skeletal muscle membrane vesicles from control and exercised rats, *Am. J. Physiol.,* 257, C1128, 1989.
37. **Castelli, W.P., Garrison, R.J., Wilson, P.W.F., et al.,** Incidence of coronary heart disease and lipoprotein cholesterol levels. The Framingham Study, *JAMA,* 256, 2835, 1986.
38. Lipid Research Clinics Program, The Lipid Research Clinics Coronary Primary Prevention Trial results II. The relationship of reduction in incidence of coronary heart disease to cholesterol lowering, *JAMA,* 251, 365, 1984.
39. **Rifkind, B.M., Tamer, I., Huss, G., et al.,** Distribution of high density and other lipoproteins in selected LRC prevalence study propulations, *Lipids,* 14, 105, 1979.
40. **Gordon, T., Castelli, W.P., Hjortland, M.C., et al.,** High density lipoproteins as a protective factor against coronary heart disease. The Framingham Study, *Am. J. Med.,* 62, 707, 1977.
41. **Haskell, W.L.,** Dose-response relationship between physical activity and disease risk factors, *Sport for All,* Oja, P. and Telama, R., Eds., Proc. World Congr. Sport All, p. 125, 1990.
42. **Leon, A.S.,** Physical activity and risk of ischemic heart disease— an update, in *Sport for All,* Oja, P. and Telama, R., Eds., Proc. World Congr. Sport All, p. 251, 1990.
43. **Duncan, J.J., Gordon, N.F., and Scott, C.B.,** Women walking for health and fitness. How much is enough? *JAMA,* 266, 3295, 1991.
44. National Center for Health Statistics: Plan and operation of the Health and Nutrition Examination Survey, U.S. 197-1973, U.S. Dept. Health, Education and Welfare publication NO(HSM) 73-1310, Vital Health Stat. (1) 1973, (10a,b).
45. Health implications of obesity: National Institutes of Health Consensus Development Conference, *Ann. Intern. Med.,* 103, 1073, 1985.
46. **Mann, J.I., Doll, R., Thorogood, M., et al.,** Risk factors for myocardial infarction in young women, *Br. J. Prev. Soc. Med.,* 30, 94, 1976.
47. **Hubert, H.B., Feinleib, M., McNamara, D.M., et al.,** Obesity as an independent risk factor for cardiovascular disease: a 26 year follow-up of participants in The Framingham Study, *Circulation,* 67, 968, 1983.
48. **Bjorntorp, P., Smith, U., and Lonnroth, P.,** Eds., Health implications of regional obesity, *Acta. Med. Scand. Suppl.,* 723, 1, 1988.
49. **Despres, J.-P., Tremblay, A., Nadeau, A., et al.,** Physical training and changes in regional adipose tissue distribution, *Acta. Med. Scand. Suppl.,* 723, 205, 1988.
50. **Wingard, ,D.L., Suarez, L., and Barrett-Connor, E.,** The sex differences in mortality from all-causes and ischemic heart disease, *Am. J. Epidemiol.,* 117, 165, 1983.

51. **Haynes, S.G., Feinleib, M., and Kannel, W.B.,** The relationship of psychosocial factors to coronary heart disease incidence in The Framingham Study. III. Eight year incidence of coronary heart disease, *Am. J. Epidemiol.,* 111, 37, 1980.
52. **Petruzzello, S.J., Landers, D.M., Hatfield, B.D., et al.,** A meta-analysis on the anxiety reducing effects of acute and chronic exercise, *Sports Med.,* 11, 143, 1991.
53. **Powell, K.E., Christenson, G.M., and Kreuter, M.W.,** Objectives for the nation: assessing the role physical education must play, *J. Phys. Ed.,* 55, 18, 1984.
54. **Caspersen, C.J., Christenson, G.M., and Pollard, R.A.,** Status of the 1990 physical fitness and exercise objectives — evidence from NHIS 1985, *Public Health Rep.,* 101, 587, 1986.
55. **Dishman, R.K.,** Compliance/adherence in health-related exercise, *Health Psychol.,* 1, 237, 1982.
56. **Dishman, R.K.,** Exercise compliance: a new view for public health. *Phys. Sportsmed.,* 14, 127, 1986.
57. **Mirotznik, J., Speedling, E., Stein, R., et al.,** Cardiovascular fitness program: factors associated with participation and adherence, *Public Health Rep.,* 100, 13, 1985.
58. **Oldridge, N.B.,** Compliance and dropout in cardiac exercise rehabilitation, *J. Cardiac Rehabil.,* 4, 166, 1984.
59. **Laporte, R.E., Montoye, H.J., and Caspersen, C.J.,** Assessment of physical activity in epidemiological research: problems and prospects, *Public Health Rep.,* 100, 131, 1985.
60. **Gordon, N.F. and Gibbons, L.W.,** *The Cooper Clinic Cardiac Rehabilitation Program,* Simon and Schuster, New York, 1990.
61. **American College of Sports Medicine,** The recommended quantity and quality of exercise for developing and maintaining cardiorespiratory and muscular fitness in healthy adults, *Med. Sci. Sports Exerc.,* 22, 265, 1990.
62. **DeBusk, R.F., Stenestrand, U., Sheehan, M., et al.,** Training effects of long versus short bouts of exercise in healthy subjects, *Am. J. Cardiol.,* 65, 1010, 1990.
63. **Blair, S.N.,** *Living with Exercise: Improving Your Health Through Moderate Physical Activity,* American Health Publishing, Dallas, 1991.
64. **Jones, B.H., Rock, P.B., and Moore, M.P.,** Musculoskeletal injury: risks, prevention, and first aid, in *Resource Manual for Guidelines for Exercise Testing and Prescription,* American College of Sports Medicine, Lea & Febiger, Philadelphia, 1988.
65. **Blair, S.N., Kohl, H.W., and Goodyear, N.N.,** Rates and risks for running and exercise injuries: studies in three populations, *Res. Q. Exercise Sport,* 58, 221, 1987.
66. **Taimela, S., Kujala, U.M., and Osterman, K.,** Intrinsic risk factors and athletic injuries, *Sports Med.,* 9, 205, 1990.
67. **Wolfe, L.A., Hall, P., Webb, K.A., et al.,** Prescription of aerobic exercise during pregnancy, *Sports Med.,* 8, 273, 1989.
68. **Caspersen, C.J., Powell, K.E., and Christenson, G.M.,** Physical activity, exercise and physical fitness: definitions and distinctions for health related research, *Public Health Rep.,* 100, 126, 1985.

Chapter 3

PHYSICAL ACTIVITY, LIPIDS, AND LIPOPROTEIN METABOLISM: THE BENEFIT OF EXERCISE AND TRAINING IN HYPERLIPIDEMIA

A. Berg, M. Halle, M. Baumstark, I. Frey, and J. Keul

TABLE OF CONTENTS

I. INTRODUCTION

Physical activity is now recognized as an important therapeutic modality in combination with changes in diet and weight loss for the treatment of impaired lipid metabolism. Pharmacological treatment is sometimes inevitable; despite the recognized beneficial effect of exercise on lipid and lipoprotein metabolism and its known value in rehabilitation following myocardial infarction,[1] physical exercise and training are still not accorded the attention they deserve in the treatment of hyperlipoproteinemia. The purpose of this review is to discuss the important aspects of physical activity on lipid metabolism and to emphasize its benefits in altering lipoprotein levels in both primary and secondary prevention of coronary heart disease.

II. NOVEL DEFINITION OF AN ATHEROGENIC LIPOPROTEIN PROFILE

The diagnostic criteria of dyslipoproteinemias have been redefined repeatedly during the last few years. They have become independent of merely recognizing elevated serum cholesterol values or lipoprotein fractions of elevated Low Density Lipoproteins (LDL) and reduced levels of High Density Lipoproteins (HDL) in particular. The assessment of the lipoprotein profile has changed since the heterogeneity of atherogenic LDL and cardio-protective HDL particles has been recognized. Among the lipoprotein fraction, LDL and HDL particles have been shown to clearly differ in lipid and apolipoprotein composition, particle size, and physico-chemical properties, and can be influenced differently by endogenous (e.g., genetic) or exogenous (e.g., nutritional, life style) factors (Figure 1).[2–5]

Coronary angiographic studies have demonstrated a direct correlation between LDL levels and, in particular, the levels of the fraction of small, dense LDL particles and a negative correlation between HDL-2 particles (the larger HDL particles) to the extent and progression of coronary atherosclerosis under cholesterol lowering therapy.[6,7] Small LDL particles correlate with a threefold elevated risk of myocardial infarction and progression of coronary atherosclerosis within 2 years.[6] Decrease of small LDL under pharmacological therapy is also accompanied by a delay in atherosclerotic progression.

Thus, today, an atherogenic lipoprotein profile is defined as a lipid constellation of elevated serum cholesterol and triglyceride levels with an elevation of small LDL particles and a reduction of HDL-2 subfraction particles.[8] This new approach to the evaluation of lipoprotein profiles is a particular reason for reconsidering and highlighting the influence of physical activity on lipoprotein metabolism.

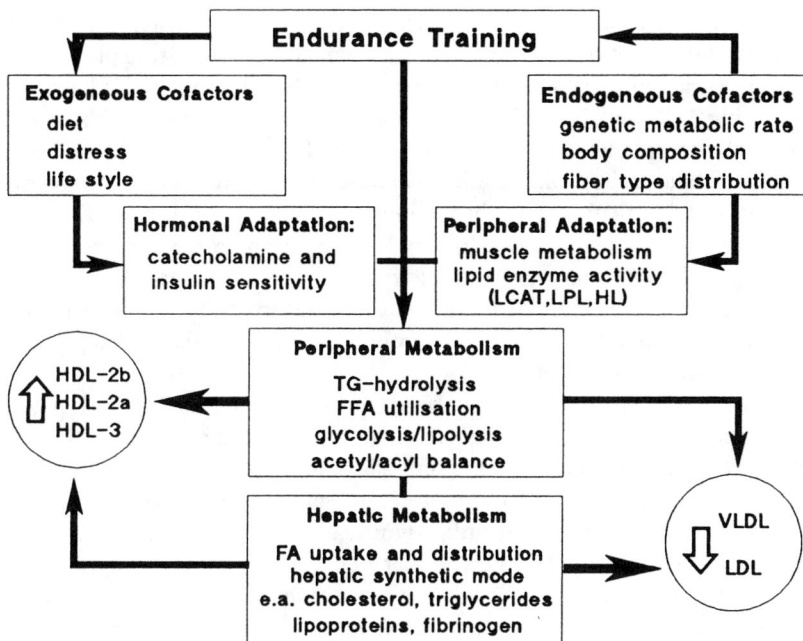

FIGURE 1. The effect of endurance training and corresponding factors on lipids and lipoprotein metabolism.

III. EFFECT OF PHYSICAL ACTIVITY ON MUSCULAR LIPID METABOLISM

Acute and chronic endurance exercise has been shown to alter lipid metabolism.[9-14] The adaptation effects induced by increased physical activity arise from the interplay of various adaptation mechanisms. Exercising skeletal muscle plays a central role in the control of these mechanisms. The increase in aerobic energy metabolism and oxygen quantity required during augmented physical activity is the basic control parameter for the adaptation processes during regular physical exercise training. Therefore, physical activity should be performed in an optimal aerobic range. From a therapeutic point of view, in order to improve the peripheral lipoprotein profile, an increment in energy metabolism of at least 1000 kcal/week is required.[15] From a preventive medical point of view, to reduce the incidence of coronary heart disease and prolong life expectancy, a minimum of an additional 2000 kcal/week of energy metabolism is necessary.[16] To achieve these effects, running at least 15 km/week for 6 to 12 months must be undertaken.[17]

Unlike anaerobic metabolism, which represents an unstable metabolic situation with elevation of lactate concentration and accumulation of inorganic phosphates, aerobic metabolism is controlled via mitochondrial feedback regulation by ADP and NADH concentrations.[18,19] In agreement with modern threshold concepts used in sports medicine and their practical application in diagnostics and training in healthy individuals and patients,[18,20,21] moderate intensities of physical activity in the range of the aerobic threshold are necessary for the new arrangement of lipid and lipoprotein metabolism[20,21] that is strived for in primary or secondary preventive medicine.[1,22] Therefore, determination of the individual aerobic threshold intensity is useful for participants in cardiac and prevention programs to ensure that an appropriate training schedule is determined.

During exercise at an intensity near the so-defined aerobic threshold, the high oxidative muscle fibers are activated. The slight increase in ADP in the muscle stimulates respiration to ensure adequate oxygen uptake. At this particular exercise intensity, NADH concentrations in the working type-I muscle fibers remain low and may even be significantly reduced below resting levels.[23] At the same time, the intracellular lipoprotein lipase activity increases in the type-I muscle fibers.[24] Muscle biopsy studies confirm this regulatory process and demonstrate a close correlation between the intramuscular ratios of free fatty acids (FFA) and lipoprotein lipase (LPL) during exercise.[24] With an adequate duration of exercise, an optimal utilization of lipids can be expected in the working muscle. The fatty acids released by adipose tissue, or via hydrolysis of circulating lipoproteins and intramuscular triglyceride stores represent the energy substrate for muscle lipid metabolism. After about 2 h of muscular exercise, plasma-free fatty acids reach a plateau of about five to six times their resting concentration. This plateau represents the balance between fatty acid hydrolysis from triglyceride stores and fatty acid conversion within the muscle.[19] In exercising muscle, approximately 50% of the energy supply is obtained from conversion of FFA after 60 min, and approximately 80% is obtained after 120 min of endurance exercise. During long-term exercise, however, more than 70% of the energy requirement is obtained by the conversion of extramuscular FFA.[19]

Following endurance training, the diminished concentrations of circulating FFA with concurrent reduction of the respiratory quotient indicate the training-induced shift in energy balance in favor of fatty acid oxidation. This training effect, frequently aimed for in sports therapy, can also be attained in healthy elderly people and patients.[21]

More than 20 years ago, the close correlations between plasma concentrations of FFA and the proportion of muscular energy obtained from FFA led to the hypothesis of passive, diffusion-mediated muscular FFA uptake dependent on plasma FFA concentrations.[19] In contrast to this hypothesis, the cellular availability and use of free fatty acids in the liver and muscle cells via an active regulatory process has recently been given increasing attention.[24] FFA are transported in the blood via albumin. Since fatty acids cannot be taken up into tissues when ligated to albumin, dissociation of the FFA-albumin-ligand complex has been postulated. Additional investigations of dissociation rates *in vitro* and cellular FFA uptake *in vivo* indicate that a specific receptor exists for the albumin complex which regulates the cleavage of the albumin-ligand complex and the subsequent cellular uptake of the ligand.[25] It has been demonstrated that the uptake of FFA in myocytes and hepatocytes fulfills the criteria for a carrier-mediated process bound to a highly specific membrane protein.[25] The presence of such an active transport and controlling system for cellular FFA metabolism could be of great importance not only in specific muscular and hepatic diseases,[26] but also for possible metabolic and hormonal modulation of FFA utilization in training and sports therapy.

IV. EFFECT OF PHYSICAL ACTIVITY ON PERIPHERAL LIPOPROTEIN METABOLISM

It has been well established that an increase in aerobic performance capacity, both in healthy subjects and cardiac patients, leads to an elevation of HDL and a reduction in VLDL and LDL cholesterol, as well as triglycerides (Figure 2).[11,15,21] With improved aerobic capacity, the variation in the calculated risk ratio of HDL cholesterol to total cholesterol or LDL to HDL cholesterol decreases and is found less frequently in endurance-trained subjects.[10,21] Likewise, serum concentrations of the LDL apolipoprotein, apo B, are usually lower, and concentrations of the HDL apolipoprotein, apo A-I, are usually higher in trained individuals. The latter is caused by efficient catabolism of triglyceride-rich lipoproteins with delivery of lipids to HDL particles and decreased apolipoprotein A-I and A-II catabolism.[27] Modifications of the other apolipoproteins, e.g., apo C-II, apo C-III, apo E, and apo (a), have not been shown in relation to physical activity.

The reduction of triglycerides and VLDL cholesterol levels and simultaneous increase in HDL cholesterol induced by physical exertion are thought to be caused by increased metabolism of triglycerides during and following physical activity. This process is catalyzed by lipoprotein lipase (LPL) activity in muscle and fatty tissue.[24] When the musuclar triglyceride stores are mobilized, the synthesis of LPL in the muscular endothelial bed is also upregulated which leads to increased metabolism of serum triglycerides and triglyceride-rich VLDL particles.[28] The improved supply and subsequent increase in metabolism of triglycerides and triglyceride-rich lipoproteins leads to the reduction in serum triglyceride levels and triglyceride-rich lipoproteins. The resulting triglyceride-poor lipoprotein remnants play an important role in the conversion of small, dense, protein-rich HDL-3 to large, lipid-loaded HDL-2 particles during acute exercise (Figure 3).[9,28] Then, the HDL-3 subfraction particles are transformed to HDL-2 by the action of lecithin-cholesterol-acyl-transferase (LCAT), thereby displacing free cholesterol to the lipophile nucleus of the lipoprotein particle. An elevated LCAT activity, which is observed immediately after physical exercise in trained and normal

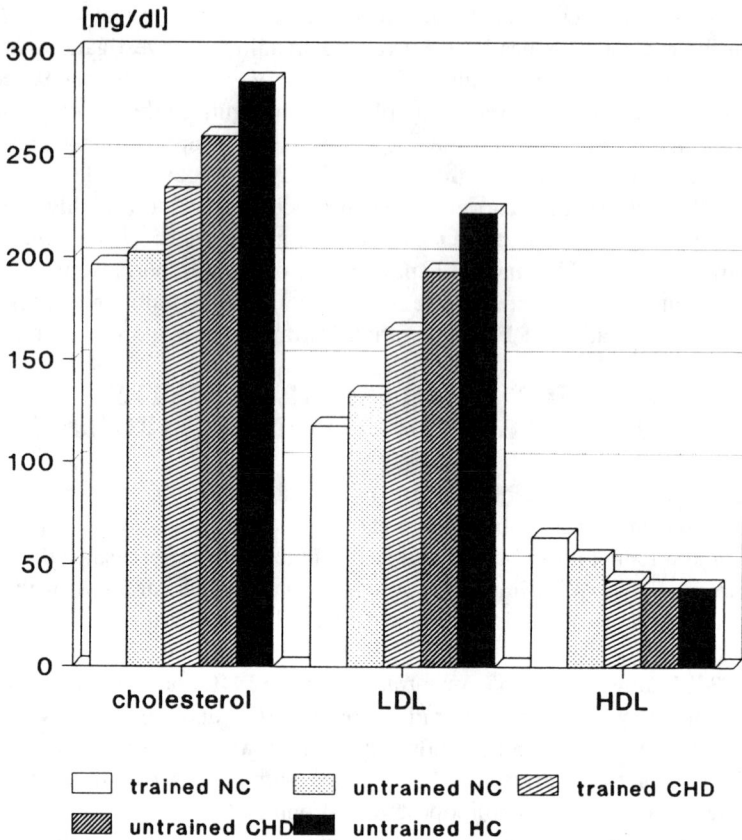

FIGURE 2. Correlation between training history and total LDL, as well as HDL, cholesterol in five groups (150 individuals at comparable ages, 48.5 ± 9.8 years) of clinically healthy normocholesterolemic (NC) and hypercholesterolemic (HC) subjects and patients with myocardial infarction (CHD). Data as mean values cited from Reference 21.

individuals,[29] can thereby essentially contribute to an increase of anti-atherogenic HDL-2 particles (Figures 3 and 4).

In contrast to acute and chronic exercise-induced increases in LPL and LCAT activity with subsequent increase in HDL-2 particles, another lipoprotein enzyme, hepatic lipase (HL), is inhibited by physical activity.[15,30] Hepatic lipase catalyses the metabolism of HDL-2 to HDL-3 particles and promotes the metabolism of smaller remnant particles formed by LPL hydrolysis. Therefore, both reduced hepatic lipase activity as well as increased activity of lipoprotein lipase, like that observed in physically active individuals, promote an increase in HDL-2, and particularly large HDL-2b particles (Figure 4).

In addition to HDL metabolism, the exercise-induced change in lipoprotein enzyme activities also appears to influence the composition and distri-

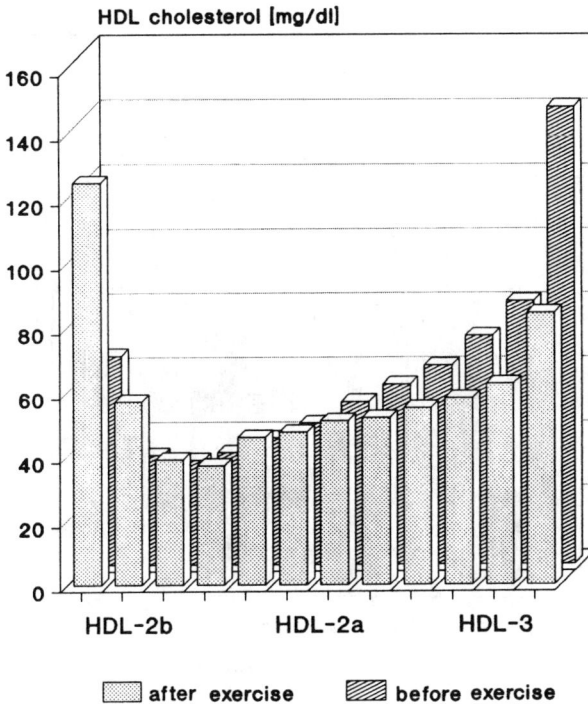

FIGURE 3. Acute change of HDL subfraction profile induced by prolonged endurance exercise (n = 9). Data as mean values cited from Reference 9.

bution of HDL and LDL subfraction particles. Investigations on the influence of lipoprotein lipase and LDL subfraction particles conclude that adipose tissue lipoprotein lipase negatively correlates with small, dense LDL subfraction particles,[31] while the inhibition of the hepatic lipase causes a reduction of the same.[32] These observations indicate that the larger the LDL particles, the better they are converted by lipoprotein lipase; the smaller they are, the better they are converted by hepatic lipase.

During acute and chronic exercise, the hepatic lipase activity is reduced and the lipoprotein lipase activity is increased, leading to an improved conversion of large to medium size LDL and a delayed conversion from medium size to small LDL particles. This may be the explanation for different LDL profiles seen in normo- and hypercholesterolemic individuals of different training conditions. Within the LDL subfraction profile of normocholesterolemic individuals, a significant reduction in triglyceride-rich LDL particles (LDL-1) in endurance athletes compared to untrained individuals is evident (Figure 5). Similar differences for LDL-1 particles are found in hypercholesterolemia, indicating an increase in LPL activity in athletes compared to untrained individuals, which promotes the metabolism from large (LDL-1) to medium size (LDL-3 and LDL-4) LDL particles. Significant differences

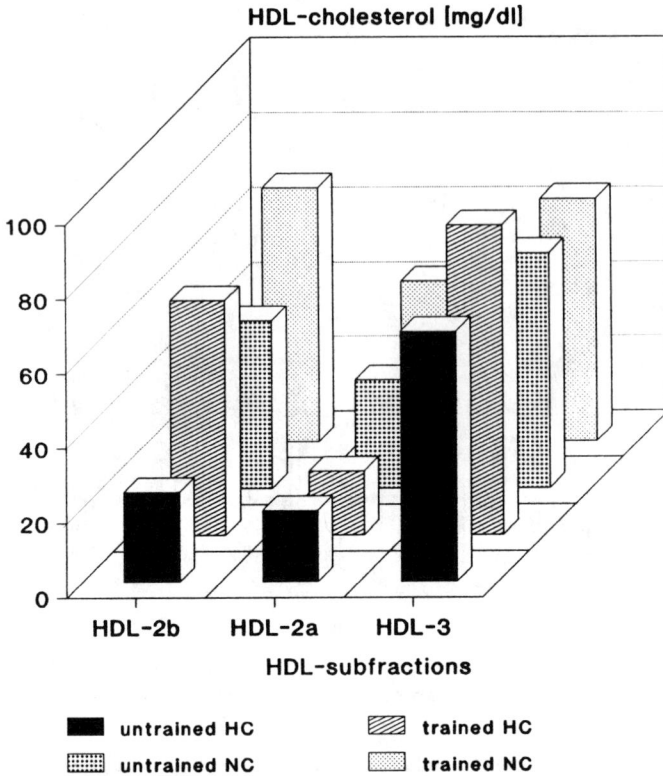

HDL-cholesterol [mg/dl]

FIGURE 4. Single observations of typical HDL subfraction profiles of untrained and endurance trained, normocholesterolemic (NC) and hypercholesterolemic (HC) males. In contrast to hypercholesterolemia, endurance training does increase the HDL pool, especially HDL-2b.

in the LDL subfraction distribution between trained and untrained hypercholesterolemic individuals can also be observed for small LDL particles (LDL-5 and LDL-6). LDL particles of trained hypercholesterolemic males show distinct differences in size compared to untrained hypercholesterolemic individuals (Figure 5). Although both groups do not differ in total LDL cholesterol levels, hypercholesterolemic athletes have significantly *less* small LDL particles and significantly *more* medium size LDL particles than untrained hypercholesterolemic subjects. This means that the number of smaller LDL particles (those LDL particles which especially favor atherogenesis) is reduced in trained individuals. It indicates that physical activity may inhibit or prolong the conversion of medium to small LDL particles via inhibition of hepatic lipase, and at the same time promote the conversion of large to medium size LDL by increased activity of lipoprotein lipase. The changes during physical activity in both HDL and LDL subfraction profiles could thus be explained by the modification of the lipoprotein enzyme activities. Thereby, a more favorable LDL subfraction profile is present in trained hypercholes-

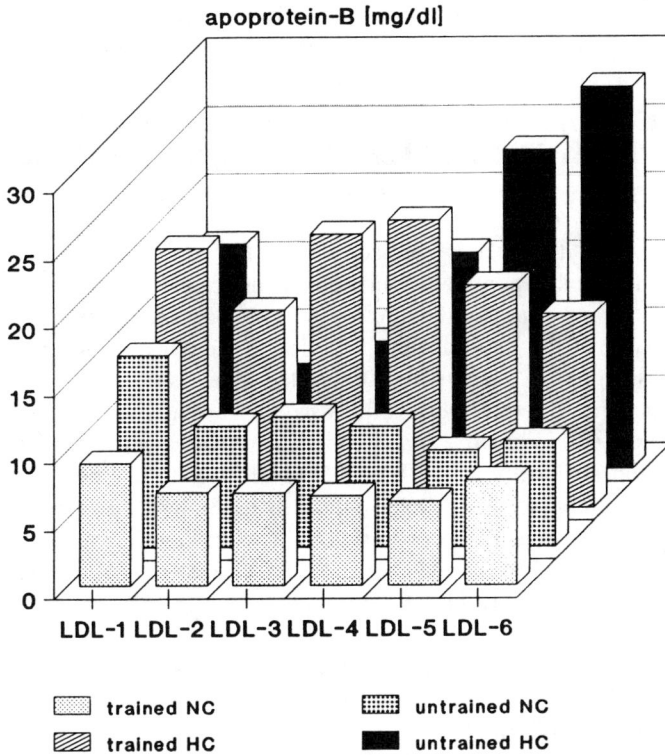

FIGURE 5. Typical LDL subfraction profiles of untrained and trained, normocholesterolemic (NC) as well as hypercholesterolemic (HC) males. Data as mean values (n = 60), endurance training does decrease the LDL pool, especially LDL-1, LDL-5, and LDL-6.

terolemic subjects in addition to an improved HDL subfraction profile and serum triglycerides and apolipoprotein constellation, as described above.

Endurance-trained individuals also reveal changes in the composition of lipoprotein particles compared to untrained individuals. The composition of the lipoprotein particles is expressed as the ratio of lipids per apolipoprotein molecules. LDL particles contain less cholesterol per particle (LDL cholesterol to apolipoprotein-B ratio), whereas HDL particle loading with cholesterol is elevated in endurance athletes (HDL cholesterol to apolipoprotein A-I ratio).[21] In addition, the phospholipid content of the HDL particles, usually reduced in advancing age and coronary heart disease patients, is maintained high in physically active individuals. In conclusion, HDL particles of endurance-trained athletes consist of significantly less protein, while phospholipid concentrations are elevated.[33]

Weight loss and weight differences as well as differences in nutrition of physically active and inactive people are frequently cited as reasons for differences in serum triglyceride and HDL levels and explained by an elevation of VLDL synthesis in overweight patients. However, triglyceride reduction and lipoprotein changes appear to be inducible by physical activity alone.[10,11,27]

V. PRACTICAL IMPORTANCE OF THE SHIFT IN THE LIPOPROTEIN PROFILE INDUCED BY PHYSICAL EXERCISE

The results and facts presented support the hypothesis of a multifactorial change in lipid and lipoprotein metabolism induced by increased physical activity. By means of physical exercise, it seems possible to favorably affect the lipid profile of the "still healthy" as well as the atherogenic lipid profile of cardiac risk groups, such as hypercholesterolemic individuals. This effect is achieved either directly, with respect to the currently known factors for atherosclerosis, or indirectly, by circumstances which are coupled with a monitored and physically active lifestyle. Overall, the differences observed in serum lipoprotein profiles between untrained and endurance-trained subjects strongly indicate adaptation mechanisms induced by physical activity. These effects cause the following metabolic processes that oppose possible progression of vascular atherosclerotic processes:

1.   Enlargement of the HDL pool responsible for reverse cholesterol transport with an elevation of the HDL-2 subfraction component that is considered cardio-protective.
2.   Acceleration of plasma triglyceride cleavage with improved metabolism of the probably atherogenic large triglyceride-rich LDL particles.[34]
3.   Reduction of the LDL pool with decrease in the certainly atherogenic small LDL particles.

VI. CONCLUSION

Aerobic physical activity — with respect to the lipid and lipoprotein metabolism — results in a reduction of triglycerides, total and LDL cholesterol, with a particular reduction in small LDL particles, and a clear increase in HDL cholesterol and particular HDL-2 subfraction particles. These changes are dependent on the intensity and frequency of physical activity. These phenomena create the condition for both the cardio-protective effect of physical activity in primary prevention, especially in hypercholesterolemia,[16] and also for the reduction of cardiac mortality rates in patients after myocardial infarction by training-oriented rehabilitation measures.[1] That extensive changes in lifestyle accompanied by changes in nutrition and eating habits can actually result in a demonstrable success of reducing coronary atherosclerosis has recently been shown in a prospective study with coronary heart disease patients.[22] This is another reason to promote physical exercise in primary and secondary prevention of dyslipoproteinemia and coronary heart disease.

REFERENCES

1. **O'Conner, G.T., Buring, J.E., Yusuf, S., et al.**, An overview of randomized trials of rehabilitation with exercise after myocardial infarction, *Circulation*, 80, 234, 1989.
2. **Baumstark, M., Kreutz, W., Berg, A., Frey, I., and Keul, J.**, Structure of human low-density lipoprotein subfractions, determined by X-ray small-angle scattering, *Biochim. Biophys. Acta*, 1037, 48, 1990.
3. **Foster, D.M., Chait, A., Albers, J.J., Failor, R.A., Harris, C., and Brunzell, J.D.**, Evidence for kinetic heterogeneity among human low density lipoproteins, *Metabolism*, 35, 685, 1986.
4. **Gordon, D.J. and Rifkind, B.M.**, High-density lipoprotein — the clinical implications of recent studies, *N. Engl. J. Med.*, 321, 1311, 1989.
5. **Teng, B., Thompson, G.R., Sniderman, A.D., Forte, T.M., Krauss, R.M., and Kwiterovich, P.O.**, Composition and distribution of low density lipoprotein fractions in hyperapobetalipoproteinemia, normolipidemia, and familial hypercholesterolemia, *Proc. Natl. Acad. Sci. U.S.A.*, 80, 6662, 1983.
6. **Levy, R.I., Brensike, J.F., Epstein, S.E., et al.**, The influence of changes in lipid values induced by cholestyramine and diet on progression of coronary artery disease: results of the NHLBI Type II Coronary Intervention Study, *Circulation*, 69, 325, 1984.
7. **Brown, G., Albers, J.J., Fisher, L.D., et al.**, Regression of coronary artery disease as a result of intensive lipid-lowering therapy in men with high levels of apoprotein B, *N. Engl. J. Med.*, 323, 1287, 1990.
8. **Austin, M.A., King, M.C., Vranizan, K., and Krauss, R.M.**, Atherogenic lipoprotein phenotype: a proposed genetic marker for coronary heart disease risk, *Circulation*, 82, 495, 1990.
9. **Berg, A., Johns, J., Baumstark, M., Kreutz, W., and Keul, J.**, HDL subfractions after a single, extended episode of physical exercise, *Atheroslerosis*, 47, 231, 1983.
10. **Berg, A. and Keul, J.**, Influence of maximum aerobic capacity and relative body weight on the lipoprotein profile in athletes, *Atherosclerosis*, 55, 225, 1985.
11. **Dufaux, B., Assmann, G., and Hollmann, W.**, Plasma lipoproteins and physical activity: a review, *Int. J. Sports. Med.*, 3, 123, 1982.
12. **Griffin, B.A., Skinner, E.R., and Maughan, R.J.**, The acute effect of prolonged walking and dietary changes on plasma lipoprotein concentrations and high-density lipoprotein subfractions, *Metabolism*, 37, 535, 1988.
13. **Williams, P.T., Krauss, R.M., Vranizan, K.M., and Wood, P.D.S.**, Changes in lipoprotein subfractions during diet-induced and exercise-induced weight loss in moderately overweight men, *Circulation*, 81, 1293, 1990.
14. **Wood, P.D., Stefanick, M.L., Dreon, D.M., et al.**, Changes in plasma lipids and lipoproteins in overweight men during weight loss through dieting as compared with exercise, *N. Engl. J. Med.*, 319, 1173, 1988.
15. **Haskell, W.**, The influence of exercise training on plasma lipids and lipoproteins in health and disease, *Acta Med. Scand.*, 711, 25, 1985.
16. **Paffenbarger, R., Hyde, R.T., Wing, A.L., and Steinmetz, C.H.**, A natural history of athleticism and cardiovascular health, *J. Am. Med. Assoc.*, 252, 491, 1984.
17. **Williams, P.T., Haskell, W.L. and Vranizan, K.**, The effects of running mileage and duration on plasma lipoprotein levels, *JAMA*, 247, 2674, 1982.
18. **Chance, B., Leigh, J.S., Clark, B.J., et al.**, Control of oxidative metabolism and oxygen delivery in human skeletal muscle: a steady-state analysis of the work/energy cost transfer function, *Proc. Natl. Acad. Sci. U.S.A.*, 82, 8384, 1985.
19. **Keul, J., Doll, E., and Keppler, D.**, Energy metabolism of human muscle, *Med. Sport (Basel)*, 7, 1972.
20. **Berg, A., Jakob, E., Lehmann, M., Dickhuth, H.H., Huber, G., and Keul, J.**, Aktuelle Aspekte der modernen Ergometrie, *Pneumologie*, 44, 2, 1990.

21. **Berg, A., Lehmann, M., and Keul, J.**, *Körperliche Aktivität bei Gesunden und Koronarkranken*, 2nd ed., Thieme Verlag, Stuttgart, Germany, 1986.
22. **Ornish, D., Brown, S.E., Scherwitz, L.W., et al.**, Can lifestyle changes reverse coronary heart disease? *Lancet*, 336, 129, 1990.
23. **Ren, J., Henriksson, J., Katz, A., and Sahlin, K.**, NADH content in type I and type II human muscle fibres after dynamic exercise, *Biochem. J.*, 251, 183, 1988.
24. **Oscai, L. and Palmer, W.**, Muscle lipolysis during exercise — an update, *Sports Med.*, 6, 23, 1988.
25. **Stremmel, W. and Diede, H.**, Fatty acid uptake by human hepatoma cell lines represents a carrier-mediated uptake process, *Biochim. Biophys. Acta*, 1013, 218, 1989.
26. **Vyska, K., Machulla, H., Stremmel, W., et al.**, Regional myocardial free fatty acid extraction in normal and ischemic myocardium, *Circulation*, 78, 1218, 1988.
27. **Thompson, P.D., Cullinane, E.M., Sady, S.P., Flynn, M.M., Chenevert, C.B., and Herbert, P.N.**, High density lipoprotein metabolism in endurance athletes and sedentary men, *Circulation*, 84, 140, 1991.
28. **Kiens, B. and Lithell, H.**, Lipoprotein metabolism influenced by training-induced changes in human skeletal muscle, *J. Clin. Invest.*, 83, 558, 1989.
29. **Frey, I., Baumstark, M.W., Berg, A., and Keul, J.**, Influence of acute maximal exercise on lecithin: cholesterol acyltransferase activity in healthy adults of differing
30. **Stubbe, I., Hansson, P.G., Nilsson-Ehle,** Plasma lipoproteins and lipolytic enzyme activities during endurance training in sedentary men: changes in high density lipoprotein subfractions and composition, *Metabolism*, 32, 1120, 1983.
31. **Haberek-Davidson, A., Stefanick, M.L., Superko, H.R., Terry, R.B., Lindgren, F., and Wood, P.D.**, Correlation of adipose tissue lipoprotein lipase (LPL) activity with plasma lipoprotein subfractions in overweight men, *Fed. Proc.*, 44, 1893, 1985.
32. **Goldberg, I.J., Le, N.A., and Paterniti, J.R.**, Lipoprotein metabolism during acute inhibition of hepatic triglyceride lipase in the cynomolgus monkey, *J. Clin. Invest.*, 70, 1184, 1982.
33. **Frey, I., Berg, A., Baumstark, M.W., Collatz, K.G., and Keul, J.**, Effects of age and physical performance capacity on distribution and composition of high-density subfractions in men, *Eur. J. Appl. Physiol.*, 60, 441, 1990.
34. **Krauss, R.M., Williams, P.T., Brensike, J., et al.**, Intermediate-density lipoproteins and progression of coronary artery disease in hypercholesterolaemic men, *Lancet*, 2, 62, 1987.

Chapter 4

EXERCISE, NATURAL IMMUNITY, AND CANCER: CAUSATION, CORRELATION, OR CONUNDRUM

Laurie Hoffman-Goetz and Brian MacNeil

TABLE OF CONTENTS

I. INTRODUCTION

Cancer is a leading cause of premature death in North America, second only to cardiovascular disease. Whereas deaths from heart disease and stroke have been declining since a peak in 1960, the age-adjusted cancer mortality has been climbing.[1] Major initiatives outlined by the National Cancer Institute (U.S.) include objectives for the year 2000 of a reduction in cancer mortality by 50% from what would occur if the 1980 rates were to prevail to the end of the century.[2] Greater focus on prevention, screening, and determination of biobehavioral risk factors has been suggested by experts to offer more promise than the development of "cures" in the war against cancer.[1,3,4] The staggering economic burden of cancer in the U.S. is estimated at over 35 billion dollars annually in direct costs;[5] this economic factor alone is a compelling argument for prevention based enabling strategies.

Against this backdrop of emphasis on prevention and determination of risk factors is the sobering realization that cancer is a complex group of more than 100 diseases. Some cancers, such as Wilms' tumor, are principally diseases of children; other cancers, such as pancreatic cancer, are largely diseases of the elderly; still other cancers have characteristic incidence patterns according to age and sex (e.g., cervical cancer). Cancers can originate in solid tissue, blood, or lymphatic glands. Because each type of cancer is associated with distinct and complex risk factors, preventive measures must be multidimensional.

This chapter considers the evidence for cancer-specific benefits and risks of physical activity and exercise. Animal studies[6-9] and epidemiologic studies (e.g., Kohl et al.[10] for review) are cautiously suggestive of relationships between physical activity and certain cancers; however, when a significant association is observed, biologically plausible mechanisms are not usually explored. In view of the numerous physiological and biochemical changes which occur with exercise, emphasis will be placed on those changes which occur in the natural immune system with chronic exercise and in the physically conditioned individual. Although current scientific opinion suggests that spontaneous tumors in humans are largely nonimmunogenic,[11] natural (nonspecific) immune mechanisms may be of relevance in tumor surveillance and in cancer therapy. Clinical trials to evaluate the efficacy of various components and products of the natural immune system in cancer immunotherapy are underway.[12] In spite of the considerable work on natural immune mechanisms against cancer, and the increasing attention to natural immune changes with exercise, the hypothesis that physical activity influences the incidence of and mortality from certain cancers consequent to the enhancement of natural immunity has not been systematically evaluated.

At this point, it may be useful to consider a review by Caspersen et al.[13] on the differences between physical activity, exercise, and physical fitness. Physical activity refers to any activity that results from muscular contraction and is best thought of as the total energy expenditure throughout a day, including sleep and occupational and leisure activity. The majority of epidemiological studies examine physical activity to varying degrees of completeness. Exercise is a portion of physical activity, but is a distinct subset due to the intention of those performing the activity to maintain or improve some aspect of physical fitness. The vast majority of studies on natural immunity examine responses to exercise only and not the broader category of physical activity. Finally, physical fitness is a set of attributes including cardiovascular and muscular endurance, muscular strength, flexibility, and body composition. Physical fitness is determined in part by a genetic element. Confusing data may evolve from these unapparent differences if epidemiological studies measure physical activity (assessed by occupational status) and cancer risks, while laboratory studies of natural immunity focus only on exercise. Improved methods of determining physical activity and its components in epidemiological studies may greatly assist interpreting results from exercise-based laboratory studies. Likewise, assessing natural immune function during various components of physical activity is warranted.

II. PHYSICAL ACTIVITY AND CANCER

A. PHYSICAL ACTIVITY AND COLON CANCER

Colon cancer is generally thought of as a disease of western, industrialized countries with the highest incidence rates in the U.S. and Canada, and the lowest in Asia, Africa, and South America. Because colon cancer is viewed as a formidable disease with limited therapeutic success, recent scientific efforts have focused on prevention with the aim of identifying lifestyle-related etiologic factors.[14]

Most of the recent etiologic hypotheses linking lifestyle to colon cancer have emphasized dietary factors, especially high fat and/or low fiber diets. These factors have been demonstrated to modify bile acid excretion, microflora constituency in the gut, and bacterial enzymatic activity, with the net result being alteration in the concentration of suspected carcinogens.[15-17] Other dietary factors, including elevated alcohol consumption[18,19] and low vitamin D intake,[20-23] have also been implicated in influencing colon cancer risk.

Another potential risk factor for colon cancer which has received considerable public attention is physical activity. Despite an increasing number of epidemiological studies, the relationship between physical activity and colon cancer risk is not straightforward. The controversy stems from a number of factors which influence the interpretation of the strength of association between physical activity and risk for colon cancer. These include the multidimensional nature of physical activity, which involves activities of daily living, occupational activity, and exercise;[13] the reliability of assessment instruments of physical activity that are used in epidemiological investigations;[24] the absence of data linking instruments for assessment of physical activity with physiological measures of fitness such as maximal oxygen uptake or body composition analysis;[13] difficulties in partitioning significant effects due to physical activity (including occupational activity) from exercise; uncertainty about the optimum levels of exercise which minimize cancer-specific risks;[25] confounding of physical activity data with body weight and fatness which also impact on colon cancer risk;[19,26] and inability to separate effects due to physical activity from dietary changes accompanying exercise, such as increased caloric intake.[27-29] A recent review by Kohl and associates[10] outlines the methodological issues inherent in epidemiological studies of physical activity and cancer.

Despite these caveats and limitations, physical activity and colon cancer incidence show significant association which argues for the importance of this potential risk factor. Several case-control studies,[30-38] using occupational activity alone or including physical activities performed in recreation or leisure, suggest an inverse relationship between sedentariness and relative risk for colon cancer; the adjusted (by age, smoking history, gender, body weight, and in some studies, diet) relative risk for sedentary males and colon cancer incidence is on the order of 1.6 to 3.0, depending upon the site (e.g., ascending vs. descending colon). An impressive study by Whittemore et al.[39] using continentally separate but ethnically related populations with different colon cancer risks supports the hypothesis that a sedentary lifestyle increases the relative risk for colon cancers; sedentary Chinese-Americans, classified by either job type or by lifestyle, had significantly elevated risk for colon cancers (*males:* odds raio (O.R.) = 1.6, 95% confidence interval (C.I.) = 1.1 to 2.4 for sedentary lifestyle; O.R. = 2.5, 95% C.I. = 1.1 to 5.9 for sedentary by job type; *females:* O.R. = 2.0, 95% C.I. = 1.2 to 3.3 for sedentary lifestyle). In China, a sedentary lifestyle was associated with increased risk for colon cancer only in females (O.R. = 2.5, 95% C.I. = 1.0 to 6.3). In contrast, a recent study by Kune and colleagues[40] did not find a significant association between physical activity and risk of colon cancer in either males or females.

Prospective studies typically provide a higher degree of methodological rigor since baseline measurement of physical activity is unlikely to be confounded by the presence of cancer or faulty recall by respondents. Wu et al.[19] reported on the association between colon cancer incidence and physical activity. This study was a 4.5 year follow-up of >11,000 males and females of a retirement community in California. Physical activity was classified in three levels (<1 h, 1 to 2 h, or >2 h/d), although the total duration of physical activity was not given. Data for males showed the most physically active group having a reduced relative risk of 0.62 (95% C.I.: 0.45 to 0.87) for colon cancer incidence relative to the physically less active group. No data were presented for females. Seversen et al.[41] conducted a study of 8,000 Japanese American men living in Hawaii. Physical activity was classified as the average time spent over 24 h in five types of activities (basal, sedentary, slight, moderate, heavy) which was linked to estimates of oxygen consumption. Both occupational and nonoccupational physical activity was included.

During an 11-year followup, 191 cases of colon cancer were detected. Although higher levels of physical activity were associated with a reduced risk of colon cancer, the risks did not decrease in a linear fashion, nor was the trend significant. Ballard-Barbash et al.[37] examined the association between self-reported physical activity and large bowel cancer in a cohort of participants of the Framingham Study. The cohort (1906 men and 2308 women) was followed for 28 years. A physical activity index, similar to that used by Seversen et al.,[41] was computed for the various levels of physical activity. An inverse association between physical activity and large bowel cancer was observed for men but not for women. The age-adjusted relative risk for inactive men, relative to highly active men, was 1.8. This association was not confounded by body mass index. However, it should be noted that the 95% C.I. was wide and included 1.0.

Animal studies have focused on the exercise component of physical activity in relation to colon cancer. Andrianopoulos et al.[42] allowed male rats voluntary access to in-cage running wheels over 20 weeks and measured the number, weight, and size of 1,2-dimethylhydrazine (DMH)-induced colon tumors. Rats given free access to running wheels had a significantly reduced incidence of DMH-induced tumors (6/11) relative to nonphysically active controls (18/20). However, because exercised rats had lower body weights than nonexercised controls, the possibility of confounding by caloric restriction cannot be ruled out. Klurfeld et al.[43] partitioned the anti-DMH tumor promoting effects of caloric restriction and exercise. Colon tumor incidence in rats given forced treadmill exercise at a relatively high intensity (24 m/min, 60 min duration, 5 d/week) was significantly lower than ad libitum fed, sedentary controls, but higher than either calorically restricted and exercised or calorically restricted and sedentary animals. Lower body weight, as well as reduced colon transit time, likely contributed to the lower incidence of colon tumors observed in the exercised animals.

B. PHYSICAL ACTIVITY AND CANCERS OF THE BREAST AND REPRODUCTIVE SYSTEM

Breast cancer currently ranks as the leading cause of cancer mortality in North American women.[44] The search for major etiologic factors in breast cancer points to age at menarche, the cumulative number of ovulatory cycles, and levels and metabolism of sex steroids, particularly estrogen, as major determinants of risk.[45,46] Dietary factors, especially high fat intake and/or low intake of cruciferous vegetables, have also been linked to risk of breast cancer. Dietary fats have been hypothesized to increase levels of physiologically active estrogen derivatives (e.g., 16 α-hydroxyestrone and estriol) and thereby enhance the risk for endocrine-responsive tumors such as cancer of the breast. Epidemiologic studies suggest that in countries where saturated fat intake is low, the incidence of breast cancer is low and, conversely, where the intake of saturated fat is high, the incidence of breast cancer is correspondingly high.[47-49] Methodological issues in epidemiologically driven studies of diet and breast cancer have been reviewed by Graham.[50] Relationships among dietary components, estrogen metabolism, and breast cancer are further complicated by the presence of obesity, which also affects levels of endogenous estrogens.[51]

The idea that exercise may have a protective effect against cancers of the breast and reproductive system was first put forward by Frisch et al.[52] Alumnae (5398) from eight colleges and two universities were surveyed concerning women's health issues. The women were classified as athletes (minimum 1 year university-level athletics team or regular volitional exercise conditioning) or nonathletes. The nonathletes had higher relative risks for cancers of the breast (1.86, 95% C.I. = 1.00 to 3.47) and the reproductive system (2.53, 95% C.I. = 1.17 to 5.47) compared with former college athletes. Potential confounding variables of age, family history of cancer, age of menarche, number of pregnancies, oral contraceptive use, exogenous estrogen use, body weight, and cigarette smoking were controlled for in the analyses. It should be noted, however, that despite the strength of the association, this study used prevalence rates. Selection bias, due to selective cancer deaths prior to the survey point, and problems related to temporal sequence (i.e., determination that athletic participation antedated cancer occurrence), need to be considered in interpreting this study. Lower prevalence (lifetime) rates for former college athletes of nonreproductive system cancers, excluding cancers of the skin and cutaneous melanoma, have been reported for this population,[53] as well as lower prevalence of benign tumors of the breast and reproductive system.[54] One hypothesized mechanism for the beneficial effect of exercise in reducing risk of breast and reproductive system cancers involves delay or interruption of ovulatory cycles.[55] Intense exercise in premenarcheal girls is associated with delays in menarche and secondary amenorrhea during adolescence;[56-58] delays in menarche and fewer cumulative number of ovulatory cycles have been reported to reduce the risk of breast cancer.[59-61]

Experimental data on exercise and mammary tumors in rodents add another level of complexity to the exercise-cancer association, namely, voluntary vs. forced exercise. Rodents given voluntary exercise prior to chemical induction of mammary tumors (e.g., N-methylnitrosourea) have reduced tumor incidence and prolonged tumor latency relative to sedentary controls.[62-65] Stimulation of rat mammary tumorigenesis occurs with forced exercise.[66-69] Unfortunately, since the intensity of physical exercise was not determined in these studies (either by oxygen consumption measurements or by end-point skeletal muscle oxidative enzyme activities indicative of training), it is difficult to titrate the effect of exercise on mammary tumorigenesis. For example, in the study by Thompson et al.,[67] rats were exercised at an absolute intensity of 20 m/min, 1 degree slope, 15 min/d, 5 d/week for 140 d; over time, however, the relative intensity of the work would drop, leading to a dilution of the exercise effects. Moreover, forced vs. voluntary exercise represent very different paradigms in terms of evoking the psychological stress response which in itself modifies experimental tumorigenesis.[70,71] Endocrine and immunologic responses were not evaluated in these forced exercise paradigms.

C. PHYSICAL ACTIVITY AND OTHER SITE-SPECIFIC CANCERS

There are only a handful of epidemiological reports evaluating the impact of physical activity and/or exercise on cancers other than of the colon and breast. The paucity of data and often conflicting direction of effects between studies limits the conclusions which can be drawn about physical activity and other site-specific cancers.

In a case-control study of prostate cancer risk and lifetime occupational physical activity, Le Marchand et al.[72] reported a significant negative association with years spent in sedentary or light activity occupations among men >70 years (O.R. = 0.5, 95% C.I. = 0.3 to 0.9), i.e., lower risk among occupationally inactive subjects. Paffenbarger et al.[73] found that individuals who were physically active in sports during college had a higher relative risk of prostate cancer than those who were less active (R.R. = 1.66, p < 0.03); however, in a subsequent analysis of a subset of this population using a more accurate measure of physical activity, no association was found between physical activity and prostate cancer risk. Seversen et al.[41] found no association between physical activity and cancer of the prostate. In contrast, a recent case-control study[38] using cases and controls drawn from the Missouri Cancer Registry showed a significantly increased risk of prostate cancer (O.R. = 1.5, 95% C.I. = 1.2 to 1.8) in individuals classified as low occupational activity (<20% time physically active). Higher relative risk (1.8, 95% C.I. = 1.0 to 3.3) for incidence of prostate cancer in the NHANES 1 population was associated with little or no recreational exercise.[74] Given that the direction of the association between physical activity and prostate cancer is inconsistent, and further, since there are no experimental studies in this area, it is impossible to draw meaningful conclusions at this time.

Scientific evidence relating lung cancer risk with physical activity is more limited. Two studies report an increased risk of lung cancer in physically inactive men, as classified by occupation;[38,74] control for second hand cigarette smoke, which is more likely to be encountered in sedentary occupations, was not included in either study. Paffenbarger et al.[73] reported a general trend for reduction in mortality rates due to lung cancers in moderately to highly active men, controlling for differences in age, smoking, and body mass index. In contrast, Seversen et al.[41] did not find a consistent association between lung cancer and level of physical activity. To date, there is only one study on experimental lung tumors and exercise.[75] Incidence of induced CIRAS 3 lung tumors in mice given treadmill exercise for 6 weeks was not significantly different from sedentary controls. The impact of voluntary exercise on the incidence and latency of experimental lung tumors in rodents has not been investigated.

D. PHYSICAL ACTIVITY AND CANCER OF ALL SITES

Several studies report on the association between physical activity and overall cancer mortality or risk. An early study[76] reported cancer deaths in a cohort of 8400 former Harvard alumni categorized as major, minor, or nonathletes; major athletes had a significantly higher cancer death rate, and early age at death relative to nonathletes. A similar association between athletics and death from neoplasia was reported by Rook[77] in a study of Cambridge University sportsmen. In contrast, three recent epidemiological investigations suggest a protective effect of physical activity on cancer (all sites) mortality. Paffenbarger et al.[73] reported a significant decline in death rates from all cancers along a gradient of physical activity (as assessed by postcollege recreational exercise) in a large cohort of Harvard alumni. In the study by Albanes et al.,[74] the relative risk of cancer in males who were physically inactive by job classification was significantly elevated relative to very active individuals; the highest relative risk for cancer was found in males who were inactive both recreationally and occupationally (R.R. = 1.9, 95% C.I. = 1.3 to 2.7). An interesting study by Blair et al.[78] evaluated physical fitness, as measured by a maximal treadmill exercise test, and the risk of cancer mortality in >10,000 men and >3,000 women. Cigarette smoking, body mass index, serum cholesterol and glucose, and blood pressure were controlled for in the analyses. Age-adjusted cancer death rates were significantly lower in both men and women who were in the most fit quintile, relative to those in the least fit quintile. Possible biological mechanisms to explain the protective effect of physical activity/exercise/fitness on risk of cancer were not presented in these studies. Such mechanisms would be systemic in nature (e.g., endocrinological, immunological) rather than unique to a given body compartment (e.g., colonic peristalis), although systemic effects would not preclude concurrent tissue specific effects. Further, these mechanisms should exhibit a dose response relationship to physical activity, exercise, and/or physical fitness, and demonstrate plausibility and coherence with existing knowledge in cancer biology.

In summary, although physical activity/exercise/physical fitness may be risk factors for cancer, the epidemiological and experimental evidence is not at all conclusive about the strength of the association. The strongest data are for sedentariness and higher incidence of cancer of the colon. Firmer conclusions regarding cancers of the breast and reproductive system await prospective studies and clinical trials. Given the methodological difficulties in assessing physical activity and exercise in epidemiological surveys, and the relative absence of animal studies in this field, exercise and physical activity are conceptually provocative but circumstantially inconclusive factors in cancer risk.

III. CANCER AND NATURAL IMMUNITY

This section presents a brief overview of natural immune mechanisms that are involved (experimentally at least) in tumor control. Natural immunity encompasses a variety of cells and biologically active secretory products from these cells. Natural immune mechanisms display neither specificity (or only partial specificity) nor immunological memory, are inducible, show self-nonself discrimination, and play important roles in resistance to disease. It is beyond the scope of this chapter to present a detailed review of natural immune components; many excellent reviews on this topic are available.[79,80] We will, instead, attempt to provide a framework for the later consideration of exercise-induced changes in natural immunity and how these may relate to cancer processes. Since the majority of spontaneously arising tumors appear to be nonimmunogenic,[11,81,82] the natural immune system may be an important initial line of defense against neoplastic cells. The focus will be on the evidence for the involvement of macrophages and natural killer (NK) cells and the secretory products of these cells, such as interleukin-1 (IL-1) and tumor necrosis factor (TNF) in tumor destruction. These components of natural immunity have been the most extensively studied in relation to exercise.

Activated macrophages appear to be cytostatic and/or cytotoxic.[83-85] Although numerous cells and products can lead to macrophage activation, of relevance here is the role of cytokines such as INF γ and macrophage activating factor (MAF).[83-85] The mechanisms by which macrophages exert their cytotoxic effects are not certain and both direct and indirect mechanisms have been reported.[83,86] The indirect pathway involves the release from activated macrophages of IL-1 and TNF.[87] Both of these cytokines have been shown to be tumorilytic.[83,86,88-90] Support for a direct mechanism of macrophage cytotoxicity stems from the ability of activated macrophages to lyse IL-1 and TNF resistant tumor cells.[83,86] This process may involve transfer of cytolytic substances such as hydrolytic enzymes, hydrogen peroxide, or complement component C3 into tumor cells at areas of direct cell to cell contact.[83,91,92] In general, the cytotoxic actions of macrophages are reduced in cancer patients[93-95] and plasma from some cancer patients has inhibitory effects on macrophage cytotoxicity.[94,96] Prostaglandin E_2 is known to down regulate macrophage cytotoxicity[97,98] and has been reported to be produced in higher quantities by tumor cells relative to nontumor cells.[99] Quite opposite to the cytolytic actions of macrophages, there are also reports of macrophages stimulating tumor growth.[100-102] The mechanism may involve IL-1, at least for fibroblast-derived tumors, or it may be that the presence of macrophages at the tumor site results in the generation of macrophage-resistant variants of the tumor that can grow more rapidly than original tumor cells.[84]

The ability of NK cells to destroy neoplastic cells is well established.[103,104] Low levels of NK activity *in vitro* have been associated with greater metastatic responses, while high levels of NK activity (due to strain characteristics or chemical inducers of NK cytotoxicity) result in reduced metastasis.[105,106]

Similar results have been reported with *in vivo* assessment of NK activity and tumor growth.[107] Indeed, tumor cells resistant to NK lysis may be more metastatic than NK-sensitive tumors.[108]

Experimental evidence for a critical role of NK cells in tumor resistance derives from studies using monoclonal antibodies to inactivate or block NK cell responses. Injection of one such monoclonal antibody (anti-asialo GM_1) enhanced pulmonary and hepatic metastasis.[109] Antimetastatic activity could be restored by injection of normal donor spleen cells presumably containing a population of NK cells; if, however, the donor spleen cells were also treated with anti-asialo GM_1, tumor metastasis was not limited. The transfer of the same number of mature T lymphocytes had no effect on tumor outcome.[110] Anti-asialo GM_1 treatment did not affect the growth of the primary tumor in the footpad, suggesting that the main location of tumor resistance offered by NK cells is in the blood.[109]

The ineffectiveness of NK cells against solid tumors has been demonstrated by the finding of reduced NK activity with increasing tumor mass.[111-115] This may partially reflect the large number of tumor cells present in a solid tumor compared to the number of NK effector cells: tumor cell growth rates overwhelm NK lytic capacity. Accompanying this is the potential for actual suppression of NK function.[113,115] Possible mechanisms of the tumor-induced NK suppression include inhibition of the production of positive regulators such as IL-2 or INF. It may be that NK cells become refractory to stimulation by cytokines and lymphokines.[116] Prostaglandin (PG) production is another possible mechanism for the reduction in NK activity in cancer patients. Macrophages can infiltrate tumors[117] and release PGs,[118] which in turn could inhibit NK activity.[119] This tumor-induced suppression of NK cells is also apparent in human cancer patients with advanced disease, as they typically exhibit low levels of NK activity.[103,113,120]

Cytokines have both direct and indirect effects in natural tumor resistance. The direct cytotoxic action has been attributed to some cytokines such as IL-1, TNF, and IFN.[83,86,88-90,121] The other aspect of cytokine anti-tumor activity is the ability to regulate other cells of the immune system which have cytotoxic functions. Interferon γ is able to enhance the cytotoxic function of macrophages.[88] One area currently receiving much attention is the use of IL-2- and lymphokine-activated killer cells (LAK) as a therapy for cancer patients with advanced disease.[12,116] Some cytokines possess autocrine effects such as the ability of TNF to enhance TNF production by macrophages.[86] Finally, it is likely that a complex network of cytokine communications exist[121,122] which may also interact with neuroendocrine factors to regulate natural tumor immunity.[123] In tumor-bearing rats, production of IL-1 and IL-2 is reduced[124] which may be a factor in successful tumor proliferation. Tumor resection was followed by a partial return of IL-2 activity toward those of control animals.

Although there is experimental support that NK cells, macrophages, and various cytokines play a role in resistance to some tumors, *in vivo* evidence has been more difficult to obtain. The central question of whether higher levels of NK activity and other components of natural immunity, prior to development of cancer, results in greater resistance to the cancer is unclear. Longitudinal prospective studies, with the aim of identifying normal population variation in natural immune reactivity and subsequent cancer development, would help clarify this issue.

IV. EXERCISE AND NATURAL IMMUNITY

The recent surge of interest in the area of exercise and immunology has revealed that many immune parameters are altered after an acute bout of physical activity. However, exercise simultaneously results in many other systemic changes, such as neuroendocrine function, blood flow patterns, and fluid and electrolyte balance. As a result, one may ask if the immune fluctuations are of any relevance to the functioning of the immune system *in vivo* in terms of host resistance. Although transient immune changes may affect the response to a pathogen if encountered within that window of time, it is most likely that meaningful effects of exercise on immunity will be those that are present in the resting state after a period of chronic exposure to exercise. Therefore, studies that examine immune parameters both at rest and after acute exercise in trained and untrained individuals provide the most useful information regarding the ability of exercise to alter immune function. A further consideration is the time past since the last bout of activity if true resting samples are to be obtained. This can be particularly important for subjects currently undergoing regular training, since resting results may be biased by a recent training session. A minimum of 24 to 48 h should be allowed for stabilization of cell numbers and body fluids.

It is well established that physical exercise results in an increase in the number of circulating white blood cells which quickly returns to pre-exercise levels.[125-131] Most studies reveal that the resting number of leukocytes and the leukocytosis following acute activity is not changed by exercise training[130-134] with the exception of a recent report by Ferry et al.[134] in which a small reduction in leukocyte number was reported in trained cyclists at rest.

A. EXERCISE AND MONOCYTE/MACROPHAGE FUNCTION

The number of monocytes and macrophages have been reported to increase with exercise in trained and untrained individuals, with an increase or no change in the relative proportions of these cells.[125,133-137] However, in samples obtained from subjects at rest, chronic exercise training did not alter the levels of monocytes/macrophages.[133,134] Interestingly, Voronina and Mayanskii[138] found that in both mice and rats, exercise reduced the absolute number of blood monocytes and peritoneal macrophages while the number of alveolar macrophages was increased. Organ-specific changes have also been reported for lymphocyte subsets after exercise.[139] Thus, the site from which the sample was obtained may influence the results.

The phagocytic function of monocytes and macrophages has been shown to be unchanged[140] or increased after acute and chronic exercise.[136,141] Again, an organ-specific effect has also been demonstrated in that peritoneal and alveolar macrophage phagocytosis was increased while hepatic phagocytosis was reduced.[138] It was suggested that the increase in phagocytosis in the lung and peritoneum was secondary to the reduction in the liver since the liver typically accounts for 80 to 95% of total blood clearance. In a very comprehensive study, and one which examined human macrophages obtained from the connective tissue of the forearm, phagocytosis was enhanced by acute exercise compared to the subjects' resting values.[142] The same study also found that endurance-trained mice had elevated phagocytic levels at rest compared to untrained controls.

Macrophage migration, chemotaxis, and enzyme content was increased in resting trained mice and in acutely exercised humans and mice.[142] Macrophage activation has also been reported after exercise as indicated by release of neopterin and elevated reactive oxygen species production (as measured by nitroblue tetrazolium reduction).[136,141,143] Monocyte activation may result in prostaglandin (PG) production[118] which can be inhibitory to several immune responses.[119,144,145] An increase in monocyte percentage[146,147] and PGE_2[146] levels has been reported 2 h after an exercise session. Prostaglandins have been shown to affect cell growth rates of normal epithelium and colonic tumors[148,149] and intestinal motility;[150] both may be important factors in colon cancer. Monocytes sampled from trained cyclists had enhanced IL-1 production for up to 2 h after submaximal exercise.[133] Finally, mouse peritoneal macrophages obtained after exhaustive treadmill running were better able to retard the growth of cultured sarcoma cells although antibody-dependent cellular cytotoxicity was not affected.[151]

B. EXERCISE AND NEUTROPHIL FUNCTION

Acute exercise increases the absolute number of circulating neutrophils; however, a reduction in neutrophil percentage is present due to a greater increase in lymphocyte numbers.[126,127,131,133-135,152-154] Chronic exercise has been reported to reduce,[134,155] increase,[131] or not change[133] the numbers of circulating neutrophils in the resting state. The bactericidal activity of neutrophils may be unchanged[133] or elevated by exercise.[156,157] Pedersen et al.[146] followed the neutrophil numbers and chemiluminescence before, at the end of exercise, and 2 h and 24 h post-exercise. Although significant increases in neutrophil numbers were present post-exercise, the greatest increase occurred 2 h after exercise. The chemiluminescence data followed the same pattern; however, no significant increases were present until 2 h after exercise. The responses had returned, for the most part, to pre-exercise levels by 24 h after exercise. Resting function in trained individuals has been reported to be unchanged from sedentary controls[158] or reduced.[133] In a more extensive study,[157] the kinetics of neutrophil microbicidal activity was unaltered between trained and untrained subjects, but trained subjects displayed a lower sensitivity to the opsonized zymosan particles at low concentration levels. At saturating stimulus levels, no differences were present between the two groups.

C. EXERCISE AND CYTOKINES

Several earlier reports indicated that the plasma level of IL-1 is increased after exercise when measured via thymocyte proliferation assay or the ability to elevate body temperature.[159-161] These studies did not make any corrections for fluid shifts which occur in exercise. After an exhaustive treadmill test, 12 to 16% of plasma volume is lost.[162] This point is illustrated in a later study in which IL-1 levels were unchanged 2 h after exercise.[163] In this study, a specific RIA to assay plasma IL-1 was used and values were corrected for plasma volume shifts. The same earlier studies did report that the supernatants from unstimulated cultured mononuclear cells had an elevated IL-1 activity,[159] and that resting levels of IL-1 were higher in trained subjects relative to sedentary controls.[161] The resting samples in the trained subjects, however, may have been biased by recent exercise since athletes refrained from exercise for 2 d and controls for 7 d. Monocytes sampled post-exercise and stimulated in culture have a greater ability to produce IL-1 than monocytes obtained prior to exercise.[133] IL-2 production from mitogen-stimulated cells has been reported to be reduced[133] or increased[164] following exercise. Pahlavani[165] found a reduced IL-2 production after exercise only in young rats with no exercise effect in older rats. Uncorrected plasma IL-2 levels following exercise have been shown to be reduced for up to 2 h with an increase above resting values by 24 h after exercise.[166] Plasma TNF and INFα have been reported to be increased following an acute bout of exercise.[143,166,167]

D. EXERCISE AND NATURAL KILLER CELLS

The effects of acute exercise on NK cell frequency are well documented. Incorporating three fitness levels of subjects and four exercise protocols, Kendall et al.[168] observed similar increases in the NK cell percentage of total lymphocytes across all conditions. These effects were present for the four different bicycle ergometer exercise tests of varying intensity and duration. Overall, a significant increase in the proportion and absolute number of NK cells was present immediately after exercise, with complete recovery to resting levels by 30 min post-exercise. No differences were observed at rest between the groups for absolute number or percentage of NK cells, with the exception of the low fitness group having an elevated proportion of NK cells apparently due to lower levels of T-helper cells. Similar reports of exercise and NK cell number and percentage have been published.[146,169,170] The increase of NK cell number and percentage was shown to be a consistent effect when low fit subjects performed the same exercise routine for 5 d.[171] It should be noted that a definitive NK cell monoclonal antibody is not yet available to permit precise quantification of NK cells.

NK cell activity is known to increase after acute exercise, followed by a reduction in cytotoxic activity which is present by 2 h post-exercise.[146,169,172-175] Return to normal levels is typically complete by 24 h post-exercise. The increase in NK activity at the end of exercise is due, for the most part, to the increased proportion of NK cells. This will effectively increase the effector to target ratio in the cytotoxicity assay. The reduction in NK function 2 h post-exercise, however, cannot be accounted for quite so easily since cell numbers have normalized by this time. The reduced cytotoxicity is probably a delayed result of the fluctuations in neuroendocrine factors during the exercise session. Using an epinephrine infusion, Kappel et al.[147] were able to mimic the exercise-induced increase in NK activity immediately following exercise as well as the reduction in NK function 2 h later. The epinephrine effect was suggested to be due to an alteration in the number of NK cells immediately after exercise and an elevation of monocyte numbers 2 h post-exercise. And, although epinephrine did not affect NK cytotoxicity *in vitro,* other endocrine and neuroendocrine factors cannot be discounted. For example, receptors for many neuroendocrine factors are present within NK cells, and the ability of these factors to alter NK activity (at least *in vitro*) has been repeatedly demonstrated.[176-179]

Long term exercise appears to enhance NK activity, but this effect has not always been consistent. Elderly women who underwent a 16-week calisthenic and aerobic exercise program three times a week had elevated baseline NK activity.[180] A greater increase in NK activity following an acute bout of exercise was present in the exercise-trained group. This study may state more about the withdrawal from exercise in the control group since prior to the study, all subjects were enrolled in an ongoing exercise program for an unspecified period of time. In another group of elderly women, those enrolled in a brisk walking program for 15 weeks showed an increase in NK activity after 6 weeks compared to controls.[181] The significance of this finding is questionable since no further increases occurred in the walking group by 15 weeks, while the control NK activity levels rose to the level of the walking group.

Seasonal changes are known to occur in immune responses[182] and this raises questions about the actual role of exercise in regulating NK activity with chronic exercise. Fifteen weeks of 60 min exercise sessions 5 d/week reduced the resting NK cytotoxicity across 46 subjects.[183] This study did not include nonexercised controls for any changes that may have occurred within this time frame, regardless of exercise condition. Pedersen et al.[184] compared the NK response of untrained controls to elite racing cyclists. The trained group (at rest) had a mean of 38% of maximal target cell lysis compared to a mean of 30% for controls. The cyclists also had higher frequencies of NK cells (8.3% vs. 3.8%). Although subjects were instructed to refrain from exercise for 20 h prior to the sampling time, this may not have been adequate time for full recovery from the last training session in the cyclists.

In mice, acute bouts of exercise were shown to depress NK activity when sampled 30 min after an exhaustive treadmill run.[185] This effect was present in trained and untrained animals. Training nonsignificantly attenuated the reduction in NK activity after exercise. No enhancement of NK function was present at rest for the trained animals. A significant reduction in splenic NK cell frequency was noted in all the exercised groups regardless of the acute or chronic nature of the exercise. It is possible that during exercise, NK cells could leave the spleen and other sites of NK cell deposition to enter the circulation. This fits with human data since exercise increases the number of circulating NK cells.[168]

In general, it appears that exercise acutely increases NK activity during and immediately following exercise due, at least partially, to an increase in the proportion of NK cells present. Within 2 h, the response is reduced below normal levels and may not recover until the next day. This portion of the response is likely due to the effects of the various neuroendocrine changes that occur with exercise. Chronic exposure to exercise may or may not increase the NK activity but appears to be highly dependent on the length of the exercise history.

V. EXERCISE, NATURAL IMMUNITY, AND CANCER

The level at which exercise-induced changes in natural immunity could affect cancer development has not been conceptually addressed in the literature. Although descriptive studies of exercise and cancer are important for establishing associations, parallel work aimed at eludicating mechanisms, immunological or other, are clearly needed. The plausibility of linkages between physical activity, natural immunity, and cancer need to be considered within the framework of theories of the molecular biology of cancer initiation, promotion, and progression. For example, endocrine changes with exercise might influence the expression of lymphocyte protooncogenes (e.g., c-fos and c-myc), the expression of which is a requirement for lymphocyte activation and regulation of cell proliferation.[186,187] At this level, exercise-induced endocrine changes might function to enhance the expression of protooncogenes or inactivate tumor suppressor gene expression in cells of the immune system; presumably, this type of action could potentially contribute to the development of the neoplastic phenotype in cells of the immune system. Alternatively, exercise-induced changes in various hormones could influence signal transduction and cellular activation within natural killer cells, for example, through second messengers (e.g., protein kinase C, phospholipase C mediated pathways); the biologic consequences of activation would include cytokine secretion, such as TNF, which is tumorilytic. It is also important to observe that if exercise has a promotion or antipromotion effect (rather than influencing cancer initiation), this should lead to a period of increased or decreased risk, followed by a compensatory period once exercise has been stopped. Certain types of cancers are known to be hormone sensitive, such as those of the breast and reproductive system.[64,188] The same hormone changes that affect the function of natural immune system components may also affect the metabolic processes of these cancers, altering growth patterns, or the sensitivity to cytotoxic mechanisms. Alternatively, exercise-induced changes in blood flow might result in greater delivery of natural killer cells, cytokines, and so on to tissue sites where tumors are proliferating; at this level, exercise would interact with the immune system to enhance cancer surveillance and decrease early tumor growth. Indirect mechanisms involving interactions between exercise and other risk factors (e.g., influence of diet on natural immune function) also need to be explored in the development of models. In contrast, there is evidence to suggest that an active immune response can accelerate (rather than retard) the growth and progression of some tumors;[189] the role of NK cells as immunostimulatory agents in tumorigenesis is an area of current investigation. Thus, although exercise may enhance some aspects of natural immunity, whether this enhancement actually results in reduced tumor growth is unclear.

VI. CONCLUSIONS

The relationships between physical activity and/or exercise and cancer are undoubtedly complex. Although evidence from epidemiological and animal studies suggests that regular, physical activity reduces the risk of some human cancers or decreases experimental tumorigenesis, the strength of the evidence is controversial. Parallel studies on exercise and natural immunity, while demonstrating significant enhancement or suppression (depending on the nature and extent of exercise) of various immunological components, have not typically been translated into clinically relevant situations. Despite the conceptual appeal of an exercise-natural immunity-cancer relationship, empirical evidence to support or contest this relationship is not available to date.

Given that cancer is a constellation of diseases having complex interactive origins involving genetic and environmental factors, a single unifying role for exercise (or exercise coupled with natural immunity) in the etiology of cancer is unlikely. Nevertheless, to the extent that cancer incidence rates are increasing in the North American population, to the extent that biobehavioral risk factors for cancer are only imperfectly understood, and to the extent that physical fitness is an important component of public health promotion strategies, the subject of physical activity, natural immunity, and cancer will continue to merit diligent research in the basic and epidemiological sciences.

ACKNOWLEDGMENTS

This work was supported by a grant from the Natural Sciences and Engineering Research Council of Canada.

REFERENCES

1. **Bailar, J.C. and Smith, E.M.**, Progress against cancer? *N. Engl. J. Med.*, 314, 1226, 1986.
2. **Greenwald, P.G. and Sondik, E.J.**, Cancer control objectives for the nation: 1985–2000, *Natl. Cancer Inst. Monogr.*, 2, 3, 1986.
3. **Cairns, J.**, The treatment of diseases and the war against cancer, *Sci. Am.*, 253, 51, 1985.
4. **Breslow, L. and Cumberland, W.G.**, Progress and objectives in cancer control, *JAMA*, 259, 1690, 1988.
5. **Brown, M.L.**, The national economic burden of cancer: an update, *J. Natl. Cancer Inst.*, 82, 1811, 1990.
6. **Rusch, H.P. and Kline, B.E.**, The effect of exercise on the growth of a mouse tumor, *Cancer Res.*, 4, 116, 1944.
7. **Hoffman, S.A., Paschkis, K.E., DeBias, D.A., Cantarow, A., and Williams, T.L.**, The influence of exercise on the growth of transplanted rat tumors, *Cancer Res.*, 22, 597, 1962.
8. **Moore, C. and Tittle, P.W.**, Muscle activity, body fat, and induced rat mammary tumors, *Surgery*, 73, 329, 1973.
9. **Baracos, V.E.**, Exercise inhibits progressive growth of the Morris hepatoma 7777 in male and female rats, *Can. J. Physiol. Pharmacol.*, 67, 864, 1988.
10. **Kohl, H.W., LaPorte, R.E., and Blair, S.N.**, Physical activity and cancer: an epidemiologic perspective, *Sports Med.*, 6, 222, 1988.
11. **Hewitt, H.B.**, The choice of animal tumors for experimental studies of cancer therapy, in *Advances in Cancer Research*, Vol. 27, Klein, G. and Weinhouse, S., Eds., Academic Press, New York, 1978, 149.
12. **Rosenberg, S.A.**, Adoptive immunotherapy for cancer, *Science*, 262, 62, 1990.
13. **Caspersen, C.J., Powell, K.E., and Christenson, G.M.**, Physical activity, exercise, and physical fitness: definitions and distinctions for health related research, *Public Health Rep.*, 100, 126, 1985.
14. **Nomura, A.**, An international search for causative factors of colorectal cancer, *J. Natl. Cancer Inst.*, 82, 894, 1990.
15. **Reddy, B.S., Weisburger, J.H., and Wynder, E.L.**, Fecal bacterial β-glucuronidase: control by diet, *Science*, 183, 416, 1974.
16. **Roberfroid, M.B.**, Dietary modulation of experimental neoplastic development: role of fat and fiber content and caloric intake, *Mutat. Res.*, 259, 351, 1991.
17. **Burkitt, D.P.**, Epidemiology of cancer of the colon and rectum, *Cancer*, 28, 3, 1971.
18. **Breslow, N.E. and Enstrom, J.E.**, Geographic correlations between cancer mortality rates and alcohol-tobacco consumption in the United States, *J. Natl. Cancer Inst.*, 53, 631, 1974.
19. **Wu, A.H., Paganini-Hill, A., Ross, R.K., Henderson, B.E.**, Alcohol, physical activity and other risk factors for colorectal cancer: a prospective study, *Br. J. Cancer.*, 55, 687, 1987.
20. **Garland, C.F., Barrett-Connor, E., Rossof, A.H., Shekelle, R.B., Criqui, M.H., and Paul, O.**, Dietary vitamin D and calcium and risk of colorectal cancer: a 19 year prospective study in men, *Lancet*, p. 307, 1985.
21. **Frampton, R.J., Omond, S.A., and Eisman, J.A.**, Inhibition of human cancer cell growth by 1,25-dihydroxyvitamin D_3 metabolites, *Cancer Res.*, 43, 4443, 1983.
22. **Gorham, E.D., Garland, C.F., and Garland, F.C.**, Physical activity and colon cancer risk, *Int. J. Epidemiol.*, 18, 728, 1989.
23. **DeLuca, H.F. and Ostrem, V.**, The relationship between vitamin D system and cancer, *Adv. Exp. Med. Biol.*, 206, 413, 1986.
24. **LaPorte, R.E., Montoye, H.J., and Caspersen, C.J.**, Assessment of physical activity in epidemiologic research: problems and prospects, *Public Health Rep.*, 100, 131, 1985.

25. **Siscovick, D.S., LaPorte, R.E., and Newman, J.N.**, The disease-specific benefits and risks of physical activity and exercise, *Public Health Rep.*, 100, 180, 1985.
26. **Albanes, D.**, Potential for confounding of physical activity risk assessment by body weight and fatness, *Am. J. Epidemiol.*, 125, 745, 1987.
27. **Slattery, M.L. and Jacobs, D.R.**, The interrelationships of physical activity, physical fitness, and body measurements, *Med. Sci. Sports Exercise*, 19, 564, 1987.
28. **Willett, W.C. and Stampfer, M.J.**, Total energy intake: implications for epidemiologic analyses, *Am. J. Epidemiol.*, 124, 17, 1986.
29. **Willett, W.C.**, Implications of total energy intake for epidemiologic studies of breast and large-bowel cancer, *Am. J. Clin. Nutr.*, 45, 354, 1987.
30. **Gerhardsson, M., Norell, S.E., Kiviranta, H., Pedersen, N.L., and Ahlbom, A.**, Sedentary jobs and colon cancer, *Am. J. Epidemiol.*, 123, 775, 1986.
31. **Gerhardsson, M., Floderus, B., and Norell, S.E.**, Physical activity and colon cancer risk, *Int. J. Epidemiol.*, 17, 743, 1988.
32. **Gerhardsson DeVerdier, M., Steineck, G., Hagman, U., Rieger, A., and Norell, S.E.**, Physical activity and colon cancer: a case referent study in Stockholm, *Int. J. Cancer*, 46, 985, 1990.
33. **Vena, J.E., Graham, S., Zielezny, M., Swanson, M.K., Barnes, R.E., and Nolan, J.**, Lifetime occupational exercise and colon cancer, *Am. J. Epidemiol.*, 122, 357, 1985.
34. **Frederiksson, M., Bengtsson, N.-O., Hardell, L., and Axelson, O.**, Colon cancer, physical activity, and occupational exposures, *Cancer*, 63, 1838, 1989.
35. **Slattery, M.L., Schumacher, M.C., Smith, K.R., West, D.W., and Abd-Elghany, N.**, Physical activity, diet, and risk of colon cancer in Utah, *Am. J. Epidemiol.*, 128, 989, 1988.
36. **Vena, J.E., Graham, S., Zielezny, M., Brasure, J., and Swanson, M.K.**, Occupational exercise and risk of cancer, *Am. J. Clin. Nutr.*, 45, 318, 1987.
37. **Ballard-Barbash, R., Schatzkin, A., Albanes, D., Schiffman, M.H., Kreger, B.E., Kannel, W.B., Anderson, K.M., and Helsel, W.E.**, Physical activity and risk of large bowel cancer in the Framingham study, *Cancer Res.*, 50, 3610, 1990.
38. **Brownson, R.C., Chang, J.C., Davis, J.R., and Smith, C.A.**, Physical activity on the job and cancer in Missouri, *Am. J. Public Health*, 81, 639, 1991.
39. **Whittemore, A.S., Wu-Williams, A.H., Lee, M., Shu, Z., Gallagher, R.P., Deng-ao, J., Lun, Z., Xianghui, W., Kun, C., Jung, D., Teh, C.-Z., Chengde, L., Yao, X.J., Paffenberger, R.S., and Henderson, B.E.**, Diet, physical activity, and colorectal cancer among Chinese in North America and China, *J. Natl. Cancer Inst.*, 82, 915, 1990.
40. **Kune, G.A., Kune, S., and Watson, L.F.**, Body weight and physical activity as predictors of colorectal cancer risk, *Nutr. Cancer.*, 13, 9, 1990.
41. **Severson, R.K., Nomura, A.M.Y., Grove, J.S., and Stemmermann, G.N.**, A prospective analysis of physical activity and cancer, *Am. J. Epidemiol.*, 130, 522, 1989.
42. **Adrianopoulos, G., Nelson, R.L., Bombeck, C.T., and Souza, G.**, The influence of physical activity in 1,2 dimethylhydrazine induced colon carcinogenesis in the rat, *Anticancer Res.*, 7, 849, 1987.
43. **Klurfeld, D.M., Welch, C.B., Einhom, E., and Kritchevsky, D.**, Inhibition of colon tumor promotion by caloric restriction or exercise in rats, *FASEB J.*, 2, A433, 1988.
44. **Wynder, E.L.**, Primary prevention of cancer: planning and policy considerations, *J. Natl. Cancer Inst.*, 83, 475, 1991.
45. **Henderson, B.E., Ross, R.K., Judd, H.L., Krailo, M.D., and Pike, M.C.**, Do regular ovulatory cycles increase breast cancer risk? *Cancer*, 56, 1206, 1985.
46. **Vihko, R. and Apter, D.**, The epidemiology and endocrinology of the menarche in relation to breast cancer, *Cancer Surv.*, 5, 561, 1986.
47. **Kelsey, J.L.**, A review of the epidemiology of breast cancer, *Epidemiol. Rev.*, 1, 74, 1979.

48. **Armstrong, B. and Doll, R.**, Environmental factors and cancer incidence and mortality in different countries, with special reference to dietary factors, *Int. J. Cancer,* 15, 617, 1975.
49. **Miller, A.B. and Bulbrook, R.D.**, The epidemiology and etiology of breast cancer, *N. Engl. J. Med.,* 303, 1246, 1980.
50. **Graham, S.**, Fats, calories, and caloric expenditure in the epidemiology of cancer, *Am. J. Clin. Nutr.,* 45, 342, 1987.
51. **Simopoulos, A.P.**, Calories and energy expenditure in carcinogenesis: conference report, *J. Am. Diet. Assoc.,* 87, 92, 1987.
52. **Frisch, R.E., Wyshak, G., Albright, N.L., Albright, T.E., Schiff, I., Jones, K.P., Witschi, J., Shiang, E., Koff, E., and Marguglio, M.**, Lower prevalence of breast cancer and cancers of the reproductive system among former college athletes compared to non-atheletes, *Br. J. Cancer,* 52, 885, 1985.
53. **Frisch, R.E., Wyshak, G., Albright, N.L., Albright, T.E., and Schiff, I.**, Lower prevalence of non-reproductive system cancers among female former college athletes, *Med. Sci. Sports Exercise,* 21, 250, 1989.
54. **Wyshak, G., Frisch, R.E., Albright, N.L., Albright, T.E., and Schiff, I.**, Lower prevalence of benign diseases of the breast and benign tumours of the reproductive system among former college athletes compared to non-athletes, *Br. J. Cancer,* 54, 841, 1986.
55. **Goldsmith, M.F.**, Will exercise help keep women away from oncologists — or obstetricians? *JAMA,* 259, 1769, 1988.
56. **Warren, M.P.**, The effects of exercise on pubertal progression and reproductive function in girls, *J. Clin. Endocrinol. & Metab.,* 51, 1150, 1980.
57. **Frisch, R.E., Von Gotz-Welbergen, A.V., McArthur, J.W., Albright, T., Witschi, J., Bullen, D., Birnholz, J., Reed, R.B., and Hermann, H.**, Delayed menarche and amenorrhea of college athletes in relation to age of onset of training, *JAMA,* 256, 1559, 1981.
58. **Bernstein, L., Ross, R.K., Lobo, R.A., Hanisch, R., Krailo, M.D., and Henderson, B.E.**, The effects of moderate physical activity on menstrual cycle patterns in adolescence: implications for breast cancer prevention, *Br. J. Cancer,* 55, 681, 1987.
59. **MacMahon, B., Trichopoulos, D., Brown, J., Andersen, A.P., Aoki, K., Cole, P., DeWaard, F., Kauraniemi, T., Morgan, R.W., Purde, M., Ravnihar, B., Stormby, N., Westlund, K., and Woo, N.-C.**, Age at menarche, probability of ovulation and breast cancer risk, *Int. J. Cancer,* 29, 13, 1982.
60. **Apter, D. and Vihko, R.**, Early menarche, a risk factor for breast cancer, indicates early onset of ovulatory cycles, *J. Clin. Endocrinol. & Metab.,* 57, 82, 1983.
61. **Moore, J.W., Clark, G.M.G., Takatani, O., Wakabayashi, Y., Hayward, J.L., and Bulbrook, R.D.**, Distribution of 17β-estradiol in the sera of normal British and Japanese women, *J. Natl. Cancer Inst.,* 71, 749, 1983.
62. **Cohen, L.A., Choi, K., and Wang, C.-X.**, Influence of dietary fat, caloric restriction, and voluntary exercise on N-nitrosomethylurea-induced mammary tumorigenesis in rats, *Cancer Res.,* 48, 4276, 1988.
63. **Benjamin, H., Storkson, J., and Pariza, M. W.**, Effect of voluntary exercise on mammary tumor development, *FASEB J.,* 2(Abstr.), A1191, 1988.
64. **Cohen, L.A.**, Fat and endocrine-responsive cancer in animals, *Prev. Med.,* 16, 468, 1987.
65. **Kritchevsky, D.**, Influence of caloric restriction and exercise on tumorigenesis in rats *Proc. Soc. Exp. Biol. Med.,* 193, 35, 1990.
66. **Thompson, H.J., Ronan, A.M., Ritacco, K.A., Tagliaferro, A.R., and Meeker L.D.**, Effect of exercise on the induction of mammary carcinogenesis, *Cancer Res.,* 48 2720, 1988.
67. **Thompson, H.J., Ronan, A.M., Ritacco, K.A., and Tagliaferro, A.R.**, Effect of typ and amount of dietary fat on the enhancement of rat mammary tumorigenesis by exercise *Cancer Res.,* 49, 1904, 1989.

68. **Magrane, D.,** Effect of exercise and caloric restriction on DMBA induced mammary tumorigenesis and plasma lipids in rats fed high fat diets, *FASEB J.,* 5, A927, 1991.
69. **White, M.T., Lane, H.W., Teer, P., Keith, R.E., and Strahan, S.,** The effect of diet and exercise on incidence of 7,12 dimethylbenz(A)anthracene-induced mammary tumors in virgin Balb/c mice, *FASEB J.,* 5, A927, 1991.
70. **Weinberg, J. and Emerman, J.T.,** Effects of psychosocial stressors on mouse mammory tumor growth, *Brain Behav. Immun.,* 3, 234, 1989.
71. **Sklar, L.S. and Anisman, H.,** Social stress influences tumor growth, *Psychosom. Med.,* 42, 347, 1980.
72. **LeMarchand, L., Kolonel, L.N., and Yoshizawa, C.N.,** Lifetime occupational physical activity and prostate cancer risk, *Am. J. Epidemiol.,* 133, 103, 1991.
73. **Paffenberger, R.S., Hyde, R.T., and Wing, A.L.,** Physical activity and incidence of cancer in diverse populations: a preliminary report, *Am. J. Clin. Nutr.,* 45, 312, 1987.
74. **Albanes, D., Blair, A., and Taylor, P.R.,** Physical activity and risk of cancer in the NHANES 1 population, *Am. J. Public Health,* 79, 744, 1989.
75. **Hoffman-Goetz, L., MacNeil, B., and Arumugam, Y.,** Differential effects of exercise and housing condition on murine natural killer cell activity and tumor growth, *Int. J. Sports. Med.,* in press, 1991.
76. **Polednak, A.P.,** College athletics, body size, and cancer mortality, *Cancer,* 38, 382, 1976.
77. **Rook, A.,** An investigation into the longevity of Cambridge men, *Br. Med. J.,* 1, 773, 1954.
78. **Blair, S.N., Kohl, H.W., Paffenberger, R.S., Clark, D.G., Cooper, K.H., and Gibbons, L.W.,** Physical fitness and all-cause mortality: a prospective study of healthy men and women, *JAMA,* 262, 2395, 1989.
79. **Lotzová, E. and Herberman, R.B.,** *Immunobiology of Natural Killer Cells,* CRC Press, Inc., Boca Raton, FL, 1986.
80. **Old, L.J.,** Tumor necrosis factor (TNF), *Science,* 230, 630, 1985.
81. **Hewitt, H.B., Blake, E.R., and Walder, A.S.,** A critique of the evidence for active host defence against cancer, based on personal studies of 27 murine tumours of spontaneous origin, *Br. J. Cancer,* 33, 241, 1976.
82. **Middle, J.G. and Embleton, M.J.,** Naturally arising tumors of the inbred WAB/Not rat strain. II. Immunogenicity of transplanted tumors, *J. Natl. Cancer. Inst.,* 67, 637, 1981.
83. **Fidler, I.J. and Ichinose, Y.,** Mechanisms of macrophage mediated tumor cell lysis: role for the monokines tumor necrosis factor and interleukin-1, in *Immunity to Cancer,* Vol. 2, Mitchell, M.S., Ed., Alan R. Liss, New York, 1987, 169.
84. **Nelson, D.S.,** Alterations in macrophage function in tumor-bearing hosts, in *Immune Responses to Metastases,* Vol. 1, Herberman, R.B., Wiltrout, R.H., and Gorelik, E., Eds., CRC Press, Boca Raton, FL, 1987, 79.
85. **Peck, R.,** Neuropeptides modulating macrophage function, *Ann. N.Y. Acad. Sci.,* 496, 264, 1987.
86. **Mace, K.F., Ehrke, M.J., Hori, K., Maccubin, D.L., and Mihich, E.,** Role of tumor necrosis factor in macrophage activation and tumoricidal activity, *Cancer Res.,* 48, 5427, 1988.
87. **Nathan, C.F.,** Secretory products of macrophages, *J. Clin. Invest.,* 79, 319, 1987.
88. **Feinman, R., Henriksen-DeStefano, D., Tsujimoto, M., and Vilcek, J.,** Tumor necrosis factor is an important mediator of tumor cell killing by human monocytes, *J. Immunol.,* 138, 635, 1987.
89. **Lachman, L.B., Dinarello, C.A., Llansa, N.D., and Fidler, I.J.,** Natural and recombinant human interleukin 1-β is cytotoxic for human melanoma cells, *J. Immunol.,* 136, 3098, 1986.

90. **Heicappell, R., Naito, S., Ichinose, Y., Creasey, A.A., Lin, L.S., and Fidler, I.J.,** Cytostatic and cytolytic effects of human recombinant tumor necrosis factor on human renal cell carcinoma cell lines derived from a single surgical specimen, *J. Immunol.,* 138, 1634, 1987.

91. **Bucana, C.D., Hoyer, L.C., Breesman, S., McDaniel, M., and Hanna, Jr., M.G.,** Morphological evidence for the translocation of lysosomal organelles from cytotoxic macrophages into the cytoplasm of tumor target cells, *Cancer Res.,* 36, 4444, 1976.

92. **Bucana, C.D., Hoyer, L.C., Schroit, A.J., Kleinerman, E., and Fidler, I.J.,** Ultrastructural studies of the interaction between liposome-activated human blood monocytes and allogeneic tumor cells *in vitro, Am. J. Pathol.,* 112, 101, 1983.

93. **Mantovani, A., Polentarutti, N., Prei, G., Shavit, Z.B., Vecchi, A., Bolis, G., and Mangioni, C.,** Cytotoxicity on tumor cells of peripheral blood monocytes and tumor-associated macrophages in patients with ascites ovarian tumors, *J. Natl. Cancer Inst.,* 64, 1307, 1980.

94. **Cameron, D.J. and Stromberg, B.V.,** The ability of macrophages from head and neck cancer patients to kill tumor cells, *Cancer,* 54, 2403, 1984.

95. **Nakahashi, H., Yasumoto, K., Nagashima, A., Yaita, H., Takeo, S., Motohiro, A., Furukawa, T., Inokuchi, K., and Nomoto, K.,** Antitumor activity of macrophages in lung cancer patients with special reference to location of macrophages, *Cancer Res.,* 44, 5906, 1984.

96. **Gerrard, T.L., Terz, J.J., and Kaplan, A.M.,** Cytotoxicity to tumor cells of monocytes from normal individuals and cancer patients, *Int. J. Cancer,* 26, 585, 1980.

97. **Schultz, R.M., Pavilidis, N.A., Stylos, W.A., and Chirigos, M.A.,** Regulation of macrophage tumoricidal function: a role for prostaglandins of the E series, *Science,* 202, 320, 1978.

98. **Taffett, S.M. and Russell, S.W.,** Macrophage-mediated tumor cell killing: regulation of expression of cytolytic activity by prostaglandin E, *J. Immunol.,* 126, 424, 1981.

99. **Bennett, A., Del Tacca, M., Stamford, I.F., and Zebro, T.,** Prostaglandins from tumours of human large bowel, *Br. J. Cancer,* 35, 881, 1977.

100. **Mantovani, A.,** *In vitro* effects on tumor cells of macrophages isolated from an early passage chemically-induced murine sarcoma and from its spontaneous metastases, *Int. J. Cancer,* 27, 221, 1981.

101. **Kadhim, S.A. and Rees, R.C.,** Enhancement of tumor growth in mice: evidence for the involvement of host macrophages, *Cell. Immunol.,* 87, 259, 1984.

102. **Gorelik, E., Wiltrout, R.H., Brunda, M.J., Holden, H.T., and Herberman, R.B.,** Augmentation of metastasis formation by thioglycollate-elicited macrophages, *Int. J. Cancer,* 29, 575, 1982.

103. **Robertson, M.J., and Ritz, J.,** Biology and clinical relevance of human natural killer cells, *Blood,* 76, 2421, 1990.

104. **Herberman, R.B. and Ortaldo, J.R.,** Natural killer cells: their role in defense against disease, *Science,* 214, 24, 1981.

105. **Hanna, N.,** Expression of metastatic potential of tumor cells in young nude mice is correlated with low levels of natural killer cell-mediated cytotoxicity, *Int. J. Cancer,* 26, 675, 1980.

106. **Kärre, K., Klein, G.O., Kiessling, R., Klein, G., and Roder, J.C.,** *In vitro* NK-activity and *in vivo* resistance to leukemia: studies of beige, beige/nude and wild type hosts on C57BL background, *Int. J. Cancer,* 26, 789, 1980.

107. **Riccardi, C., Santoni, A., Barlozarri, T., Puccetti, P., and Herberman, R.B.,** *In vivo* natural reactivity of mice against tumor cells, *Int. J. Cancer,* 25, 475, 1980.

108. **Hanna, N. and Fidler, I.J.,** Relationship between metastatic potential and resistance to natural killer cell-mediated cytotoxicity in three murine tumor systems, *J. Natl. Cancer Inst.,* 66, 1183, 1981.

109. **Gorelik, E., Wiltrout, R.H., Okumura, K., Habu, S., and Herberman, R.B.,** Role of NK cells in the control of metastatic spread and growth of tumor cells in mice, *Int. J. Cancer.,* 30, 107, 1982.
110. **Barlozarri, T., Leonhardt, J., Wiltrout, R.H., Herberman, R.B., and Reynolds, C.W.,** Direct evidence for the role of LGL in the inhibition of experimental tumor metastases, *J. Immunol.,* 134, 2783, 1985.
111. **Lala, P.K., Santer, V., Libenson, H., and Parhar, R.S.,** Changes in the host natural killer cell population in mice during tumor development: kinetics and *in vivo* significance, *Cell. Immunol.,* 93, 250, 1985.
112. **Wei, W.-Z. and Heppner, G.,** Natural killer activity of lymphocytic infiltrates in mouse mammary lesions, *Br. J. Cancer,* 55, 589, 1987.
113. **Pross, H.F. and Baines, M. G.,** Alterations in natural killer cell activity in tumor-bearing hosts, in *Immune Responses to Metastases,* Vol. 1, Herberman, R.B., Wiltrout, R.H., and Gorelik, E., Eds., CRC Press, Boca Raton, FL, 1987, 57.
114. **Rowse, G.J., Rowan, R.E., Weinberg, J., and Emerman, J.T.,** Alterations in splenic natural killer cell activity induced by the Shionogi mouse mammary tumor, *Cancer Lett.,* 54, 81, 1990.
115. **Pollack, R.E., Babcock, G.F., Romsdahl, M.M., and Nishioka, K.,** Surgical stress-mediated suppression of murine natural killer cell cytotoxicity, *Cancer Res.,* 44, 3888, 1984.
116. **Lefor, A.T., Mulé, J.J., and Rosenberg, S.A.,** Lymphokine-activated killer cells: biology and therapeutic efficacy, in *Functions of the Natural Immune System,* Reynolds, C.W. and Wiltrout, R.H., Eds., Plenum Press, New York, 1989, 39.
117. **Mantovani, A., Bottazzi, B., Allavena, P., Balotta, C.,** Tumor-associated leukocytes in metastasizing tumors, in *Immune Responses to Metastases,* Herberman, R.B., Wiltrout, R.H., and Gorelik, E., Eds., CRC Press, Boca Raton, FL, 1987, 105.
118. **Chandler, D.B. and Fulmer, J.D.,** Prostaglandin synthesis and release by subpopulations of rat alveolar macrophages, *J. Immunol.,* 139, 893, 1987.
119. **Brunda, M.J., Herberman, R.B., and Holden, H.T.,** Inhibition of murine natural killer cell activity by prostaglandins, *J. Immunol.,* 124, 2682, 1980.
120. **Lotzová, E., Savary, C.A., Pollock, R.E., and Fuchshuber, P.,** Immunologic and clinical aspects of natural killer cells in human leukemia, *Nat. Immun. Cell Growth Regul.,* 9, 173, 1990.
121. **Meager, A.,** Antiviral, antimicrobial, and antitumour cytokines, in *Cytokines,* Open University Press, Buckingham, 1990, 179.
122. **Scales, W.E. and Kunkel, S.L.,** Regulatory interactions between interleukin-1, tumor necrosis factor, and other inflammatory mediators, in *Interleukin-1, Inflammation and Disease,* Bomford, R. and Hendersen, B., Eds., Elsevier, New York, 1989, 163.
123. **Nakamura, H.,** Neuroendocrine interactions with interleukin-1 in inflammation, in *Interleukin-1, Inflammation and Disease,* Bomford, R. and Henderson, B., Eds., Elsevier, New York, 1989, 229.
124. **Ravikumar, T., Rodrick, M., Steele, Jr., G., Marrazo, J., O'Dwyer, P., Dodson, T., and King, V.,** Interleukin generation in experimental colon cancer of rats: effects of tumor growth and tumor therapy, *J. Natl. Cancer Inst.,* 74, 893, 1985.
125. **Andersen, K.L.,** Leukocyte response to brief, severe exercise, *J. Appl. Physiol.,* 7, 671, 1955.
126. **McCarthy, D.A. and Dale, M.M.,** The leukocytosis of exercise: a review and a model, *Sports Med.,* 6, 333, 1988.
127. **Keast, D., Cameron, K., and Morton, A.R.,** Exercise and the immune response, *Sports Med.,* 5, 248, 1988.
128. **Galun, E., Burstein, R., Assia, E., Tur-Kaspa, I., Rosenblum, J., and Epstein, Y.,** Changes of white blood cell count during prolonged exercise, *Int. J. Sports Med.,* 8, 253, 1987.

129. **Gimenez, M., Mohan-Kumar, T., Humbert, J.C., De Talance, N., and Buisine, J.,** Leukocyte, lymphocyte and platelet response to dynamic exercise, *Eur. J. Appl. Physiol.,* 55, 465, 1986.

130. **Gimenez, M., Mohan-Kumar, T., Humbert, J.C., De Talance, N., Teboul, M., and Belenguer, F.J.A.,** Training and leukocyte, lymphocyte and platelet response to dynamic exercise, *J. Sports Med.,* 27, 172, 1987.

131. **Oshida, Y., Yamanouchi, Y., Hayamizu, S., and Sato, Y.,** Effect of acute physical exercise on lymphocyte subpopulations in trained and untrained subjects, *Int. J. Sports Med.,* 9, 137, 1988.

132. **Soppi, E., Varjo, P., Eskola, J., and Laitinen, L.A.,** Effect of strenuous physical stress on circulating lymphocyte number and function before and after training, *J. Clin. Lab. Immunol.,* 8, 43, 1982.

133. **Lewicki, R., Tchórzewski, H., Majewska, E., Nowak, Z., and Baj, Z.,** Effect of maximal physical exercise on T-lymphocyte subpopulations and on interleukin 1 (IL 1) and interleukin 2 (IL 2) production *in vitro, Int. J. Sports Med.,* 9, 114, 1988.

134. **Ferry, A., Picard, F., Duvallet, A., Weill, B., and Rieu, M.,** Changes in blood leukocyte populations induced by acute maximal and chronic submaximal exercise, *Eur. J. Appl. Physiol.,* 59, 435, 1990.

135. **Tvede, N., Pedersen, B.K., Hansen, F.R., Bendix, T., Christensen, L.D., Galbo, H., and Halkjær-Kristensen, J.,** Effect of physical exercise on blood mononuclear cell subpopulations and *in vitro* proliferative responses, *Scand. J. Immunol.,* 29, 383, 1989.

136. **De La Fuente, M., Martin, M.I., and Ortega, E.,** Changes in the phagocytic function of peritoneal macrophages from old mice after strenuous physical exercise, *Comp. Immunol. Microbiol. Infect. Dis.,* 13, 189, 1990.

137. **Landmann, R.M.A., Müller, F.B., Perini, C.H., Wesp, M., Eme, P., and Bühler, F.R.,** Changes of immunoregulatory cells induced by psychological and physical stress: relationship to plasma catecholamines, *Clin. Exp. Immunol.,* 58, 127, 1984.

138. **Voronina, N.P. and Mayanskii, D.N.,** Effect of intensive physical exercise on macrophage functions, *Bull. Exp. Med. Biol.,* 104, 1120, 1987.

139. **Hoffman-Goetz, L., Thorne, R., Randall Simpson, J., and Arumugam, Y.,** Exercise stress alters murine lymphocyte subset distribution in spleen, lymph nodes and thymus, *Clin. Exp. Immunol.,* 76, 307, 1989.

140. **Skornik, W.A. and Brain, J.D.,** Effect of sulfur dioxide on pulmonary macrophage endocytosis at rest and during exercise, *Am. Rev. Respir. Dis.,* 142, 655, 1990.

141. **Fehr, H.-G., Lötzerich, H., and Michna, H.,** The influence of physical activity on peritoneal macrophage function: histochemical and phagocytic studies, *Int. J. Sports Med.,* 9, 77, 1988.

142. **Michna, H.,** The human macrophage system: activity and functional morphology, *Bibl. Anat.,* 31, 1, 1988.

143. **Dufaux, B. and Order, U.,** Plasma elastase-α 1-antitrypsin, neopterin, tumor necrosis factor, and a soluble interleukin-2 receptor after prolonged exercise, *Int. J. Sports Med.,* 10, 434, 1989.

144. **Goodwin, J.S. and Webb, D.R.,** Regulation of the immune response by prostaglandins, *Clin. Immunol. Immunopath.,* 15, 106, 1980.

145. **Rappaport, R.S. and Dodge, G.R.,** Prostaglandin E inhibits the production of human interleukin 2, *J. Exp. Med.,* 155, 943, 1982.

146. **Pedersen, B.K., Tvede, N., Klarlund, K., Christensen, L.D., Hansen, F.R., Galbo, H., Kharazmi, A., and Halkjær-Kristensen, J.,** Indomethacin *in vitro* and *in vivo* abolishes post-exercise suppression of natural killer cell activity in peripheral blood, *Int. J. Sports Med.,* 11, 127, 1990.

147. **Kappel, M., Tvede, N., Galbo, H., Haahr, P.M., Kjær, M., Linstow, M., Klarlund, K., and Pedersen, B.K.,** Evidence that the effect of physical exercise on NK cell activity is mediated by epinephrine, *J. Appl. Physiol.,* 70, 2530, 1991.

148. **Narisawa, T., Sato, M., Tani, M., Kudo, T., Takahashi, T., and Goto, A.,** Inhibition of development of methylnitrosourea-induced rat colon tumors by indomethacin treatment, *Cancer Res.,* 41, 1954, 1981.

149. **Tutton, P.J.M. and Barkla, D.H.,** Influence of prostaglandin analogues on epithelial cell proliferation and xenograft growth, *Br. J. Cancer.,* 41, 47, 1980.

150. **Thor, P., Konturek, J.W., Konturek, S.J., and Anderson, J.H.,** Role of prostaglandins in intestinal motility, *Am. J. Physiol.,* 248, G353, 1985.

151. **Lötzerich, H., Fehr, H.-G., and Appell, H.-J.,** Potentiation of cytostatic but not cytolytic activity of murine macrophages after running stress, *Int. J. Sports Med.,* 11, 61, 1990.

152. **Hanson, P.G. and Flaherty, D.K.,** Immunological responses to training in conditioned runners, *Clin. Sci.,* 60, 225, 1981.

153. **Deuster, P.A., Curiale, A.M., Cowan, M.L., and Finkelman, F.D.,** Exercise-induced changes in populations of peripheral blood mononuclear cells, *Med. Sci. Sports Exercise,* 20, 276, 1988.

154. **Cannon, J.G., Orencole, S.F., Fielding, R.A., Meydani, M., Meydani, S.N., Fiatarone, M.A., Blumberg, J.B., and Evans, W.J.,** Acute phase response in exercise: interaction of age and vitamin E on neutrophils and muscle enzyme release, *Am. J. Physiol.,* 259, R1214, 1990.

155. **Dorner, H., Heinold, D., and Hilmer, W.,** Exercise-induced leukocytosis — its dependence on physical capability, *Int. J. Sports Med.,* 8(Abstr.), 152, 1987.

156. **Pincemail, J., Camus, G., Roesgen, A., Dreezen, E., Bertrand, Y., Lismonde, M., Deby-Dupont, G., and Deby, C.,** Exercise induces pentane production and neutrophil activation in humans. Effect of propranolol, *Eur. J. App. Physiol.,* 61, 319, 1990.

157. **Smith, J.A., Telford, R.D., Mason, I.B., and Weidemann, M.J.,** Exercise, training and neutrophil microbicidal activity, *Int. J. Sports Med.,* 11, 179, 1990.

158. **Green, R.L., Kaplan, S.S., Rabin, B.S., Stanitski, C.L., and Zdziarski, U.,** Immune function in marathon runners, *Ann. Allergy,* 47, 73, 1981.

159. **Cannon, J.G. and Kluger, M.J.,** Endogenous pyrogen activity in human plasma after exercise, *Science,* 220, 617, 1983.

160. **Cannon, J.G., Evans, W.J., Hughes, V.A., Meredith, C.N., and Dinarello, C.A.,** Physiological mechanisms contributing to increased interleukin-1 section, *J. Appl. Physiol.,* 61, 1869, 1986.

161. **Evans, W.J., Meredith, C.N., Cannon, J.G., Dinarello, C.A., Frontera, W.R., Hughes, V.A., Jones, B.H., and Knuttgen, H.G.,** Metabolic changes following eccentric exercise in trained and untrained men, *J. Appl. Physiol.,* 61, 1864, 1986.

162. **Senay, L.C. and Pivarnik, J.M.,** Fluid shifts during exercise, *Exercise Sport Sci. Rev.,* 13, 335, 1985.

163. **Randall Simpson, J. and Hoffman-Goetz, L.,** Exercise, serum zinc, and interleukin-1 concentrations in man: some methodological considerations, *Nutr. Res.,* 11, 309, 1991.

164. **Shechtman, O., Elizondo, R., and Taylor, M.,** Exercise augments interleukin-2 induction, *Med. Sci. Sports Exercise,* 20(Abstr.), S18, 1988.

165. **Pahlavani, M.A., Cheung, T.H., Chesky, J.A., and Richardson, A.,** Influence of exercise on the immune function of rats of various ages, *J. Appl. Physiol.,* 64, 1997, 1988.

166. **Espersen, G.T., Elbæk, A., Ernst, E., Toft, E., Kaalund, S., Jersild, C., and Grunnet, N.,** Effect of physical exercise on cytokines and lymphocyte subpopulations in human peripheral blood, *APMIS,* 98, 395, 1990.

167. **Viti, A., Muscettla, M., Paulesi, L., Bocci, V., and Almi, A.,** Effect of exercise on plasma interferon levels, *J. Appl. Physiol.,* 59, 426, 1985.

168. **Kendall, A., Hoffman-Goetz, L., Houston, M., MacNeil, B., and Arumugam, Y.,** Exercise and blood lymphocyte subset responses: intensity, duration and subject fitness effects, *J. Appl. Physiol.,* 69, 251, 1990.

169. **Pedersen, B.K., Tvede, N., Hansen, F.R., Andersen, V., Bendix, T., Bendixen, G., Galbo, H., Haahr, P.M., Klarlund, K., Sylvest, J., Thomsen, B.S., and Halkjær-Kristensen, J.,** Modulation of natural killer cell activity in peripheral blood by physical exercise, *Scand. J. Immunol.,* 27, 673, 1988.

170. **Targan, S., Britvan, L., and Dorey, F.,** Activation of human NKCC by moderate exercise: increased frequency of NK cells with enhanced capability of effector-target lytic interactions, *Clin. Exp. Immunol.,* 45, 352, 1981.

171. **Hoffman-Goetz, L., Randall Simpson, J., Cipp, N., Arumugam, Y., and Houston, M.,** Lymphocyte subset responses to repeated submaximal exercise in men, *J. Appl. Physiol.,* 68, 1069, 1990.

172. **Brahmi, Z., Thomas, J.E., Park, M., and Dowdeswell, I.R.G.,** The effect of acute exercise on natural killer cell activity of trained and sedentary human subjects, *J. Clin. Immunol.,* 5, 321, 1985.

173. **Fiatarone, M.A., Morley, J.E., Bloom, E.T., Benton, D., Solomon, G.F., and Makinodan, T.,** The effect of exercise on natural killer cell activity in young and old subjects, *J. Gerontol.,* 44, M37, 1989.

174. **Mackinnon, L.T., Chick, T.W., van As, A., Tomasi, T.B.,** Effects of prolonged intense exercise on natural killer cell number and function, in *Exercise Physiology: Current Selected Research,* Dotson, C. and Humprey, J., Eds., AMS Press, New York, 1988, 77.

175. **Berk, L.S., Nieman, D.C., Youngberg, W.S., Arabatzis, K., Simpson-Westerberg, M., Lee, J.W., Tan, S.A., and Eby, W.C.,** The effect of long endurance running on natural killer cells in marathoners, *Med. Sci. Sports Exercise,* 22, 207, 1990.

176. **Blalock, J.E.,** A molecular basis for bidirectional communication between the immune and neuroendocrine systems, *Physiol. Rev.,* 69, 1, 1989.

177. **Plaut, M.,** Lymphocyte hormone receptors, *Annu. Rev. Immunol.,* 5, 621, 1987.

178. **Rabin, B.S., Cohen, S., Ganguli, R., Lysle, D.T., and Cunnick, J.E.,** Bidirectional interaction between the central nervous system and the immune system, *Crit. Rev. Immunol.,* 9, 279, 1989.

179. **Hellstrand, K., Hermodsson, S., and Strannegård, Ö.,** Evidence for a β-adrenoceptor-mediated regulation of human natural killer cells, *J. Immunol.,* 134, 4095, 1985.

180. **Christ, D.M., Mackinnon, L.T., Thompson, R.F., Atterbom, H.A., and Egan, P.A.,** Physical exercise increases natural cellular-mediated tumor cytotoxicity in elderly women, *Gerontology,* 36, 66, 1989.

181. **Nieman, D.C., Nehlsen-Cannarella, S.L., Markoff, P.A., Balk-Lamberton, A.J., Yang, H., Chritton, D.B.W., Lee, J.W., and Arabatzis, K.,** The effects of moderate exercise training on natural killer cells and acute upper respiratory tract infections, *Int. J. Sports Med.,* 11, 467, 1990.

182. **Haus, E., Lakatua, S.J., Swoyer, J., and Sackett-Lundeen, L.,** Chronobiology in hematology and immunology, *Am. J. Anat.,* 168, 467, 1991.

183. **Watson, R.R., Moriguchi, S., Jackson, J.C., Werner, L., Wilmore, J.H., and Freund, B.J.,** Modification of cellular immune functions in humans by endurance exercise training during β-adrenergic blockade with atenolol or propranolol, *Med. Sci. Sports Exercise,* 18, 95, 1986.

184. **Pedersen, B.K., Tvede, N., Christensen, L.D., Klarlund, K., Kragbak, S., and Halkjær-Kristensen, J.,** Natural killer cell activity in peripheral blood of highly trained and untrained persons, *Int. J. Sports Med.,* 10, 129, 1989.

185. **Randall Simpson, J. and Hoffman-Goetz, L.,** Exercise stress and murine natural killer cell function, *Proc. Soc. Exp. Biol. Med.,* 195, 129, 1990.

186. **Finkel, T.H., Kubo, R.T., and Cambier, J.C.,** T-cell development and transmembrane signalling: changing biological responses through an unchanging receptor, *Immunol. Today,* 12, 79, 1991.

187. **Cooper, R.M.,** *Oncogenes,* Jones & Bartlett Publishers, Boston, 1990.

188. **Newbold, R.R., Bullock, B.C., and McLachlan, A.,** Uterine adenocarcinoma in mice
     following developmental treatment with estrogens: a model for hormonal carcinogenesis,
     Cancer Res., 50, 7677, 1990.
189. **Outzen, H.C. and Prehn, R.T.,** The concept of the immune reaction in oncogenesis:
     a host tumor interaction, in *Etiology of Cancer in Man,* Levine, A.S., Ed., Kluwer
     Academic Publishers, Dordrecht, The Netherlands, 1989, 180.

Chapter 5

THE ROLE OF EXERCISE IN CANCER THERAPY

Maryl L. Winningham

TABLE OF CONTENTS

I. INTRODUCTION

As a result of improvements in detection techniques and intensive therapies, cancer survivors now number over five million. The quality of their survival is often tempered by long-term physiological, psychological, and socioeconomic impairments resulting from disease and its attendant therapies. Specifically, occupational pursuits may be hindered by job discrimination, and "energy loss."[1-3] Social consequences may include high divorce rates[1] and decreased energy for leisure time activities.[3] Psychological after-effects may include depression,[1,4] adjustment to physical compromise,[4-6] fear and anxiety,[6] as well as fear of recurrence.[4,6] Finally, physiological effects include decreased pulmonary functioning,[5,6] chronic cardiomyopathy, pericarditis, latent myocardial infarction, and neurological, gastrointestinal, and urological disorders.[5,6]

The use of "whole body" exercise to address some of the above problems in cancer patients is a relatively new component of rehabilitation. Traditionally, in oncology, exercise has been limited to physical therapy which addresses specific impairments caused by amputation or surgery. In the past decade, the need for a new, more vigorous approach to the rehabilitation of cancer patients has been recognized. Indeed, results from several studies suggest the application of aerobic exercise in promoting functional capacity, and the well-being of select groups of cancer patients has great promise. This chapter will review research related to cancer and exercise, then discuss guidelines and recommendations for using exercise as a rehabilitative intervention in cancer patients.

II. THE EXERCISE-CANCER INTERACTION

There have been relatively few controlled studies investigating the interactive effect of physical activity and neoplastic diseases. Several animal studies involving rats or mice with induced malignancies indicated that exercising animals showed inhibited tumor growth, extended survival time, and even occasional complete tumor regression when compared with sedentary, control animals.[7-12] Although ethical issues preclude controlled human studies, some researchers have offered epidemiological evidence that sedentarism is a risk factor for colon cancer in males[13-15] and breast and reproductive cancers in women.[16] However, there are some problems with interpreting these data, particularly with respect to the influence of dietary fat on the risk of these cancers.

III. EXERCISE FOR PEOPLE WITH CANCER

It is remarkable that several decades of exercise research supports widespread cardiac rehabilitation programs. Cancer is the leading cause of death behind heart disease; yet, the application of exercise principles to oncology rehabilitation has been tested by relatively few controlled studies. Dietz suggested that oncology rehabilitation should begin as early as possible and continue throughout the convalescence.[17]

In response to a moderate-intensity, supervised, exercise pilot program using the Winningham Aerobic Interval Training (WAIT) protocol for the cycle ergometer, breast cancer patients undergoing chemotherapy exercised three times a week for 10 to 12 weeks. The exercising patient group showed an improvement in functional capacity and feelings of internal control, compared with a nonexercising group. In fact, the response of the exercise group was comparable to that achieved by a group of healthy women.[18] The significant improvement in functional capacity in breast cancer patients participating in this program was substantiated in a subsequent study by MacVicar et al.[19]

Select distressing symptoms often associated with breast cancer and treatment may be mitigated by an intervention such as the WAIT protocol, which utilizes fixed ratios of higher and lower workloads to stimulate biochemical adaptation without stimulating fatigue. MacVicar and Winningham investigated changes in psychological status measured by the Profile of Mood States in exercising patients vs. a control group. The control (nonexercise) group showed an overall worsening of mood states while the exercise group showed improvements in tension/anxiety, depression/dejection, fatigue and feelings of vigor.[20] Further, Winningham and MacVicar noted an improvement in somatization, in general, and nausea, in specific, in the exercise group compared with the control group as measured on the Symptom Checklist-90-Revised.[21]

In contrast to the often reported cachexia found in cancer patients, women undergoing treatment for breast cancer gain weight. The mechanism for this gain is unknown. In a report by Winningham et al., the skinfold body fat profile changes in breast cancer patients in the WAIT exercise program were similar regardless of whether the women were initially obese or not; exercising subjects moderated fat gain and increased lean body weight compared with the increase in body fat of control subjects.[22]

IV. EXERCISE FOR CANCER PATIENTS: PROBLEMS OF DISEASE AND THERAPY

What is commonly called "cancer" actually consists of many different types of malignancies. The primary characteristic of malignancies is an abnormal, unrestricted growth of body cells that compress, invade, and destroy contiguous body tissues. When the malignant cells break away from the original mass and are carried by the blood or lymph to distant sites in the body, they set up secondary colonies or metastases that invade, subvert, and destroy organs in the new site.[23,24]

Each type of cancer has a unique course of disease and combination of treatments. Regardless of type of cancer or treatment, many patients experience profound fatigue and activity-limiting symptoms. Patients are often advised by health professionals to rest; furthermore, severe effects of treatment often result in periods of bedrest. The bedrest and immobility literature clearly shows the deleterious effects of too much bedrest; particularly, problems resulting from an imbalance between activity and rest.[25-27] However, there has been no research on differentiating the effects and symptoms of reduced activity and bedrest from those of disease and treatment. Although bedrest may impair select immune processes,[26] it is not known to what extent activity programs may maintain or promote immunological health in cancer patients.

Therapy for cancer can be considered under four categories: surgery, radiation therapy, chemotherapy, and immunotherapy. Treatment usually consists of a combination of interventions; in addition, chemotherapy usually involves multiple pharmacological agents. The object of most pharmacologic treatments is to kill cells. This cytotoxic effect, unfortunately, does not discriminate between tumor cells and host cells. For this reason, rapidly dividing normal cells such as hair follicles, gastrointestinal tract mucosal cells, and bone marrow cells are most easily affected. Each drug has a distinctive *nadir;* that is, a period after administration when bone marrow depression is expressed. This can result in anemia, thrombocytopenia, and leukopenia, making the patient more vulnerable to dyspnea and hypoxia, hemorrhage, and infection.

Disease, as well as treatment, can limit or interfere with normal physiological responses to activity. In addition, after-effects of treatment may impair the oxygen uptake and transport system long after the disease has been treated and the treatment has ceased, contributing to impairment and disability. Exercise leaders should be aware of antineoplastic agents the patient has received which may have this effect, and screen accordingly. In developing exercise prescriptions and programs for people with cancer, it is essential to account for all these factors. Above all, it is crucial to develop the exercise prescription so patients start slowly and progress at a pace that will not result in muscular stiffness or pain, dyspnea, or feelings of fatigue.

With appropriate precautions, people with cancer should be able to benefit with individualized exercise programs as do many other clinical populations. The following guidelines and precautions may serve in adapting existing programs to the needs of people with cancer.

V. GUIDELINES AND PRECAUTIONS: EXERCISE FOR CANCER PATIENTS

Existing cardiopulmonary rehabilitation programs provide a model for the development of oncology rehabilitation programs. When developing safe exercise programs or research protocols for cancer patients, it is critical to consider the following issues and adjust the exercise test and/or prescription accordingly.

Are there limitations to activity based on pre-existing conditions? — Smoking and high fat intake are risk factors for cardiopulmonary disease shared by many cancer, as well as cardiac, patients. In addition, patients may suffer from such pre-existing conditions as low fitness level, orthopedic injuries, arthritis, and other musculoskeletal disorders. Guidelines developed by the American College of Sports Medicine provide an excellent basis for pre-exercise screening:[28] Cancer patients should be screened for exercise clearance as any other population, with particular attention paid to risk factor assessment. Patients with pre-existing cardiac, vascular, or pulmonary disease may benefit from referral to established cardiopulmonary rehabilitation programs for appropriate supervision. Finally, specific contraindications to exercise and exercise testing developed by the American College of Sports Medicine should be adhered to in working with cancer patients.

Are there limitations to activity based on medical procedures undergone by the patient? — For many with cancer, surgical treatment is followed by radiation therapy, chemotherapy, or immunotherapy. Sufficient recovery time is necessary to accommodate the effects of surgery. In addition, patients may have catheters or ports implanted as a means of delivering drugs and/or nutrients, or obtaining blood samples. The surgeon should be consulted about the amount of time needed to promote healing of these sites. During this time, care must be taken that they are not dislodged by vigorous activity.

Are there limitations in mobility as a result of disease or treatment? — Patients with a sedentary lifestyle or recovering from a prolonged illness may suffer from limited flexibility. In addition, chemotherapeutic agents such as vincristine, which have neurotoxic side effects, can result in limited muscular function and poor coordination, especially in hands and feet. It is not uncommon for metastases to be found in bone, affecting skeletal integrity and presenting a risk for fractures. The pelvis, femur, humerous, skull, and vertebrae are common sites of metastasis. Bone, neck, or back pain of recent origin should be evaluated. Where specific musculoskeletal problems exist, a physical therapy referral may be appropriate to prevent further functional loss or deterioration.

Are there limitations in oxygen delivery as a result of disease or treatment? — Patients with head and neck malignancies, as well as those with lung cancer, may have difficulty with airway obstruction or gas exchange. Further, many head and neck, as well as lung, cancer patients are current or former smokers, meaning they may have chronic obstructive lung disease as well as coronary artery disease. Pleural and pericardial effusions may be contributing factors to dyspnea. It is not uncommon for patients receiving radiation therapy or certain chemotherapeutic agents to develop pneumonitis resulting in permanent pulmonary fibrosis. Patients who receive thoracic radiation have been known to develop accelerated or premature coronary artery disease and possible myocardial infarction. Finally, drugs such as doxorubacin and cyclophosphamide can be cardiotoxic, resulting in damage to cardiac tissue. The development of an irregular or resting pulse above 100 beats per minute should be evaluated. The hematologic system may be affected by primary disease, metastases, or treatment; thus, oxygen transport may be jeopardized in several ways. Most chemotherapeutic agents have a nadir of 7 to 14 d, during which time patients are most susceptable to hemorrhage, infection, and anemia.

Are there limitations in activity as a result of nutritional and fluid deficits? — Nutrient and fluid intake is often compromised as a result of nausea and vomiting, as well as diarrhea and malabsorption associated with treatment. It is not uncommon for patients to suffer fatigue and confusion, especially in hot, humid weather, as a result of fluid volume deficits. Discourage vigorous activity within 24 h of vomiting and diarrhea to allow patients time to rehydrate. In addition to encouraging fluid intake, discourage patients from restricting salt intake unless there is a specific medical indication justifying it.

Are there limitations based on risk for anemia, bleeding, and infection? — Where appropriate, laboratory values should be monitored to evaluate risk of activity: platelet count should be above 50,000/mm^3 to prevent the possibility of hemorrhage. Hemoglobin should be above 10 g/dl; however, higher levels, such as 12 g/dl, may be more appropriate for those living at higher altitutdes. Infection is a common risk during treatment for cancer. As a general rule of thumb, patients should avoid exposure to infection if their white blood count is lower than 3,000/mm^3; however, an absolute granulocyte count above 2,500/mm^3 is a better indicator of immune competence, when available. Patients can be taught to monitor their own temperatures. A persistent resting temperature in excess of 100°F or 37.8°C should be evaluated. Finally, laboratories and exercise facilities should be scrupulously careful about hand washing and disinfecting equipment. Pulmonary function and respiratory gas collection equipment should be sterilized according to established standards.[28]

VI. SUMMARY

Organizations such as the American Cancer Society, the National Cancer Institute, and the National Institutes of Health are good sources of information for exercise leaders and researchers who have not had prior experience working with cancer patients. An oncology rehabilitation team should include a medical, surgical, and radiation oncology specialist as consultants; and an exercise physiologist, an oncology clinical nurse specialist, a nutritionist/dietician, and a physical therapist as core members.

Exercise shows promise in promoting functioning and feelings of well-being in cancer patients. There are challenging opportunities for clinical research and practice. By incorporating guidelines and precautions specific to cancer and cancer treatment into existing cardiopulmonary programs, the quality of life of many individuals living with cancer could be enriched.

REFERENCES

1. **Fobair, P., Hoppe, R.T., Bloom, J., Cox, R., Varghese, A., and Spiegel, D.,** Psychosocial problems among survivors of Hodgkin's disease, *J. Clin. Oncol.,* 4(5), 805, 1986.
2. **Bloom, J.R., Hoppe, R.T., Fobair, P., Cox, R.S., Varghese, A., and Spiegel, D.,** Effects of treatment on the work experience of long-term survivors of Hodgkin's disease, *J. Psychosoc. Oncol.,* 6(3/4), 65, 1988.
3. **Bloom, J.R., Gorsky, R.D., Fobair, P., Hoppe, R., Cox, R.S., Varghese, A., and Spiegel, D.,** Physical performance at work and leisure: validation of a measure of biological energy in survivors of Hodgkin's disease, *J. Psychosoc. Oncol.,* 8(1), 49, 1990.
4. **Welch-McCaffrey, D., Hoffman, B., Leigh, S.A., Loescher, L.J., and Meyskens, Jr., F.L.,** Surviving adult cancers. II. Psychosocial implications, *Ann. Intern. Med.,* 111, 517, 1989.
5. **Loescher, L.J., Welch-McCaffrey, D., Leigh, S.A., Hoffman, B., and Meyskens, Jr., F.L.,** Surviving adult cancers. I. Physiologic effects, *Ann. Intern. Med.,* 111, 411, 1989.
6. **Loescher, L.J., Clark, L., Atwood, J.R., Leigh, S., and Lamb, G.,** The impact of the cancer experience on long-term survivors, *Oncol. Nurs. Forum.,* 17(2), 223, 1990.
7. **Yun, J.,** Influence of fatigue upon growth of rat tumors, *Chin. Med. J.,* 45, 247, 1931.
8. **Rusch, H.P. and Kline, B.E.,** The effect of exercise on the growth of a mouse tumor, *Cancer Res.,* 4, 116, 1944.
9. **Rashkis, H.A.,** Systemic stress as an inhibitor of experimental tumors in swiss mice, *Science,* 116, 169, 1952.
10. **Hoffman, S.S., Paschkis, K.E., DeBias, D.A., Cantarow, A., and Williams, T.L.,** The influence of exercise on the growth of transplanted rat tumors, *Cancer Res.,* 22, 597, 1962.
11. **Rigan, D.,** Exercise and cancer: a review, *J. Am. Osteopath. Assoc.,* 62(3), 54, 1963.
12. **Moore, C. and Tuttle, P.W.,** Muscle activity, body fat, and induced rat mammary tumors, *Surgery,* 73(3), 329, 1973.
13. **Garabrant, D.J., Peters, J.M., Mark, T.M., Bernstein, L.,** Job activity and colon cancer risk, *Am. J. Epidemiol.,* 119, 1005, 1986.
14. **Gerhardsson, M., Norell, S.E., Kiviranta, H., Pedersen, N.L., and Ahlbom, A.,** Sedentary jobs and colon cancer, *Am. J. Epidmiol.,* 123, 775, 1986.
15. **Vena, J.E., Graham, S., Zielezny, M., Brasure, J., and Swanson, M.K.,** Occupational exercise and risk of cancer, *Am. J. Clin. Nutr.,* 45, 318, 1987.
16. **Frisch, R.E., Wyshak, G., Albright, N.L., Albright, T.E., Schiff, I., Jones, K.P., Witschi, J., Shiang, E., Koff, E., and Marguglio, M.,** Lower prevalence of breast cancer and cancers of the reproductive system among former college athletes compared to non-athletes, *Br. J. Cancer,* 52, 885, 1985.
17. **Dietz, Jr., J.H.,** *Rehabilitation Oncology,* John Wiley & Sons, New York, 1981.
18. **Winningham, M.L.,** Effects of a Bicycle Ergometry Program on Functional Capacity and Feelings of Control in Women with Breast Cancer, Dissertation, Ohio State University, Columbus, 1983.
19. **MacVicar, M.G., Winningham, M.L., and Nickel, J.L.,** Effects of aerobic interval training on cancer patients' functional capacity, *Nurs. Res.,* 38, 348, 1989.
20. **MacVicar, M.G. and Winningham, M.L.,** Promoting the functional capacity of cancer patients, *Cancer Bull.,* 38, 235, 1986.
21. **Winningham, M.L. and MacVicar, M.G.,** The effect of aerobic exercise on patient reports of nausea, *Oncol. Nurs. Forum,* 15, 447, 1988.
22. **Winningham, M.L., MacVicar, M.G., Bondoc, M., Anderson, J., and Minton, J.,** Effect of aerobic exercise on body weight and composition in breast cancer patients, *Oncol. Nurs. Forum,* 16(5), 683, 1989.

23. **del Regato, J.A. and Spjut, H.J.**, *Cancer: Diagnosis, Treatment, and Prognosis*, 5th ed., C. V. Mosby, St. Louis, 1977.
24. **Pitot, H.C.**, *Fundamentals of Oncology*, 3rd ed., Marcel Dekker, New York, 1986.
25. **Kraus, H. and Raab, W.**, *Hypokinetic Disease*, Charles C Thomas, Springfield, IL, 1961.
26. **Greenleaf, J. and Kozlowski, S.**, Physiological consequences of reduced physical activity during bed rest, in *Exercise and Sports Science Review*, Terjung, R., Ed., Franklin Institute Press, Philadelphia, 1982, 84.
27. **Nicogossian, A., Huntoon, C., and Pool, S., Eds.**, *Space Physiology and Medicine*, 2nd ed., Lea & Febiger, Philadelphia, 1989.
28. American College of Sports Medicine, Guidelines for Exercise Testing and Prescription, 4th ed., Lea & Febiger, Philadelphia, 1991.

Chapter 6

SHORT-TERM EXERCISE AND IMMUNE FUNCTION

Tony J. Verde

TABLE OF CONTENTS

I. INTRODUCTION

In general, two questions are asked regarding physical activity and immune function: (1) Does prudent physical activity enhance immune function, and (2) Does intense training diminish the body's immune defenses? These questions have been speculated upon for years; some authors have offered answers with little substantiation. Only recently has there been a collaborative scientific effort to attempt to answer these questions.

Exercise immunology is in its infancy. Like all new areas of investigation, more questions arise than are answered. The following chapter will review some of the questions and research that has ventured to supply answers.

The most common method of assessing human immune function is the enumeration of peripheral blood leukocytes, lymphocytes, subpopulations of lymphocytes, and natural killer cells. Lymphocyte proliferative capacity *in vitro,* in response to a mitogenic stimulant, is the second most commonly employed measurement, while the analysis of salivary and mucosal IgA levels has recently become a common methodology of studies on long-term exercise and immune function.

There very well may be no single standardized measure of *in vivo* immune function, since the immune system is a complex network of neural, hormonal, cellular, psychological, and physiological interactions. Likewise, the function of an automobile cannot be determined by only testing the brakes. This lack of a common denominator, both in terms of immunological assessment and exercise protocols, limits valid comparisons among studies and the ability to draw meaningful interpretations. Such a predicament underlies the very nature of the developmental stage of exercise immunology.

Alterations in the immune response to short-term exercise are usually quite transient; thus, most of the reported exercise-induced alterations are observed in blood samples taken immediately or soon after exercise. Considering that most effects are transient, short-term exercise is likely to have only a minor impact upon the normal defense reactions against bacteria, viruses, and neoplastic cells.[1] The tendency of acute exercise to provoke transient alterations in immune parameters seems partially due to both the fitness level of the subject and the relative intensity of the exercise bout.

The objective of this chapter is to focus on the most commonly used measures of immune function and discuss the immune response to short-term exercise which, for the purpose of this chapter, is presented as bouts of exercise that are 60 min or less in duration. When possible, the exercise intensity will be expressed in relation to maximal capabilities. The discussion will be limited to interpretation of data derived from human experimentation.

II. LYMPHOCYTES AND IMMUNITY

Unlike the general processes of innate immunity, the processes of acquired immunity are directed at specific disease organisms. Much of the human body's ability to resist almost all types of invading organisms or toxins is dependent upon acquired immunity. The acquired immune system provides the body with the ability to develop specific resistance against individual invading agents such as lethal bacteria, viruses, toxins, and "foreign" tissues (whether endogenous, in the form of necrotic tissue, transplants, or from other animals).

There are two basic types of acquired immunity. The first, humoral immunity, involves the production and/or retrafficking of circulating antibodies which are capable of attacking the invading agent. The second type of acquired immunity, cell-mediated immunity, relies on the formation of large numbers of specialized lymphocytes that are specifically sensitized against the foreign agent and have the capability of attaching to the foreign agent and destroying it, either directly through the release of lysozymes or indirectly by stimulating the phagocytic activity of macrophages.

Clearly, the immunological information for the cell-mediated immune response is carried by the different populations of T-lymphocytes. There are three general categories of lymphocytes: T-cells, B-cells, and null cells. The lymphocytes whose specific functions are coded in the thymus are called T-lymphocytes; they include helper T-cells, cytotoxic T-cells, and suppressor T-cells. These three populations of sensitized T-lymphocytes are responsible for providing cell-mediated immunity through their specific functions. Helper T-cells recognize an abnormal body cell or an intruder. If such a cell is detected, they send out a chemical messenger to the cytotoxic T-cells (also called killer T-cells), and the latter actively attack the abnormal cell. Helper T-cells also play a regulatory role in humoral immunity by activating B-cells and plasmocytes to release antibodies. On the other hand, suppressor T-cells are the necessary feedback mechanism to control the destructive process initiated by the helper T-cells.

The second general category of lymphocytes, B-cells, are responsible for providing humoral immunity through their role in the synthesis of antibodies. B-cells possess surface immunoglobulins and eventually mature into plasmocytes. B-lymphocytes remain dormant in bone marrow and peripheral lymphoid tissue when not exposed to a specific antigen. However, upon exposure, the B-cells begin maturing into plasmocytes. The mature plasmocytes, through a combination of accelerated proliferation of the precursor B-cells and increased activity, then produce antibodies at an extremely rapid rate. Antibodies are a subgroup of gamma globulins called immunoglobulins; the five major classes are IgG, IgM, IgA, IgD, IgE.

The third general category of lymphocytes, the null cells, comprises any lymphocyte not identifiable as T-cells or B-cells. One representative of this group is a specific cell type called the natural killer cell (NK), which is believed to play an active role in cell-mediated immunosurveillance by actively recognizing and destroying the first few neoplastic cells that develop.[2] These neoplastic cells have the potential for developing into a malignant cancer. Discussion of the effects of short-term exercise on NK cells will be purposely omitted from this chapter, as such discussion is included in Chapter 7.

An essential feature of the healthy immune system is its ability to distinguish "self" from "non-self" and differentiate normal from diseased and damaged cells. This distinction is ultimately made by T- and B-lymphocytes — the only immunologically specific components of the immune mechanism. It is believed that lymphocytes are the most important link in the relationship between exercise and immune function.[1] Consequently, they are the primary focus of this review.

III. EFFECTS OF EXERCISE ON LEUKOCYTE AND LYMPHOCYTE ENUMERATION

Short-term exercise results in an increase in the number of lymphocytes (lymphocytosis) and neutrophils in peripheral blood sampled immediately following exercise.[3-8] These increases have been found to be related to the relative intensity (% of maximal work capacity) and duration of exercise, with a given absolute workrate resulting in a lesser increase in leucocyte numbers in trained than in untrained subjects. In subjects with high work capacity, the leukocytosis was attributable mainly to increases in neutrophils,[9] whereas in subjects with a low work capacity, it was due mainly to increases in lymphocytes.[8] These observations on subjects of differing fitness levels have been documented with longitudinal evaluation.[10,11] In highly trained competitive cyclists, 5 months of seasonal training resulted in decreased mobilization of lymphocytes and increased mobilization of neutrophils during maximal exercise.[10] Similarly, in 17 young sedentary men, a 6-week training period resulted in an attenuation of the lymphocytosis induced by an exhausting exercise test on a cycle ergometer.[11] The latter authors suggested the decreased lymphocytosis was due to a weaker mobilization of lymphocytes into the circulation than before training. The speculation was that fewer immunocompetent cells are required to produce a normal immune response when physical fitness is high, suggesting that improved fitness compensates for the influence of physical stress on the immune system.

Exercise-induced leukocytosis (35.4%) and lymphocytosis (19.7%) also occurs during bouts of acute high intensity cycle exercise to exhaustion (30 sec Wingate tests).[12] These increases cannot be fully accounted for by the exercise-induced decrease (-14.5%) in plasma volume. Quick recovery from exercise-induced lymphocytosis occurs following short-term exercise.[5] By 30 min post-exercise, resting lymphocyte, B-cell, and T-cell counts and/or proportions are reestablished.[5,13]

The underlying mechanism of exercise-induced lymphocytosis is unclear. The total number of leukocytes in the circulation at any given time has been shown to depend on a multitude of factors[14] including:

1. alpha and beta adrenoceptor activation
2. location of the noncirculating leukocyte pool
3. rates of sequestration, margination-demargination of leukocytes

4. leukocyte-endothelium interations
5. hemodynamics of cardiac output and blood flow
6. hormonal (catecholamines and cortisol)
7. sympathetic and parasympathetic neural input at the spinal cord and hypothalamus levels

While the roles of these individual factors have been sketched with regard to total leukocytes, their specific roles in exercise-induced lymphocytosis are less clear.

The margination, mobilization, distribution, and pooling of leukocytes with exercise have been reviewed elsewhere.[14] The reviewers proposed a model for the leukocytosis of exercise and discussed the location of the noncirculating lymphocyte pool. In brief, noncirculating lymphocytes have been found to localize mainly in the liver and spleen, but the mobilization of these noncirculating lymphocytes is less clear. The reviewers indicated that splenectomy had relatively little influence on the exercise-induced leukocytosis, which was in agreement with previous observations[3] showing that the number of leukocytes leaving the spleen is increased minimally by exercise. Likewise, the lungs have been shown not to be the major source of the leukocytes mobilized by exercise.[14] There have been no reports in the literature on the possible exercise-induced mobilization of the noncirculating lymphocytes from liver.

A. T- AND B-LYMPHOCYTE ENUMERATION

In blood samples taken immediately after exercise, earlier investigators attributed the lymphocytosis to increased numbers of both T-cells and B-cells.[3-5] While the absolute numbers of T-cells and B-cells, calculated per cubic millimeter of blood, increased immediately after 15 min of stationary cycling, the resultant lymphocyte population exhibited an increase in the percentage of B-cells and a decrease in the percentage of T-cells[3,5] compared to pre-exercise values. The disproportionate increase in B-cells is transient, as the percentages of T-cells and B-cells return to pre-exercise levels within 6 to 15 min of recovery.[5,11]

Unlike these earlier investigations, most experiments carried out since 1985 have employed monoclonal antibodies in conjunction with laser flow cytometry for cell enumeration and have yielded contradictory results with regards to exercise-induced alterations in B-lymphocytes. Flow cytometry methodologies showed that acute maximal treadmill exertion resulted in a decrease in the percentage of peripheral blood B-cells, but no change in their absolute number.[15,16] Similar decreases in B-cell percentage with no change in absolute numbers has also been observed following acute moderate exercise (45 min of walking).[8] Pre flow cytometry era, earlier investigators identified B-cells by the cell's possession of specific surface immunoglobulins. Clearly, the earlier technique for distinguishing B-cells could incorrectly classify NK cells as B-cells[15] and NK cells have been shown to increase with exercise.[17]

The more recent use of fluorescence-activated cell sorting allows differentiation of 10,000 or more cells per sample, which intuitively is more accurate than counting 100 or 200 cells under a microscope. Accordingly, bouts of maximal or submaximal short-term exercise appear to result in a decrease in the percentage of B-cells without a concomitant change in absolute numbers. Therefore, it appears that B-cells are not mobilized during short-term exercise.

Although modern technology has led to contradictory results of B-cell changes, monoclonal antibodies in conjunction with flow cytometry has reaffirmed the earlier observations on T-cell changes. Immediately following acute maximal exercise, the percentage of T-cells are reduced,[18] with this transient decrease no longer evident 15 min post-exercise.[16] However, if the acute bout of exercise is of moderate vs. maximal intensity, there appears to be an increase in both the percentage and number of T-cells. T-cells represent approximately one-third of the lymphocytosis induced by moderate intensity exercise, with natural killer cells accounting for most of the remaining two-thirds.[8]

1. Training Effect on T- and B-Lymphocyte Enumeration

A recent cross-sectional study[19] designed to assess the effects of fitness level and exercise intensity on exercise-induced alterations in lymphocyte counts, showed sharp reductions in the percentage of T-cells immediately after subjects performed three separate bouts of short-term submaximal exercise on a cycle ergometer (ride #1 — 65% $\dot{V}O_2$ max for 30 min; ride #2 — 30% $\dot{V}O_2$ max for 60 min; ride #3 — 75% $\dot{V}O_2$ max for 60 min). Across all fitness levels (low, moderate, and high) ride #2 (lowest relative intensity) elicited the significantly smallest decrease in T-cells. The reductions in the percentage of T-cells was significant, and of the greatest magnitude following the higher intensity ride #3, in both the moderate and high fit subject groups. There was no significant decrease in the percentage of T-cells in either the control or low fit subject groups, regardless of exercise intensity. In contrast, the absolute number of T-cells tended to increase after exercise and significantly so in the high fit subjects.

Longitudinal studies also suggest that physical training influences lymphocyte counts measured at rest.[20] In young, healthy, previously sedentary men who were trained aerobically 40 to 50 min/d (5 days/week for 15 weeks) the percentage of T-lymphocytes significantly increased from 65 to 74%.[20] In contrast, a 15-week walking program (five 45-min sessions per week) resulted in a significant decrease in absolute number and percentage of lymphocytes and in absolute number of T-cells with no significant effect on total number of leukocytes.[21] The reported differences are likely due to the varied immunological methodology and exercise design. The reported increase in the percentage of T-cells with physical training was observed on isolated lymphocytes using the E-rosetting technique for differentiation of lymphocyte type.[20] In the second study, investigators used whole blood and differentiated lymphocyte type with monoclonal antibodies and flow cytometry.[21] Furthermore, the walking program failed to elicit any improvement in $\dot{V}O_2$ max. Since such a training program had no impact on maximal aerobic power, it is not surprising that its impact on immune function was negligible.

In highly trained athletes, 5 months of normal seasonal training resulted in decreases in the absolute and relative number of neutrophils at rest, with no change in the absolute number or relative percentage of lymphocytes.[10] In elite runners, reversion to normal training patterns following three weeks of heavy training resulted in a significant lowering of the percentage of T-lymphocytes in resting blood samples,[22] suggesting that periods of heavy training are more detrimental to the immune function of athletes than periods of normal training.

B. RESPONSE OF HELPER AND SUPPRESSOR CELLS TO ACUTE EXERCISE

A number of studies have reported on the effect of exercise on subpopulations of peripheral blood lymphocytes. In 12 males (mean age 45 years), maximal treadmill exercise resulted in a significant increase in the percentage of suppressor T-cells (from 32.7 to 36.4).[16] These increases were associated with a significant decrease in the percentage of helper T-cells (from 53.8 to 43.4) and a significant 30% decrease of the helper/suppressor ratio (from 1.94 to 1.36). In the study, the absolute lymphocyte count significantly increased in response to the exercise bout (from 2.4 to 2.9 $\times$ $10^3/mm^3$). In untrained subjects, a bout of maximal exercise has been reported to elevate the absolute number of virtually all types of lymphocyte subsets with increased mobilization of suppressor cells being most evident.[10]

Similar trends seem to be evident in response to acute moderate intensity exercise.[8] In 12 sedentary women (mean age 37 years), a 45-min walk (60% $\dot{V}O_2$ max) resulted in an increase in the percentage of suppressor cells (from 28.6 to 33.2) and a decrease in the proportion of helper cells (from 51.3 to 43.9) yielding a corresponding significant decrease in the H/S ratio (1.76 to 1.26). The author noted the increase in suppressor cells was predominantly of the dimly fluorescent variety, a subpopulation of suppressor cells which are thought to function primarily as natural killer cells.[23] In untrained subjects, submaximal exercise of shorter duration (15 min) resulted in an increase in both T-suppressor and T-helper cells.[25] However, there was an associated decrease in H/S ratio (1.79 to 1.38) due to a proportionately larger increase in T-suppressor cells than in T-helper cells. An earlier study,[24] which did not differentiate lymphocyte subsets with monoclonal antibodies and flow cytometry, reported the exercise-induced (15 min submaximal) decrease in H/S ratio was due solely to a reduction in percentage of helper cells with no change in the proportion of suppressor cells.

In light of the previously mentioned regulatory feedback, changes in these lymphocyte subsets may have varying physiological effects on immunosurveillance. A reduction of the Th/Ts ratio below 1.5 has been suggested to be associated with a decrease in the proliferative response of lymphocytes to mitogenic stimulants.[2]

1. Effect of Training on Helper and Suppressor Cells
a. Cross-Sectional Studies

Regardless of fitness level, sharp reductions in the percentages of T-helper lymphocytes are observed immediately after exercise.[19] This reduction seems dependent on exercise intensity with greatest reductions occurring after bouts of higher intensity (75% — 60 min). While the percentage of T-helper cells seems to decrease with acute exercise, changes in the absolute number appear to be influenced by fitness level, such that a 15 min bout of submaximal exercise for the untrained individual[25] would elicit a response comparable to that of the trained individual following acute maximal exercise.[26] In both cases, there is a significant increase in the number of T-helper cells with a proprotionately greater increase in the number of T-suppressor cells. These unequal increases in absolute numbers of helper and suppressor cells is associated with a significant decrease in the H/S ratio. If the exercise challenge is maximal for both the trained and untrained subject, there is no change in the absolute number of T-helper cells[16] in the untrained subject compared to the significant increase in the trained subject.[26] A research design which adjusted for fitness level[19] also showed significantly greater exercise-induced increases in absolute numbers of helper cells in high fit subjects.

This same research design which controlled for fitness level and exercise intensity found no significant effect of subject fitness category or varying submaximal intensity of short-term exercise on the percentage of T-suppressor cells, although numbers of this subset increased significantly after exercise in subjects with low fitness levels.[19] Exercise-induced increases in the absolute number of suppressor cells have also been documented in highly trained athletes following acute maximal exercise.[26] Irrespective of whether the changes are expressed as a percentage or absolute numbers, recovery to baseline occurs within 30 min of ceasing exercise.[19]

Only one study has failed to report any difference between trained and untrained subjects with regard to the changes in the proportion of helper and suppressor cells in blood samples taken immediately following a bout of acute maximal exercise.[18] These investigators compared observations made on five trained men with those made on five untrained men and five untrained women. Perhaps the small sample size and gender difference masked any response difference between the untrained and trained individual.

b. Longitudinal Studies

Very few longitudinal studies have investigated the effects of training on subsets of T-lymphocytes.[10,21,22] Two have been carried out with highly trained male athletes,[10,22] whereas previously sedentary women were subjects in the other investigation.[21]

At rest — In the previously sedentary women, moderate exercise training (in the form of a 15-week walking program — five 45-min sessions per week), had no significant effect on total numbers of helper cells, suppressor cells or the H/S cell ratio.[21] In the highly trained athletes, regimens of normal training did not effect the percentages of helper cells, suppressor cells, or the H/S ratio observed in blood samples taken at rest.[10,22] However, there is evidence to suggest that when athletes engage in periods of heavy training, the proportion of helper cells may decrease and the proportion of suppressor cells increase, thus, decreasing the H/S ratio at rest.[22] Three weeks of recovery following a regimen of heavy training resulted in a significant increase in the H/S ratio, primarily due to a significant decrease in the percentage of suppressor cells.[22]

Acute exercise — Following 5 months of normal seasonal training for competitive cyclists, acute maximal exercise induced significantly lower increases in the absolute number of helper cells when compared to before training observations.[10] Thirty minutes of submaximal exercise (80% of $\dot{V}O_2$ max) resulted in similar decreases in the H/S ratio following regimens of normal training and heavy training in elite runners.[22]

IV. EFFECTS OF EXERCISE ON LYMPHOCYTE FUNCTION

The morphological transformation of T-lymphocytes to blast cells has been observed during the induction of graft vs. host disease and during the sensitization of normal guinea pigs to chemical allergens.[27] Thus, lymphocytes are transformed morphologically and functionally in response to antigenic stimulation. The fact that lymphocytes can be transformed *in vitro* by specific antigens or many nonspecific mitogens provides a useful system for studying mechanisms of immunoregulation and control in mammalian cells. Mitogen-induced cell proliferation is a useful, *in vitro,* diagnostic measure of cell-mediated immune function.[29] The *in vitro* proliferative response of lymphocytes when cultured in the presence of mitogens and antigens is generally agreed to reflect global *in vivo* immunological function.[27]

As an assessment of cell-mediated immunity, it is common to place isolated peripheral blood mononuclear cells (PBMC) in culture, and incubate them in the presence of a nonspecific mitogenic stimulus such as the plant lectin concanavalin A (Con A) or phytohemagglutinin (PHA). Such nonspecific mitogens interact with receptors on the surfaces of the various T-cells that are different from the antigen-specific T-cell receptor. The nonspecific stimulus elicits an overall (i.e., all subsets of T-cells) response. Under these conditions, the overall increase in lymphocyte transformation (blastogenesis) can be quantitated by the incorporation of radioisotopes such as tritiated thymidine into the DNA of proliferating lymphocytes. Although the proliferative response of a single antigen-specific T-cell clone is not tested by this method, the overall proliferative response of PBMC to a nonspecific mitogen, nevertheless, provides a rough measure of T-cell function. This proliferative response is blunted or absent in patients with T-cell defects (imbalance among the subpopulations of T-cells) and in pharmaceutically immunosuppressed patients.[28]

Is there an association between lymphocyte counts and function? Shifts within the proportion of T-lymphocyte subsets (specifically the H/S ratio) have been postulated to account for the observed exercise-induced alterations in lymphocyte proliferation.[2,25,30,31] Our endeavors to document any such correlation between H/S ratio and lymphocyte proliferation have failed.[22] Furthermore, it is not known whether exercise-induced alterations in numbers and subpopulations of circulating lymphocytes have any clinical significance on *in vivo* immune function, since circulating lymphocytes represent only a small percentage of the body's total lymphocyte pool.[31] Alternative suggestions have implied that the relocation of lymphocytes from tissues to the blood may decrease resistance to infection by removing cells from the local sites where the immune response is initiated.[25] As yet, the question of whether the changes in lymphocyte counts reflect functional alterations remains unanswered.

Although a number of studies have investigated the effects of exercise on leukocyte and lymphocyte counts, few have dealt with its effect on lymphocyte function. Exercise studies that have addressed the issue of function have led to a confusing picture, due to vast differences in methodology. Experimental subjects have ranged from sedentary individuals to top level, nationally ranked athletes. The reported differences in exercise-induced alterations in lymphocyte counts are primarily due to the interinvestigator difference in the timing of post-exercise blood sampling. However, exercise duration and relative intensity add to the reported differences regarding the effects of short-term exercise on lymphocyte function. Further apparent discrepancies in findings regarding exercise and lymphocyte function are often the result of different methods of expressing data (for example, relative or absolute terms).

In healthy individuals, the immediate peripheral blood lymphocyte response to a bout of exercise appears to be an increase in the number of cells, per cubic millimeter of blood, which proliferate in response to mitogen stimulation.[5,11] If lymphocyte function is expressed as a percentage of total lymphocytes, a depressed response to mitogen stimulation has been observed following exercise.[5] During exercise, however, due to the concurrent lymphocytosis, there was a greater than 60% increase in the absolute number of cells responsive to mitogen stimulation. Likewise, other investigators[11] have reported a depressed response when expressing their results in relative terms, but an enhanced response when expressed in absolute terms.

It is most common for immunological methodologies to employ a fixed number of cells per culture when investigating the *in vitro* proliferative response to mitogen stimulation. Therefore, expression of results in relative terms is common practice. In 15 healthy men (aged from 22 to 30 years), a suppressed response of lymphocytes to polyclonal mitogen stimulation has been reported following 15 min of submaximal cycle ergometer work.[3] The methodology used isolated highly purified blood lymphocytes vs. the more frequently reported response of unsorted peripheral blood mononuclear cells. The role of monocytes in the *in vitro* proliferative response was, therefore, excluded in their laboratory. In normal, healthy, sedentary volunteers, 10 min of submaximal exercise did not result in any proliferative changes in either heparinized or defibrinated blood.[32] If time elapses and blood samples are taken later in recovery from short-term exercise, lymphocyte function may return to or exceed pre-exercise levels.[5,22] Exercise-induced alterations in lymphocyte function may not have a lasting effect on host defense function because, like lymphocyte counts, the changes are sufficiently transient in nature that there is no substantial impact on viral or bacterial multiplication.[1]

V. EFFECTS OF TRAINING ON LYMPHOCYTE FUNCTION

A. CROSS-SECTIONAL STUDIES
At rest — Cross-sectional studies have indicated that the conditioned athlete exhibits a normal, healthy immune function while maintaining a normal pattern of training.[33-36] In fact, in blood specimens sampled at rest,[37] significantly higher PHA-induced lymphocyte proliferation has been reported in a group of competitive athletes compared to an age-matched sedentary control group. A positive association between fitness level and lymphocyte transformation at rest has been documented with a more elaborate research design which stratified subjects of similar age by fitness level.[38] Subjects with low fitness levels had significantly lower proliferative response to Con A at rest than did subjects of either the moderate or high fitness groups. These findings would suggested that a high fitness level does not provide any further benefit than a moderate fitness level.

Acute exercise — Despite the lower resting level of proliferation in the subject group of low fitness, acute exercise resulted in a suppression of proliferation which was still evident 2 h after exercise in all fitness groups.[38] The magnitude or the reduction was not affected by an increase in exercise duration. A trend toward greater reduction was present in the highly fit group when exercise intensity was increased.

B. LONGITUDINAL STUDIES
At rest — In blood samples taken at rest, two longitudinal training studies reported enhanced lymphocyte proliferation in response to mitogen stimulation following physical training.[11,20] In one study,[11] the physical training program consisted of 6 weeks basic training for 17 incoming naval conscripts, while in the other study,[20] 52 students attending the University of Arizona trained aerobically 40 to 50 min/d, 5 d/week for 15 weeks. Moderate exercise training (15 weeks walking program) in mildly obese women, which did not elicit an

improvement in $\dot{V}O_2$ max, had no significant effect on spontaneous blasto-genesis.[21] The failure of the latter study to document increases in immune function may also be a partial reflection of the different methodological assessment of proliferation. It is possible that spontaneous blastogenesis (in the absence of mitogenic stimulation) of lymphocytes is less sensitive in measuring change over time than the optimal response of lymphocytes to mitogenic stimulation.

In addition to the enhanced immune function at rest, observed in athletes compared to untrained subjects,[37] a further deliberate increase in training volume for a 3-week period resulted in a further elevation of resting levels of lymphocyte proliferation in response to both PHA (from an average of 37,087 cpm to 46,218 cpm) and Con A (from an average of 29,060 cpm to 38,433 cpm).[22]

Acute exercise — Following physical training of the previously sedentary individual, the exercise-induced decrease of lymphocyte transformation was attentuated in comparison with pretraining observation.[11] On the other hand, the exercise-induced decrease in lymphocyte proliferation was exacerbated in elite runners following 3 weeks of heavy training.[22] Such findings suggest that moderate amounts of physical training improve the immune response to short-term exercise, most likely by decreasing the relative stress associated with the bout of exercise. However, the fatigue associated with regimens of heavy training decreases one's tolerance to physical stress, resulting in a further suppression of the immune response to a given bout of exercise.

VI. EFFECTS OF SHORT-TERM EXERCISE ON OTHER IMMUNOLOGICAL PARAMETERS

A. IMMUNOGLOBULINS

Most of the published reports describing exercise-induced changes in serum concentrations of immunoglobulins have investigated the response to bouts of long-term exercise.[39-41] Similarly, other studies have reported the effects of endurance events on salivary IgA levels.[31,42,43] Relatively few pub-lished reports are available describing short-term exercise-induced changes in immunoglobulin levels.[44,45] In trained individuals, no significant change in serum immunoglobulin levels was observed 10 min following a 13-km sub-maximal run.[34] Nevertheless, the average serum concentration of IgM tended to a 34% rise. Likewise, in untrained subjects, short-term exercise did not significantly alter levels of serum immunoglobulins.[46]

Assessing the effects of short-term exercise on the synthesis of IgG and IgM vs. serum concentrations has rarely been reported. Highly purified blood lymphocytes obtained from blood sampled immediately after 15 min of sub-maximal exercise produced less IgG (from 2015 to 1623 ng/ml) and IgM (from 984 to 390 ng/ml) compared to pre-exercise production, following 7 d in culture with pokeweed mitogen.[24] In contrast, this exercise-induced de-crease in immunoglobulin production was not evident in highly trained subjects. Thirty minutes of submaximal exercise (80% $\dot{V}O_2$ max) did not alter IgG of IgM production in elite runners.[22]

A longitudinal training study evaluated the influence of moderate physical activity on resting serum concentrations of immunoglobulins.[21] The 15 week training study of 36 sedentary, mildly obese women (five 45-min walking sessions per week) resulted in a modest (net increase of 20% — IgG, IgM, IgA) increase which was not statistically significant. Through cross-sectional evaluations, athletes have been reported to have resting levels of serum immunoglobulins comparable to those of sedentary controls,[33] but significantly lower resting salivary IgA levels compared with age-matched controls.[43]

B. SOLUBLE FACTORS

Soluble components of the immune system include complement, interferon, and interleukins. Complement is a nonspecific complex of humoral factors, which react with antibodies to form opsonins (substances that enhance macrophage function as part of the repair process). There are no data to suggest that exercise induces functionally important alterations in the complement system of athletes. Similarly, in untrained individuals, Hanson and Flaherty[34] did not observe any changes in resting levels of serum complement C3 and C4 10 min after a submaximal run.

Inferferons are produced by certain types of activated T-cells, and by cells that have become virally infected. They induce viral resistance in uninfected cells, in part by enhancing the antigen-presenting function of macrophages. In eight untrained men, 1 h of submaximal exercise on a cycle ergometer has been shown to elevate plasma alpha interferon levels from 3 to 7 IU.[47] The clinical significance is doubtful since viral infections produce interferon levels which may be 10- to 20-fold higher.[48]

Twenty minutes of stationary cycling at 220 W indicated that strenuous physical work had a negative effect on nonspecific immunity of the organism.[46] In the seven healthy men performing this bout of acute exercise, there was a mean 26% decline of phagocytic function, 50% decrease in the mean opsonin titre, a mean 14% increase of complement titre, and no change in the properdin level. On the other hand, blood samples taken at rest indicated that phagocytic function of monocytes was significantly higher in competitive athletes than in age-matched controls.[37]

While a number of investigations have assessed the effects of long-term exercise on other populations of leukocytes,[49-53] significant increases in granulocytes and monocytes have been observed in untrained subjects following short-term submaximal exercise (15 min).[25] Acute moderate exercise of longer duration (45-min walk, 60% $\dot{V}O_2$ max) results in increased neutrophils and little or no change in granulocytes and monocytes.[8] Acute exercise does not seem to alter the numbers of basophils or eosinophils.[14]

The most consistently observed changes in other immune indices following exercise have been an increase in antibody-dependent cytotoxic and NK activity[17] and an increase in plasma interleukin-1 (1 h at 60% $\dot{V}O_2$ max).[54]

The clinical and biological significance of the effects of exercise on various host defense mechanisms are not known. These effects have been extensively reviewed elsewhere.[1,2,31,55-58]

VII. VARIATION AND LIMITATIONS

Most exercise immunology studies measure immune function at rest or following exercise. While efforts are usually made to test subjects at the same time of day to control for diurnal variations of hormones, methodologies seldom address the possibility of intra-subject day-to-day variation in their immune response to exercise. While physiological responses to a given sub-maximal workrate are fairly consistent, the effects of submaximal exercise on proportions of T-lymphocyte subsets vary over time.[6] In 18 healthy men, 60 min of cycling (65% $\dot{V}O_2$ max) repeated on days 1, 3, and 5 showed decreases in the percentage of T-cells occurring on days 1 and 3 (but not 5); decreases in the percentage of helper cells were observed only on day 3, with no effect of exercise on percentage of suppressor cells on any day. In contrast, exercise-induced leukocytosis and lymphocytosis have been shown to be re-producible over four repeat 30-sec Wingate tests, each separated by 7 d.[12]

Individuals can vary widely with regard to their *in vitro* response to polyclonal mitogens. Day-to-day variations have been noted within some individuals who might on one day produce peripheral blood lymphocytes post-exercise that exhibited a suppressed response to mitogens and on another day produced lymphocytes with an enhanced response.[2] These same authors observed that, overall, the number of tests showing post-exercise suppression of responsiveness to the mitogens was greater than the number showing enhanced activity. The biological significance of the transient changes with exercise is unknown.

Very few studies employ control groups, and changes have been observed in controls spending equal experimental time in the laboratory.[8] Statistical adjustment for this interaction would allow clearer differentiation between the effects of exercise, exercise training, and laboratory setting. Longitudinal studies may also run into effects of seasonal variation.[59]

The methodologies of several investigators[11,13,21] used whole blood for the assessment of *in vitro* lymphocyte transformation in place of isolated lymphocytes or mononuclear cells. Whole blood methodologies lend com-plexity to interpretation, due to the presence in plasma of a plethora of molecules which possibly play a role in the immune response.[60] Unpublished data by Sabiston and colleagues[61] exhibited opposite effects of exercise on mitogen-induced proliferation when using whole-blood cultures vs. isolated mononuclear cell cultures. An exercise-induced suppression of lymphocyte transformation was observed with the whole-blood cultures while an enhance-ment was evident with the isolated mononuclear cell cultures. While most other studies use suspensions of isolated mononuclear cells (lymphocytes/ monocytes), other investigators have made specific efforts to separate lymphocytes from monocytes prior to preparing their immunological assays for proliferation measures.[3,24]

It is possible, although not documented, that food intake may influence the *in vitro* proliferation capacity of isolated lymphocytes. As a precaution, some exercise immunology studies have incorporated a 12-h fast in their methodologies.[3,8,11,21] Although the response of lymphocytes to PHA has been shown to decrease after caloric restriction,[37] actual diet composition does not seem to alter immune function if the subject is not in a state of caloric deficit.[62] Further studies are needed to assess the possible interaction of diet on the immune response to exercise.

VIII. SUMMARY

The literature is not clear on whether physical training has a positive or a negative effect on immune function, although the longitudinal studies which resulted in increased $\dot{V}O_2$ max of their subjects[11,20] suggest that a moderate regular physical activity regimen is beneficial to one's immune function. Fifteen weeks of more moderate physical training, paralleled by no change in $\dot{V}O_2$ max, was not associated with an improvement of immune function.[21] Isolated cross-sectional studies have indicated that the conditioned athlete exhibits a normal, healthy immune function while maintaining a normal pattern of training,[33-36] which would not indicate any negative effects of more intensive training on the immune function of individuals who are accustomed to such habits.

If blood samples are taken soon after exercise and results are expressed in relative terms, the literature suggests that a single bout of short-term exercise is accompanied by some transient degree of suppressed lymphocyte proliferation in response to a nonspecific mitogen. This exercise-induced suppression appears to be reversible, as mononuclear cells isolated from blood sampled later on in recovery exhibit pre-exercise levels of stimulated blastogenesis or even levels which exceed pre-exercise values.

Provided that subjects are healthy and not overly fatigued, the small changes in circulating numbers of immune system variables following short-term exercise are also transient and most likely not of clinical significance. Enumeration of leukocytes, lymphocytes, and subpopulations of lymphocytes may be a limited approach to exercise immunology since changes in counts do not necessarily reflect changes in function. There is great need for a standard measure of immune function in healthy individuals to provide a common denominator for comparison among studies.

REFERENCES

1. **Simon, H.B.,** Exercise and infection, *Phys. Sportsmed.,* 15(10), 134, 1987.
2. **Keast, D., Cameron, K., and Morton, A.R.,** Exercise and immune response, *Sports Med.,* 5, 248, 1988.
3. **Hedfors, E., Holm, G., and Ohnell, B.,** Variations of blood lymphocytes during work studied by cell surface markers, DNA syntheses and cytotoxicity, *Clin. Exp. Immunol.,* 24, 328, 1976.
4. **Yu, D.T.Y., Clements, P.J., and Pearson, C.M.,** Effects of corticosteroids on exercise-induced lymphocytosis, *Clin. Exp. Immunol.,* 28, 326, 1977.
5. **Robertson, A.J., Ramesar, K.C., Potts, R.C., Gibbs, J.H., Browning, M.C., Brown, R.A., Hayes, P.C., and Swanson-Buck, J.,** The effect of strenuous physical exercise on circulating blood lymphocytes and serum cortisol levels, *J. Clin. Lab. Immunol.,* 5, 53, 1981.
6. **Hoffman-Goetz, L., Simpson, J.R., Cipp, N., Arumugam, Y., and Houston, M.E.,** Lymphocyte subset responses to repeated submaximal exercise in men, *J. Appl. Physiol.,* 68, 1069, 1990.
7. **Tvede, N., Pedersen, N.K., Hansen, F.R., Bendix, T., Christensen, L.D., Galbo, H., and Haljær-Kristensen, J.,** Effect of physical exercise on blood mononuclear cell subpopulations and *in vitro* proliferative responses, *Scand. J. Immunol.,* 29, 383, 1989.
8. **Neiman, D.C., Nehlsen-Cannarella, S.L., Donohoue, K.M., Chritton, D.B.W., Haddock, B.L., Stout, R.W., and Lee, J.W.,** The effects of acute moderate exercise on leukocyte and lymphocyte subpopulations, *Med. Sci. Sports Exercise,* 23, 578, 1991.
9. **Dorner, H., Heinold, D., and Hilmer, W.,** Exercise-induced leucocytosis — its dependence on physical capability, *Int. J. Sports. Med.,* 8, 152, 1987.
10. **Ferry, A., Picard, F., Duvallet, A., Weill, B., and Rieu, M.,** Changes in blood leucocyte populations induced by acute maximal and chronic submaximal exercise, *Eur. J. Appl. Physiol.,* 59, 435, 1990.
11. **Soppi, E., Varjo, P., Eskola, J., and Laitinen, L.A.,** Effect of strenuous physical stress on circulating lymphocyte number and function before and after training, *J. Clin. Lab. Immunol.,* 8, 43, 1982.
12. **Bailey, F., Mareesh, C.M., Hoffman, J.R., Gabaree, C.L., Hannon, D., Deschenes, M.R., Abraham, A., Kraemer, W.J., and Armstrong, L.E.,** Immune factor responses to wingate anaerobic power testing, *Med. Sci. Sports Exercise,* 23(4), S62, 1991.
13. **Eskola, J., Ruuskanen, O., Soppi, E., Viljanen, M.K., Jarvinen, M., Toivonen, H., and Kouvalainen, K.,** Effect of sport stress on lymphocyte transformation and antibody formation, *Clin. Exp. Immunol.,* 32, 339, 1978.
14. **McCarthy, D.A. and Dale, M.M.,** The leucocytosis of exercise: a review and model, *Sports Med.,* 6, 333, 1988.
15. **Deuster, P.A., Curiale, A.M., Cowan, M.L., and Finkelman, F.D.,** Exercise-induced changes in populations of peripheral blood mononuclear cells, *Med. Sci. Sports Exercise,* 20, 276, 1988.
16. **Berk, L.S., Nieman, D., Tan, S.A., Nehlsen-Cannarella, S., Kramer, J., Eby, W.C., and Owens, M.,** Lymphocyte subset changes during acute maximal exercise, *Med. Sci. Sports Exercise,* 18(Abstr.), 706, 1986.
17. **MacKinnon, L.T.,** Exercise and natural killer cells: what is the relationship? *Sports Med.,* 7, 141, 1989.
18. **Brahmi, Z., Thomas, J.E., Park, M., Park, M., and Dowdeswell, I.R.G.,** The effect of acute exercise on natural killer-cell activity of trained and sedentary human subjects, *J. Clin. Immunol.,* 5, 321, 1985.
19. **Kendall, A., Hoffman-Goetz, L., Houston, M., MacNeil, B., and Arumugam, Y.,** Exercise and blood lymphocyte responses: intensity, duration, and subject fitness effects, *J. Appl. Physiol.,* 69, 251, 1990.

20. **Watson, R.R., Moriguchi, S., Jackson, J.C., Werner, L., Wilmore, J.H., and Freund, B.J.,** Modification of Cellular immune functions in humans by endurance training during B-adrenergic blockade with atenolol or propanolol, *Med. Sci. Sports Exercise,* 18, 95, 1986.
21. **Nehlsen-Cannarella, S.L., Nieman, D.C., Balk-Lamberton, A.J., Markoff, P.A., Chritton, D.B.W., Gusewitch, G., and Lee, J.W.,** The effects of moderate exercise training on immune response, *Med. Sci. Sports Exercise,* p. 64, 1991.
22. **Verde, T.J., Thomas, S.G., Moore, R.W., Shek, P., and Shephard, R.J.,** Immune responses and increased training in the elite athlete, *J. Appl. Physiol.,* in press, 1992.
23. **Lanier, L.L., Le, A.M., Philips, J.H., Warner, N.L., and Babcock, G.F.,** Subpopulations of human natural killer cells defined by expression of the Leu-7 (HNK-1) and Leu-11 (NK-15) antigens, *J. Immunol.,* 131, 1789, 1983.
24. **Hedfors, E., Holm, G., Ivansen, M., and Wahren, J.,** Physiological variation of blood lymphocyte reactivity: T-cell subsets, immunoglobulin production, and mixed-lymphocyte reactivity, *Clin. Immunol. Immunopath.,* 27, 9, 1983.
25. **Landmann, R.M.A., Muller, F.B., Perini, C.H., Wesp, M., Erne, P., and Buhler, F.R.,** Changes of immunoregulatory cells induced by psychological and physical stress: relationship to catecholamines, *Clin. Exp. Immunol.,* 58, 127, 1984.
26. **Lewicki, R., Tchorzewski, H., Majewska, E., Nowak, Z., and Baj, Z.,** Effect of maximal physical exercise on T-lymphocyte subpopulations and on interleukin 1 (IL1) and interleukin 2 (IL2) production *in vitro, Int. J. Sports Med.,* 9, 114, 1988.
27. **Bloom, B.R.,** *In vitro* approaches to the mechanism of cell mediated immune reactions, *Adv. Immunol.,* 13, 101, 1971.
28. **Claman, H.N.,** The biology of the immune response, *JAMA,* 285, 2834, 1987.
29. **DeShazo, R.D., Lopez, M., and Salvaggio, J.E.,** Use and interpretation of diagnostic immunologic laboratory tests, *JAMA,* 258, 3011, 1987.
30. **Hoffman-Goetz, L., Keir, R., Thorne, R., Houston, M.E., and Young, C.,** Chronic exercise stress in mice depresses splenic T lymphocyte mitogenesis *in vitro, Clin. Exp. Immunol.,* 66, 551, 1986.
31. **MacKinnon, L.T. and Tomasi, T.B.,** Immunology of exercise, in *Sports Medicine Fitness, Training, Injuries,* 3rd ed., Appenzeller, O., Ed., Urban and Schwarzenberg, Baltimore, 1989, 273.
32. **Edwards, A.J., Bacon, T.H., Elms, C.A., Verardi, R., Felder, M., and Knight, S.C.,** Changes in the populations of lymphoid cells in human peripheral blood following physical exercise, *Clin. Exp. Immunol.,* 58, 420, 1984.
33. **Green, R.L., Kaplan, S.S., Rabin, B.S., Stanitski, C.L., and Zdziarski, U.,** Immune function in marathon runners, *Ann. Allergy,* 47, 73, 1981.
34. **Hanson, P.G. and Flaherty, D.K.,** Immunological responses to training in conditioned runners, *Clin. Sci.,* 60, 225, 1981.
35. **Busse, W.W., Anderson, C.L., Hanson, P.G., and Folts, J.D.,** The effect of exercise on the granulocyte response to isoproterenol in the trained athlete and unconditioned individual, *J. Allergy Clin. Immunol.,* 65, 358, 1981.
36. **Oshida, Y., Yamanouchi, K., Hayamizu, S., and Sato, Y.,** Effect of acute physical exercise on lymphocyte subpopulations in trained and untrained subjects, *Int. J. Sports Med.,* 9(2), 137, 1988.
37. **Kono, I., Matsuda, H.K.M., Haga, S., Fukushima, H., and Kashiwagi, H.,** Weight reduction in athletes may adversely affect the phagocytic function of monocytes, *Phys. Sportsmed.,* 16(7), 56, 1988.
38. **MacNeil, B., Hoffman-Goetz, L., Kendall, A., Houston, M., and Arumugam, Y.,** Lymphocyte proliferation responses after exercise in men: fitness, intensity, and duration effects, *J. Appl. Physiol.,* 70, 179, 1991.
39. **Bosenberg, A.T., Brock-Utne, J.G., Gaffin, S.L., Wells, M.T.B., and Blake, G.T.W.,** Strenuous exercise causes endotoxemia, *J. Appl. Physiol.,* 65, 106, 1988.
40. **Israel, S., buhl, B., Krause, M., and Neumann, G.,** Die konzentration der immunoglobuline A, G and M im serum bei trainierten und untrainerten sowie nach verschiedenen sportlicken ausdauerleistungen, *Medizin and Sport,* 22, 225, 1982.

41. **Poortmans, J.R., and Haralambie, G.,** Biochemical changes in a 100 km run: proteins in serum and urine, *Eur. J. Appl. Physiol.,* 40, 245, 1979.
42. **Muns, G., Leisen, H., Reidel, H., and Bergmann, K.-Ch.,** Einfluss von langstreckenlauf auf den IgA-gehalt in nasensekret und speichel, *Dtsch. Z. fur Sportmedzin,* 40, 63, 1990.
43. **Tomasi, T.B., Trudeau, F.B., Czerwinski, D., and Erredge, S.,** Immune parameters in athletes before and after strenuous exercise, *J. Clin. Immunol.,* 2(3), 173, 1982.
44. **Neiman, D.C., Tan, S.A., Lee, J.W., and Berk, L.S.,** Complement and immunoglobulin levels in athletes and sedentary controls, *Int. J. Sports Med.,* 10, 124, 1989.
45. **Poortmans, J.R.,** Serum protein determination during short exhaustive physical activity, *J. Appl. Physiol.,* 30, 190, 1970.
46. **Eberhardt, A.,** Influence of motor activity on some serologic mechanisms of non-specific immunity of the organism. II. Effect of strenuous physical effort, *Acta. Physiol. Pol.,* 22, 185, 1971.
47. **Viti, A., Muscettola, M., Paulesu, L., Bocci, V., and Almi, A.,** Effect of exercise on plasma interferon levels, *J. Appl. Physiol.,* 59, 426, 1985.
48. **Simon, H.B.,** Exercise, infection and immunity, in *Exercise in the Practice of Medicine,* 2nd ed., Fletcher, G., Ed., Futura Publishing, Mount Kisco, NY, 1988.
49. **Wells, C.L., Stern, J.R., and Hecht, L.H.,** Hematological changes following a marathon race in male and female runners, *Eur. J. Appl. Physiol.,* 48, 41, 1982.
50. **Lijnen, P., Hespel, P., Fagard, R., Lysens, R., Vanden Eynde, E., Goris, M., Goosens, W., Lissens, W., and Amery, A.,** Indicators of cell breakdown in plasma on men during and after a marathon race, *Int. J. Sports Med.,* 9, 108, 1988.
51. **Neiman, D.C., Berk, L.S., Simpson-Westerberg, M., Arabatzis, K., Younberg, W.S., Tan, S.A., Lee, J.W., and Eby, W.C.,** Effects of long endurance running on immune system parameters and lymphocyte function in experienced marathoners, *Int. J. Sports Med.,* 10, 317, 1989.
52. **Dickson, D.N., Wilkinson, R.L., and Noakes, T.D.,** Effects of ultra-marathon training and racing on hematologic parameters and serum ferritin levels in well-trained athletes, *Int. J. Sports Med.,* 3, 111, 1982.
53. **Davidson, R.J.L., Robertson, J.D., Galea, G., and Maughan, R.J.,** Hematological changes associated with marathon running, *Int. J. Sports Med.,* 8, 19, 1987.
54. **Cannon, J.G., Evans, W.J., Hughes, V.A., Meredith, C.N., and Dinarello, C.A.,** Physiological mechanisms contributing to increased interleukin-1 secretion, *J. Appl. Physiol.,* 61, 1869, 1986.
55. **Simon, H.B.,** The immunology of exercise: a brief review, *JAMA,* 252(19), 2735, 1984.
56. **Nash, H.L.,** Can exercise make us immune to disease? *Phys. Sportsmed.,* 14(3), 250, 1986.
57. **MacKinnon, L.T. and Tomasi, T.B.,** Immunology of exercise, *Ann. Sports Med.,* 3(1), 1, 1986.
58. **Shephard, R.J., Verde, T.J., Thomas, S.G., and Shek, P.,** Physical activity and the immune system, *Can. J. Sport Sci.,* 16(3), 169, 1991.
59. **Levi, F.A., Canon, C., Touitou, Y., Reinberg, A., and Mathe, G.,** Seasonal modulation of the circadian time structure of circulating T and natural killer lymphocyte subsets from healthy subjects, *J. Clin. Invest.,* 81, 407, 1988.
60. **Keller, R.H. and Calvanico, N.J.,** Suppressor macromolecules, *CRC Crit. Rev. Immunol.,* 5, 149, 1982.
61. **Sabiston, B.H., Myles, W.S., and Radomski, M.W.,** Stress-induced changes in the immune system during prolonged physical work, Defence and Civil Institute of Environmental Medicine, Downsview, Ontario, Canada, unpublished data.
62. **Richter, E.A., Kiens, B., Raben, A., Tvede, N., and Pedersen, B.K.,** Immune parameters in male athletes after a lacto-ovo vegetarian diet and a mixed Western diet, *Med. Sci. Sports Exercise,* 23, 517, 1991.

Chapter 7

LONG-TERM EXERCISE AND IMMUNE FUNCTIONS

David Keast and Alan R. Morton

TABLE OF CONTENTS

I. INTRODUCTION

It is now quite clear that in order to increase athletic performance, there are two distinct training requirements: training to refine skills and training to improve the cardiorespiratory endurance energy systems and the physical and physiological capacities required for the particular sport. In order to achieve these improvements, athletes have to enter into long-term training programs. The requirements of these programs can vary from several consecutive years of training to macro- and micro-training cycles. It is well established that training programs must stress the importance of the athlete in order to provide stimuli for the adaptation necessary for improved performance.[1] It is also a training process requirement that the athlete is continuously exposed to increasing workloads to induce maximal and enduring increases in the capacity to perform. This has been termed overload training.[2,3] However, large and unscheduled increases in training workload have to be avoided.[1,3] A rest component, essential for the maintenance of continued development of athletic fitness, is slowly being accepted. Because fatigue is a natural consequence of training, a recovery period is then required before the athlete can proceed to another training bout. However, it has only been recognized recently that during the rest period, homeostatic adaptations to the new higher level of exercise stress occur. If inadequate rest and/or too great an exercise stress has been applied over the training period, then the athlete may reach a state of failing adaptation or overreaching, which is characterized in the first instance by more serious fatigue and nonrecovery from the training sessions within the expected times.[2,3] Should this type of training be continued, then there is an increasing chance that the athlete will extend the overreaching into a more advanced phase of chronic fatigue, where there will be a serious deterioration of performance, often accompanied by increased susceptibility to injury and infectious disease. If left uncontrolled, the athlete can develop what is now being recognized as an important chronic clinical condition termed the overtraining syndrome.[3] The development and recognition of these various stages in the training process has led to some confusion of terms to describe the training process. This has recently been clarified[3] and allows a spectrum of training to be proposed. The transition from one stage to another is through ill-defined zones where some characteristics of the two distinct stages exist concurrently (Figure 1).

Improvements in an athlete's ability to tolerate and adapt to training stress are functions of the intensity, the duration, and the frequency of the stressors applied through the training program.[1-8] Part of the adaptation process is the acceptance by the body of a particular level of stress into its normal homeostatic mechanisms. Following this adaptation, the athlete is then capable of doing more work for an equivalent homeostatic displacement.[1,7,9] This so called supercompensation, which is considered to occur mainly over rest periods, is naturally accompanied by fatigue to give a "fatigue valley"[5] from which the athlete is not allowed to fully recover before the next training stress

Overload training | Too heavy an overload schedule or too large an increase in work | Gross overload ▶

Recovery time:-
Adequate ▲ Inadequate ▲ grossly inadequate ▲ Requires weeks/months ▲ ▶

Increasing state | of fatigue ▶

The Training | Continuum ▶

Increasing symptoms of homeostatic imbalance. ▶

Untrained | Balanced Training | Overreached state | Overtrained state | Overtraining Syndrome

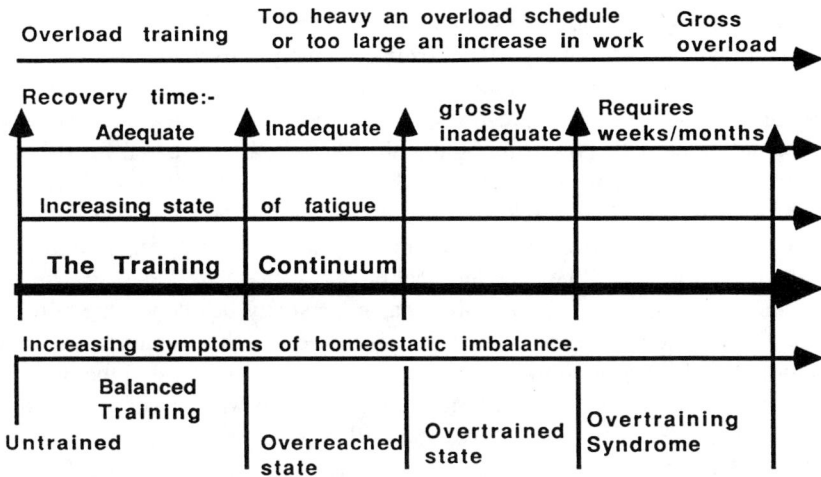

FIGURE 1. The training continuum and its properties.

is applied. This process applied sensibly leads to the development of the highly trained and often elite athlete. Probably the best known example of fatigue-induced supercompensation is that of the storage of glycogen.[10] Supercompensation can also be seen in the concentration of enzymes and in anaerobic power.[11,12] After exercise, these processes often take 2 to 3 d to occur and it has been demonstrated that it is best achieved in periods of reduced training in running[13] and swimming,[14] and in arm strength and power sports.[15] There is no reason to doubt that the adaptive processes of training may also be reflected in other systems of the body not immediately associated with sports performance. Surkina[16] has stated that the immune system is subjected to the effects of both the physical and the emotional requirements of the training process, and plays an essential role in maintaining the body's health and homeostasis. However, Surkina[16] also stressed that excessive workloads could displace the homeostatic mechanisms of the immune system such that athletes become increasingly susceptible to opportunistic infections.

Relatively recently, there has been a series of observations on the metabolism of the immune system that is likely to have far reaching effects on the association of immunity and sports training. The accepted dogma of immune reactivity has been that the cells of the immune system are, for the most part, in a resting state, with cells exhibiting an inordinately long G_0 phase of the cell cycle, awaiting antigenic stimulation to be activated both immunologically and metabolically. This activity involves antigen processing, cell interactions, population expansions, and the production of a large series of communication molecules which are essential to the final development of specific immunity, whether it be cell mediated or humoral.[17] It was assumed, therefore, that the resting cells would be in a low metabolic state and, therefore, uninteresting, and early metabolic studies tended to support this conjecture.[18] However, Ardawi and Newsholme[19] showed that the so called "resting lymphocyte" was metabolically extremely active and that these cells had an absolute requirement for glutamine,[20] the requirement for which is rapidly activated *in vitro,* in response to mitogenic challenge.[21] Subsequently, Newsholme et al.[22] showed that glutamine was equally essential for the metabolism of macrophages. Recently, Griffiths and Keast[23] have shown that both T-cells and B-cells require glutamine to generate their respective responses *in vitro* to mitogens. Furthermore, macrophages are unable to synthesize interleukin-1, the first interleukin of the interleukin cascade, in the absence of glutamine.[24] Newsholme has extensively developed the concept that the essential external source of glutamine for the immune system is muscle.[18,25] He has gone so far as to suggest that the muscles and the immune system should be considered as an integrated group with respect to metabolism.[25] Parry-Billings et al.[26] have shown that the level of glutamine in the blood does not have to approach that of the Michaelis Constant [K_m] for glutaminase, the first crucial enzyme associated with glutamine metabolism, before immunological responsiveness can be affected. It has also been shown recently that while blood glutamine concentrations rise significantly after an acute set of exercise in the well-trained athlete, the levels of glutamine in overtrained athletes are significantly reduced and remain so for at least 6 weeks of a recovery period.[27] Parry-Billings et al.[27] have suggested that serum-glutamine status may be a good predictor of overtraining.

Understanding the effects of long-term training programs on the immune system, therefore, is important as on the one hand there is the opportunity in training to fine tune immunity to enhance resistance to infection, while on the other, overtraining may lead to increased susceptibility to infectious and other disease states. One of the problems, to date, has been the almost complete lack of regard for the various types and amounts of exercise stress applied to subjects in the studies designed to investigate the immunomodulation that may be occurring as the result of exercise.[28] This is a problem that has to be addressed in future studies in this area, if any meaningful coordination of results is to be expected.

II. LONG-TERM TRAINING AND IMMUNE ENHANCEMENT

There are now several reports by athletes that moderate training programs appear to enhance their immunity.[29–36] It is beyond dispute that one of the main functions of the immune system is to maintain the body's health and to control infectious disease.[17] Surkina[16] suggested that the immune system also plays an important role in homeostasis and that both the physical and the emotional stresses of sports performance subjects the immune system to training effects which enhance immunity. This concept had support from the work of Ivanova and Talko,[37] which they interpreted to illustrate that exercise was capable of disrupting immunological homeostasis by increasing base line values of a number of important features of the immune repertoire. They also considered that these disruptions in immunological parameters provided the stimuli for immunological compensation and supercompensation during recovery periods. However, these improvements were only seen within defined limits and when exercise workloads became excessive, the athletes became more susceptible to opportunistic infections.[37] There is also evidence that judicial training programs can enhance nonspecific and innate components of the immune system. Several studies have shown that the numbers of circulating monocytes increase and that under moderate training schedules, the number of insulin receptors on them also increases.[38-43] While this suggests that the cells have greatly increased their potential for energy metabolism to occur in response to such stimuli as phagocytosis and antigen processing, there has been some evidence that the affinity binding for insulin to the receptors may be bidirectional.[44] Thus, moderate exercise induced enhanced binding while exhaustive exercise could induce decreased binding efficiency of insulin to the receptors. In well-trained athletes, the ability of neutrophils to synthesize antimicrobially active molecules, such as reactive oxygen, hydrogen peroxide, and perchlorate, appears to be enhanced on demand even though there may be some general reduction in their total capacity to synthesize these immunologically important molecules.[35]

It also appears that in highly trained racing cyclists, the number of natural killer (NK) cells circulating in the peripheral blood is significantly higher than that in untrained individuals.[45] There have also been reports that the acute response to exercise of well trained individuals leads to increased activity of NK cells in peripheral circulation.[46-48] However, it has also been reported that the number of NK cells in circulation drops following acute exercise in the well-trained athlete, but recovers within 24 h.[49] Animal experiments have suggested that long-term training using daily treadmill protocols enhances the cytolytic activity for tumor cells of splenic natural killer cells *in vitro*.[50] However, if these animals were given an acute exhaustive bout of exercise superimposed onto their training program, then the splenic capacity of natural killer cell tumor cytotoxicity was reduced. Significant increases in the levels of splenic epinephrine occurred, following the acute exhaustive exercise, and may have led to the mobilization of the NK cells to the peripheral blood, thus providing a possible explanation for the reduced splenic capacity to kill tumor cells *in vitro*.[50] Other animal trials have indicated that significant immunological resistance to tumor growth can be induced by exercise training,[51] suggesting that long-term exercise has a beneficial effect on either immunological surveillance mechanisms[52] or specific antitumor activity. There has also been some evidence that NK cell activity is enhanced in elderly people who enter into long-term exercise programs.[34,53]

On the other hand, the lowering of dietary fat appears to enhance the activity of NK cells[54] and this type of change may well be important in athletes under long-term training schedules, where diet modification is playing an ever increasing role in exercise-fitness training. However, a vegetarian diet, per se, did not appear to induce any significant changes in either subpopulations of leukocytes obtained from the peripheral blood of male athletes from a variety of sports, or in their *in vitro* activity.[55]

It is quite clear from the literature that, in the past, there has been a lack of understanding as to the roles of the energetics of various training programs on the immune system.[28] This has been particularly obvious in assessing the effects of acute exercise on immunological parameters, often using *in vitro* tests. It appears that, for the most part, long-term training schedules do not prevent acute exercise responses in all the parameters measured.[28] Both intensity and duration of physical exercise influence the levels of catecholamines induced in the body.[56,57] Epinephrine, in particular, has been shown to increase the number of leukocytes in circulation, while its influence, and that of norepinephrine, on *in vitro* responses to mitogens appears to be controversial. Claims of both enhanced and suppressed activity resulting from epinephrine injections *in vivo* or additions of epinephrine or norepinephrine, to cultures of mitogen stimulated leukocytes *in vitro,* exist.[3,28,58–62] The *in vivo* consequences of higher than normal levels of the catecholamines may well be responsible for the enhanced levels of peripheral blood leukocytes seen following acute exercise.[28] However, Ivanov and Talko[37] have demonstrated that long-term training raises base-line levels of a number of immunological parameters. There is also no doubt that long-term endurance exercise, such as marathon running, can lead to elevated leukocyte levels in circulation which then remain high for at least 3 h.[63] Cameron et al.[64] explored the effects of acute exercises, designed to stress the ATP/Creatine phosphate system and the anaerobic or the aerobic energy systems, on the changes in peripheral blood leukocytes and their responses to both T- and B-cell mitogens *in vitro,* using well-trained rugby union players, hockey players, and triathletes. The results suggested that acute anaerobic exercise, in well-trained individuals, might induce the more major changes seen in both cell poopulations in peripheral circulation and their activity *in vitro.* Our more recent studies[65] suggest that it is only at or above the lactate threshold, or more usually at or above 100% $\dot{V}O_2$ max, that major population and subpopulation changes occur in the peripheral blood leukocytes. These changes explain many of the *in vitro* responses recorded and it is unlikely that these *in vitro* responses reflect the true *in vivo* situation.

Some athletes have indicated that their general immunity appears to be enhanced with moderate levels of training.[31,32] Nieman et al.[33] studied the incidence of infectious disease in 273 runners over a 2-month training period and following competitions up to a half-marathon. Their results indicated that the athletes committed to the more serious training programs reported less infectious episodes over their training period and there was no increased incidence of flu-like infections in the week immediately following the race.[33] They suggested that the training might have been beneficial to their health status and that the added acute effect of competition in a half-marathon did not result in any added risk at the time. Shouten et al.,[66] in a retrospective study, found no increased incidence of infection or duration of infection in men that could be related to their exercise patterns. There was a weak relationship which suggested that women in the study may have reacted adversely to exercise levels; however, the authors suggested that this relationship was probably not so significant as to present a clinical problem. In a study of 68 elite track and field athletes,[67] serum antibodies to Coxsackie viruses 1 through 5 were measured, and the participants were asked to subjectively assess their infection status over a winter-training period. Once evidence of past viral infections had been removed, there was no suggestion that performance was related to current antibody status. Midtvedt and Midtvedt[68] have suggested that while athletes appear to be susceptible to some infections more than others, they are also more aware of their bodies than untrained individuals and, therefore, may anticipate changes more often which may or may not be related to infection. However, there is epidemiological evidence available that suggests that even within acceptable ranges of exercise training, there is some as yet undefined relationship between intensity of the exercise and increased numbers of infections.[69,70] On the other hand, animal studies do suggest that an ongoing infection may be aggravated by exercise,[71] possibly through a rerouting of strategically important lymphocytic cells. This in itself could lead to the development of secondary, undesirable features, such as severe myocardial calcification, in the case of Coxsackie virus infection. It has also been shown that chemical prophylaxis for one infectious agent may make an individual more susceptible to a second infection, if coupled with an ongoing exercise program.[72]

III. LONG-TERM TRAINING AND HUMORAL IMMUNITY

The effects of long-term training on humoral immunity in humans has again yielded variable results. There has been no evidence in marathon runners that levels of IgM, IgG, or IgA vary from normal,[29] and marathon runners immunized with tetanus toxoid immediately following a race showed no impairment of their abilities to produce antibody.[63] Animal studies have mimicked these responses with exercised animals yielding 2.76 times the amount of antibody, directed against *Salmonella typhi,* when compared to unexercised controls.[73] Moderate long-term exercise in the form of brisk walking has been shown to significantly enhance the levels of IgG, IgM, and IgA, although significant changes in peripheral blood leukocytes were not seen.[74] On the other hand, salivary levels of IgA in cross country skiers has been shown to be reduced immediately after a race.[75] It was suggested that the breathing of the cold air was responsible for the recorded reduction in salivary IgA. In these studies, there was little attempt at relating the changes in immunoglobulin levels to that of specific antibody. This is of particular importance with respect to salivary immunoglobulins, as it is known that much of the IgA secreted into the saliva appears to be unrelated to specific antibody and may result from nonspecific mitogen stimulation induced by the bacterial polysaccharides that abound in the oral cavity.[76]

Animal studies have also indicated that the primary response to antigen is not influenced by long-term exercise.[77,78] Earlier studies suggested that, while primary responses were not influenced by exercise training, secondary humoral responses could be enhanced.[79] At this time, there is no clear evidence that humoral immunity is affected significantly by moderate long term exercise, although some experimentation suggests that secondary immune responses may be enhanced. There is room for more definitive research in this area of sports immunology.

A. HERD IMMUNITY

One confounding aspect of studies on susceptibility to infection is associated with herd immunity and spread of infection through closely grouped members of a community. There are well documented examples of the spread of disease through sports people and their immediate contacts which represent classical examples of herd immunity.[80-86] In several instances, the infections have been shown to be more severe in the athletes than in closely associated members of the community.[81,82] It has been suggested that in these cases the increased susceptibility was as a direct result of the training programs.

IV. LONG-TERM TRAINING AND ASTHMATICS

Asthma is one of the most common respiratory diseases, with general prevalence estimates ranging from approximately 5% of the population in the U.S. and the U.K., to approximately 10% or higher in Australia and New Zealand.[87] It is a long established fact that classical asthmatics (atopics)[17] often take to sport to increase their lung capacity which has been compromised by their asthmatic condition. In some athletes, exercise induces an asthmatic attack which does not appear to be related to the immunological sensitivities associated with the classical asthmatic.[17,88] The relationship of asthma to exercise can be described, therefore, as paradoxical. Most asthmatics will experience a transient increase in airway resistance following a bout of moderate to vigorous exercise; this is referred to as exercise-induced bronchospasm (EIB) or exercise-induced asthma (EIA). Conversely, current opinion considers regular exercise to be an integral component of the total management of asthma. Asthma is believed to be an inflammatory condition, the consequence of the release of potent pharmacological mediators.[89] Recent information suggests that some exercise-induced asthmatics may possess neutrophils which are triggered to release mediators in response to osmotic changes. These changes affect mast cells and lead to the release of histamine and other vasoactive substances which play a crucial role in an ensuing bout of "exercise-induced" asthma.[90] The final outcome of the asthmatic attack is airflow limitation principally caused by contraction of airway smooth muscle compounded by mucosal oedema and impaired mucociliary function.

Despite the early recognition of the association between exercise and asthma and extensive research into EIA during the last 40 years, no mechanism which satisfactorily explains its occurrence has been proposed and received general acceptance. The inhibition of EIA after administration of medication, which effectively inhibits the release of mast cell mediators of asthma, suggests that the mast cell plays a pivotal role in the induction of the airway obstruction seen in EIA.[91-94] However, the mechanism by which exercise precipitates the release of the reactive mediators from the mast cells and/or epithelial cells has not been elucidated. Early work indicated that there was no relationship between levels of IgE in subjects and the intensity of EIA experienced.[95,96] More recently, it has been shown that activation of the classical pathway of complement and increased synthesis of both C3a and C4a anaphylatoxins may play a role in EIA.[97] These observations, along with those suggesting that exercise-induced asthmatics may or may not have a propensity to release neutrophil mediators of mast cell histamine release,[90,98] continue to add to the complex aetiology of EIA.

Several wide-ranging pharmacological therapies, including beta-adrenergic stimulants, methylxanthines, anti-cholinergics, alpha-adrenergic antagonists, and corticosteroids have been studied to determine their effects on EIA.[99-101] In general, beta-adrenergic stimulants have proved efficacious in inhibiting the EIA response.[93] Orally administered beta-sympathomimetic drugs have also been studied with contrasting reports on their success or otherwise in the control of EIA. Cholinergic blockade of EIA was found to have little effect in preventing increased airway resistance following exercise in asthmatic patients.[102] As a result of these types of studies, a number of nonimmunological initiating stimuli of EIA have been postulated and rejected, including metabolic acidosis, hypoxemia, hypocapnia from hyperventilation, abnormal catecholamine metabolism and other autonomic nervous system abnormalities, release of bradykinin during sweating, fluid leaking from pulmonary capillaries, and exercise hypernea per se.

We believe the best current hypothesis suggests that EIA is caused by the release of some broncho-constrictive substance(s) (i.e., classical pharmacological bronchoconstrictors or some as yet undefined substances from unexpected sources such as the neutrophils or monocytes), probably in response to the changes in osmolarity of the periciliary fluid. These changes are thought to occur as a result of the loss of fluid from the airways during the conditioning (warming and humidification) of inspired air.[103] The body attempts to modify the inspired air regardless of volume and temperature such that it will be warmed to 37°C and completely saturated with water vapor before reaching the delicate alveolar tissue. This saturation of alveolar air occurs mainly by absorbing water from the airways, which effectively become ''dry'', thus concentrating any active ions in the periciliary fluid. These ions become the mediators for the release of further broncho-active mediators which may include histamine, leukotrienes, prostaglandins, etc. These substances then act directly on smooth muscles, stimulate lung irritant receptors, which in turn causes bronchoconstriction via vagal influences and/or induces an inflammatory reaction via constituents such as neutrophil chemotactic factor. These types of reactions usually peak within 2 to 10 min after cessation of exercise and usually reverse spontaneously. The resistance to airflow gradually returns to pre-exercise levels in 45 to 60 min.[104,105]

Another exercise response that some asthmatics (particularly children) display is termed the late or second reaction.[106] This may not develop for 3 to 4 h after the cessation of exercise and may take 3 to 9 h to peak. This late response is probably due to an inflammatory reaction initiated by mediators such as neutrophil chemotactic factor.[107] About 50% of asthmatics exhibit a refractory period after exercise. During this period, a second bout of exercise will provoke an airway response which is less than half that of the initial response.[108-110] This refractory period may last for more than 1 h but is usually lost within 2 to 4 h. This most probably results from an insufficiency of mediators following the initial mast cell degranulation and represents the time required for resynthesis and/or recruitment of fresh mast cells to the reactive sites.

The long term use of regular and frequent aerobic exercise (training) of moderate to heavy intensity has proved to provide physiological benefits and is an important component in the general management of asthma. This type of training increases cardiac output and the stroke volume of the heart, thus lowering the heart rate at rest at any given submaximal workload. This is associated with an increased oxygen diffusion capacity at the lungs and increased oxygen extraction rate for any given workload. These changes result in an increase in both physical exercise capacity, as determined by the measurement of maximal oxygen consumption ($\dot{V}O_2$ max), and the oxygen uptake ($\dot{V}O_2$) at which exercise can be undertaken, before lactic acid begins to accumulate in the blood. Thus, the ventilation required to perform at a given level of work decreases as a result of training while the maximum attainable ventilation rate is increased. All of these training-induced changes benefit the asthmatic, in particular, as it allows the performance of a given task with a smaller disturbance to the internal environment. This ensures that the aerobically trained asthmatic can cope better than the untrained asthmatic with the same degree of mild or moderate airway obstruction. Research has indicated that an increase in aerobic fitness increases the tolerance and threshold levels of asthmatics so that a higher level of provocation is required to produce the symptoms of EIA,[111-116] and that lower levels of medication are required to control asthmatic attacks.[112,117] Thus, while there may be occasions when training has to be suspended by asthmatics, there is considerable evidence that world class performances can be achieved by athletes who are susceptible to asthma.[118-121]

Asthma appears to be induced as the result of pharmacologically active compounds which can be released from host cells by a wide variety of means. Some of these, in humans, are easily shown to result from immunologically driven allergen/IgE; IgG_4 interactions between the mast cell, basophil, eos-

TABLE 1
Hormones and their Immunomodulatory Properties[129]

Hormone	Action	Target cell or reaction
Glucocorticoids	S	Antibody production, NK cell activity, cytokine production
Sex hormones	S/E	Lymphocyte transformation, mixed lymphocyte cultures
Thyroxine	E	Plaque-forming cell, T-cell activation
Prolactin	E	Macrophage activation, IL-2 modulation
Growth hormone	E	Antibody synthesis, macrophage activation, IL 2 modulation
Catecholamines	?S/E	Lymphocyte proliferation to mitogens
ACTH	S/E	Cytokine production, NK activity, antibody synthesis, macrophage activation
Somatostatin	S/E	Plaque forming cells, mitogen responses

Note: S, suppression; E, enhancement. In many cases, the action varies depending on the concentration of the hormone, the target cell, and its immune function.

inophil, and possibly the monocyte[17] while in EIA other provocators play a predominant role. Thus, while there is no doubt that exercise can, in some individuals, induce asthmatic attacks, the true role, if any, of any subtle innate or specific immunological "drivers" of these attacks has yet to be determined. Some cytokines, such as the interleukins (see later), are now being shown to have far reaching properties outside of their more traditional roles within the immune system. It is tempting to suggest that these molecules may play a role in EIA which has yet to be defined.

V. LONG-TERM TRAINING AND ENHANCEMENT OF THE NEUROENDOCRINE SYSTEM

It is well known that increased workloads can give rise to increased levels of stress hormones such as adrenalin (epinephrine), noradrenalin (norepinephrine), vasopressin, glucagon, growth hormone, adrenocorticotrophic hormone (ACTH), cortisol, and thyroid stimulating hormone (TSH) as a natural consequence of the stress response.[57,122] It has been suggested, however, that long term training leads to an adaptation to stress as workloads increase, due to an increased stability of the pituitary-adrenocortical system.[123-126] Immunocompetent cells have been shown to possess surface receptors for several of the above hormones and under certain circumstances, these cells may also be able to synthesize small amounts of some of these hormones.[127-129] Under normal levels of training, some of these hormones can stimulate the immune system.[129-131] Table 1 illustrates some of the immunomodulatory properties currently believed to exist for hormones modified by exercise.

Several of the hormones can also function through or as neurotransmitters suggesting that there is likely to be links between the "neuroendocrine" system and immunity. Some of these interactions may be subtle ones that relate to exercise-induced products of physiological and/or biochemical stress.[18,25] It will be seen later that hormones may play a more significant role in modulating the immune system when athletes become overtrained.

VI. LONG-TERM TRAINING AND THE CYTOKINES

It is now clear that while the basic functions of the immune system involve the recognition and processing of antigen, this is only a small part of the overall immune response. Once the basic mechanisms often associated with major histocompatibility complex (MHC II) restriction have become established such that a specific adaptive immunity can develop, there is the crucial need for cellular interactions on a large scale before amplification of the response can be established. Part of this network of cooperation is governed by a series of cytokines; the interleukins, interferons, tumor necrosis factor, and the prostaglandins. The impact these cytokines may have on specific immunity is by no means fully understood, nor are the factors which may control their synthesis or suppression.

A. THE INTERLEUKIN CASCADE

The cooperation between a series of interleukins, or soluble communication molecules, is now known to be essential for the development of the populations of cells and the differentiation of these cells to provide for the specific immune response. The interleukins, to some degree, function in what may be termed the interleukin cascade. The first interleukin of this cascade is interleukin 1 (IL1), which is now known to exist in two closely related forms. These have been termed IL1-α and IL1β.[132] The final biological outcome of these two forms of IL1 appears to be similar although they may have access to different cell populations. There are strong but by no means universal views at present that IL1β acts as a soluble mediator while IL1-α remains mostly cell associated.[132] It is now clear that IL1 is produced by a wide array of cells, but the most potent source appears to be the antigen presenting cell (APC), a macrophage, as it is induced to process antigen to provide the immunogen for MHC II restricted specific immune responses.[17,132] IL1 then stimulates T-lymphocytes to synthesize both the next interleukin (IL2) of the cascade, IL1 and IL2 receptors, and to upregulate the production of MHC class II antigens on the lymphocytes committed to the antigen. Further, interleukins of the cascade are then initiated, along with other lymphokines such as interferon ¥ (IFN¥) and tumor necrosis factor (TNF) (Table 2).

Long-term exercise, per se, might not be expected to give rise to increased levels of the interleukins, as these are more often than not synthesized specifically as a response to immune or mitogen challenge of macrophages and lymphocytes. However, there are some wide ranging cellular sources of several of these cytokines and also an ever increasingly wide range of properties

TABLE 2
Summary of the Main Features of the Interleukins, Interferon ¥, and Tumor Necrosis Factor

Lymphokine	Mol. wt.	Cell sources	Main target cells	Main actions
IL 1-α	33,000	Monocytes	Thymocytes	Immunoregulation and
IL 1β	(precursor)	Dendritic cells	Neutrophils	inflammatory mediator
	17,500	B cells	T- and B-cells	
IL 2	15,000	Fibroblasts	Tissue cells	
IL 2	15,000	T-cells	T-cells	Proliferation activation
		NK-cells	B-cells	
			Monocytes	
IL 3	15,000	T-cells	Stem cells	Pan specific colony stim-
			Progenitors	ulating factor
IL 4	15,000	T-cells	B-cells	Division and differentia-
				tion
IL 5	?15,000	T-cells	B-cells	Differentiation
	(153 amino		Eosinophils	
	acids)			
IL 6	20,000	T-cells	B-cells	Differentiation
		Fibroblasts	Thymocytes	
		Macrophages		
IF N ¥	40–50,000	T-cells	Lymphocytes	Immunoregulation B cell
	(dimer)	NK-cells	Monocytes	differentiation
			Tissue cells	
TNF-α	65–69,000	Macrophages		Activation
		Lymphocytes	Macrophages	Adhesion
TNF β (LT)		T-cells	Granulocytes	Cachexia
			Tissue cells	Enhanced MHC expression

associated with these communication molecules, for cells and organs outside of the immune system.[17] Several of these properties are associated with central hormone control centers and cachexic type reactions. Therefore, long-term exercise may well lead to tissue damage and the mobilization of these soluble communication factors with wide ranging effects both within and without of the immune system. Tantalizing reports along these lines exist in the literature and need to be investigated in some detail. Simon[133] reviewed the literature which indicated that exercise increased levels of pyrogen in circulation. This pyrogen was shown to be closely related, if not identical, to IL1. The IL1 appeared to increase for at least 3 h post exercise, and although it may have been associated in part with the increased temperature associated with extensive exercise, the IL 1 did not appear to function at the anterior hypothalamus as the set point of the temperature control center of the body remained unchanged. However, this conclusion may not have been correct as more recently IL 1, IL 6, and TNF have all been considered to contribute significantly to the temperature increases associated with athletic exertion. Whatever the true pyrogenic function of the IL 1 might be, the fact remains that it was induced in the apparent absence of a specific immune driver. It may well be that the exercise had induced tissue damage, which in turn had stimulated localized inflammatory reactions, part of the outcome of which was cytokine release to the blood.

This may also be the case with respect to the detection of IL6 in blood, following exercise.[134,135] IL 6, which is also known as IFNβ$_2$, is released from a variety of cells and may initiate and induce acute phase proteins, following localized tissue damage and early inflammatory reactions.[134] As well as being involved in the differentiation and replication of B-cells, it also has a wide array of properties that can lead to several disease states.[135] Relatively high levels of IL 6 have been found in athletes, particularly marathon runners, and may well be predictive of localized tissue damage for which there is currently no other non-invasive predictors. Chronic exercise has been shown to give rise to muscle tissue breakdown.[136–138]

There are varied reports on the interleukin responses of long-term trained athletes. The responses to acute exercise of well-trained cyclists suggested that, *in vitro,* there was an increase in IL 1 production concomitant with decreased IL 2 production and IL 2 receptor synthesis. However, this apparent aberration appeared to return to normal within 2 h of the exercise bout.[139] In well-conditioned middle distance runners training over some 80 to 150 km/week, although there was a significant decrease in circulating levels of IL 2 immediately after exercise, there was a significant increase in IL2 present in the peripheral blood 24 h later.[140] These changes were accompanied by characteristic subpopulation changes with respect to circulating lymphocytes, monocytes, and NK cells. Furthermore, TNF-α, which is a cytokine that has pyrogenic as well as cytolytic effects, was significantly increased 2 h after the exercise bout, but had returned to pre-exercise levels by 24 h.[140]

The role of the prostaglandins in the immune suppression, seen after exercise, has been controversial. Prostaglandins of the E series can be synthesized by macrophages.[141] While we have been unable to show any significant role for prostaglandins in the T-cell responses to mitogens *in vitro* post exercise,[64] others have.[141–144] PGE$_2$ has been shown to inhibit both B-lymphocyte proliferation and the production of B-cell proliferation factor, in *Staphylococcus aureus* stimulated cultures.[145,146] Recently, prostaglandins have been shown to suppress the activity of NK cells *in vitro* post exercise.[36] However, there is still no clear evidence that sustained changes in prostaglandin production occur in response to long-term training.

It can be seen, therefore, that there are some major changes that can occur in long-term trained athletes, in the levels of circulating lymphokines and closely related cytokines and in the *in vitro* production of these in response to mitogen stimulation. Large discrepancies still exist in the data, and no concensus can be arrived at as to the true effects, if any, on these parameters in the healthy but long-term trained athlete. Some of the *in vitro* changes in cytokine production may simply reflect changes in the subpopulations of cells that have occurred in the individual following exercise and, as such, would not reflect any intrinsic changes that might be associated with either immune enhancement or immune suppression in the host, following long term exercise.

VII. LONG-TERM TRAINING AND IMMUNE SUPPRESSION

We have seen that there is now a well established training continuum which results from the increasing level of training effort that occurs as athletes, and others, attempt to build up their cardiorespiratory endurance, strength, and skills, for top performance (Figure 1). Provided the athletes gradually increase their intensity of training and leave sufficient rest periods for the establishment of new homeostatic levels, well-balanced athletes will develop.[3] However, when insufficient recovery periods occur between training, or an acute large increase of exercise workload is undertaken in an attempt to push training adaptation to the limit, athletes can enter into an overreached state or move to a more serious condition now known as the overtraining syndrome.[2,3,28,147]

An athlete may also undertake a heavy training schedule for many months without any apparent side effects, only to develop over a few days all the symptoms of the fully blown overtraining syndrome. It has been recognized from the early 1920s that certain athletes appear to become susceptible to chronic infections which reduce performance at the time when top achievement levels are required. From these early observations, the view has developed that at some level of exercise stress, which is more likely to be associated with heavy long term training, there is compromisation of the immune system.[2,3,28,147,148] Rarely has it been accepted that along with the physical stress of training there is also neurologic stress, which is now being investigated with regard to its ability to contribute to immune modulation and, in particular, to induce immune-suppression.[129] Often in the chronic overtraining syndrome, central fatigue appears to be the crucial component for the extended incapacity to perform even at a minimal level of exercise.[3] Quite often, the symptoms of the exercise-induced overtraining syndrome closely mimic those of another baffling clinical syndrome, that of post viral or, simply, chronic fatigue syndrome.[149,150]

The first symptoms of overtraining occur as the result of a deliberate or unintentional extension of an acceptable training program, to a new level of exertion or due to inadequate recovery periods that lead to failing adaptation. As a consequence, extended tiredness and a loss of performance standards occurs, and these are usually the first physical signs that the athlete recognizes as the beginning of overtraining. Experienced athletes learn to recognize these symptoms, and by resting and allowing for a longer than normal regeneration period between bouts of exercise, they recover rapidly with no apparent long-term effects. If these symptoms are ignored, then the athlete will progress to a more serious state of overtraining which may lead eventually to the overtraining syndrome. There then appears to be a large array of symptoms which can manifest themselves in a wide range of patterns which has, to date, made a classical diagnosis of the overtraining syndrome virtually impossible (Table 3).[3]

Currently, there is evidence that some athletes in heavy training programs do become more susceptible to minor and/or chronic infections than athletes undertaking less demanding training schedules.[3,148] However, there is an apparent lack of hard data on individuals that can be defined as overreached, which provide evidence to suggest that a significant down regulation of immunity has occurred as a result of the overreaching. Much of the earlier information, which suggested that some compromisation to immunity occurs with long-term training, is based on the responses to mitogens *in vitro* following a single bout of acute exercise. We and others have shown that after exercise, the *in vitro* responses to mitogens are lower than pre-exercise levels, particularly if the exercise is exhausting and anaerobic in nature. These results along with a reduction in the T-helper lymphocyte/T-suppressor, cytotoxic lymphocyte (CD4/CD8) ratio now appear to reflect population shifts that occur, *in vivo,* with exercise and do not indicate down regulation of the immune system.[140,151–153]

If we accept that the overtraining syndrome represents the ultimate breakdown of the athlete to unsustainable overload stress, then most of the information to date concerning an apparent increased susceptibility to infection which has been interpreted to stem from down regulation of the immune system, must be developing in overreached athletes and the earlier stages of overtraining. Athletes at all levels of performance appear to be at risk of overtraining, with the more highly motivated ones probably being more prone.[154–157] Of general concern is the fact that the athlete's level of performance is not the sole determining factor, indicating that athletes from all skill levels may become seriously overtrained if they coach themselves or are trained by inexperienced coaches.[3,156–160] As stated previously, the most outstanding feature that is related to overtraining is the failure of the athlete to program sufficient regeneration time within the training program.[1–3,157,161]

Epidemiological studies have formed the main basis to suggest that overtraining leads to a higher incidence of infectious disease than would be normally expected.[3,28,148] Probably the first documented association between overtraining and increased incidence of infectious disease comes from the 1928 winter Olympics at St. Moritz.[162] Since that time, there have been additional reports that athletes can become progressively more susceptible to infection as a seasons training progresses and intensity of training remains high.[75,163–65] More recently, situations of abnormal and/or increasing psychological stress have also been implicated with increased susceptibility to infection.[129,166] It may well be that interactions between the physical training and associated mental stress required for elite performance provide the final mechanism for overtraining and down regulation of immunity. Surkina[16] clearly showed that when workloads imposed on marathon runners (running two marathons in

TABLE 3
The Major Symptoms of Overtraining

Performance related
  Decreased performance
  Increased aches and pains
  Inability to meet previous standards
    or training times
  Reduced skills/increased injuries
  Inability to correct technical
    errors
  Loss of coordination
  Reappearance of old mistakes

Physiological
  Abnormal T-wave pattern on ECG
  Reduced tolerance to loading
  Decreased muscle strength
  Decreased work capacity
  Increased difference between
    lying and standing heartrate
  Heart discomfort on slight
    exertion
  Changes in blood pressure
  Changes in heartrate at rest and
    exercise
  Increased respiration
  Decreased body fat
  Increased oxygen consumption
    at submaximal workloads
  Elevated basal metabolic
    rate
  Chronic fatigue
  Insomnia with night sweats
  Feels thirsty
  Anorexia nervosa
  Loss of appetite
  Bulima
  Reactivation of latent herpes
    infection
  Headaches
  Nausea
  Gastrointestinal disturbances
  Muscle soreness/pains
  Tendon problems
  Muscle damage
  Elevated C-reactive proteins
  Perfuse respiration

Psychological
  Feelings of depression
  General apathy
  Recovery prolonged
  Decreased self esteem
  Emotional instability
  Fear of competition
  Gives up when the going gets
    tough
  Decreased ability to narrow
    concentration
  Increased internal and external
    distractability
  Decreased capacity to process
    information

Immunological
  Increased susceptibility to and
    severity of colds/minor
    infections/allergies
  Unconfirmed glandular fever
  Swollen lymphnodes and one-day
    colds
  Wounds heal slowly
  Decreased lymphocyte numbers,
    neutrophils and eosinophils
  Reduced *in vitro* response to
    mitogens
  Amenorrhea/oligomenorrhea
  Significant variations in CD4/CD8
    lymphocyte ratio

Biochemical
  Negative nitrogen balance
  Hypothalamic dysfunction
  Flat glucose tolerance curves
  Depressed muscle glycogen
  Decreased bone mineral content
  Delayed menarche
  Decreased hemaglobin
  Decreased serum iron; ferritin
  Increased urea
  Elevated cortisol levels
  Decreased plasma glutamine
  Increased ketosteroids in urine
  Low free testosterone
  Increased serum hormone
    binding globulin
  Increased uric acid production
  Decreased glutamine levels

two days) were excessive, there was a marked increase in susceptibility to infection. There are also many athletes who have reported that they feel more prone to infection with excessive workloads.[31,32,66,167-169] We have recently reviewed these observations and others in some detail.[3]

Problems become apparent when we begin to define precisely whether or not the immune system is compromised by overreaching and/or the over-training syndrome and, if so, which components are the most compromised. Here we find that much of the data comes from *in vitro* tests on peripheral blood leukocytes immediately following the imposition of a further bout of acute exercise on the "overtrained" athlete. Often, under these conditions, there is little difference seen from that of the *in vitro* leukocyte responses of well-trained athletes.

Surkina[16] followed top Soviet athletes over a 4-month period of intense competitions and found that they suffered a significant drop in the number and function of their T-cells compared with the precompetition period. Three of the athletes then became ill. However, these observations were not borne out in other studies. The athletes came from different sports and, therefore, it is likely that their metabolic/hormonal stress levels may have been significantly different. We have shown that, in the short term, the type of exercise stress placed on the athlete may well influence the populations of cells available in peripheral circulation post exercise.[48,64,151,152] In one ski athlete of Surkina's studies, major T-cell variations were seen which were accompanied by a series of six illnesses over the ensuring 5 months. In follow up studies,[16] it was found that high intensity load training appeared to influence T-cell immunity most and, as a result, Surkina advocated monitoring long term training loads for their effects on immunity as part of the routine of training. Matvienko[170] found that athletes that became "stale" in their training program had lower than normal leukocyte counts which became lower if training was continued. Umarova[171] has shown that children may fall into a special category with respect to the effect of training on their immunity. Special care has to be taken when administering heavy training loads on children, as greater depression in immunity seems to occur in this age bracket, following training.

In animal studies, long-term training has been shown to depress the phagocytic capacity of Kupffer cells of the liver while at the same time the phagocytic capacity of lung alveolar macrophages was enhanced.[172] Physical exercise has been shown to cause neutrophils to release their lysozyme into the blood and, following prolonged exercise (10,000 meters), phorbol-stimulated chemiluminescence was decreased suggesting that the cells had lost some capacity to synthesize oxygen radicals.[173-175] These observations have been interpreted as extended exercise inducing suppression of the cells innate functional activity; however, they can also occur in association with suppression of indicators of specific immunity, such as secretory antibodies.[173]

Long-term endurance training has been shown to lead to suppression of NK-cell killing capacity *in vitro*.[62]

A. THE ROLE OF HORMONES

There is now substantial evidence that hormones play a significant role in immunoregulation and that exercise leads to significant hormonal variations.[56,129,176–178] However, most of the studies have involved the effects of acute exercise on blood hormone levels superimposed onto the general background levels of hormone of well-trained athletes. It is more difficult to find information on how long-term training leads to changes in normal homeostatic hormonal patterns. Overtraining has been associated with increased resting levels of cortisol and thyroid hormones.[179,180] These observations are by no means universal.[181,182] Although it is not clear as to the major contributor, a reduced ratio of free serum testosterone to cortisol has been suggested as a good indicator of overtraining.[183,184] However, we have found this also changes significantly with acute exercise stress.[151]

B. THE CATECHOLAMINES

It appears that the catecholamines (epinephrine and norepinephrine) can enhance and suppress immunological reactivity depending on concentration.[28] They have been shown to increase adenyl cyclase activity, thus increasing intracellular cAMP.[185] This has been found to decrease both T- and B-cell responses to mitogens.[59,60,186] If epinephrine was injected into subjects prior to blood being collected, the mitogen responses to phytohemagglutinin (PHA), concanavalin A (CON A) and poke weed mitogen (PWM) were significantly suppressed in vitro.[61] However, when added at physiological concentrations directly to leukocyte cultures, T-cell responses were not inhibited;[58] on the other hand, Ig synthesis can be enhanced in vitro.[187]

While it has been shown that adrenalin levels can be varied significantly by exercise, the outcome of which can influence the mobilization of leukocytes into circulation,[56,57] there is little or no information to date on the lasting consequences of these types of reactions in long-term overreaching and overtraining, although it has been suggested that catecholamine levels are reduced with overtraining.[188] The site of mobilization of leukocytes after adrenalin infusion or exercise is unclear. The lymphocytosis may result from increased emptying of lymph into the blood via the thoracic duct, while neutrophils were originally thought to come from the bone marrow, due simply to increased blood flow.[189] However, these ideas have proved to be controversial.[191,192] Subsequently, it was suggested that the cells were being mobilized from the peripheral marginated pool, the lungs, and the spleen, where cells were known to adhere to the walls of the smaller venules and capillaries.[61,192] Changes seen in the subsets of cells mobilized were explained by differences in basic circulation times and of their stickiness or sensitivity to adrenalin.[61,193,194] There is a need to explore changes in the populations of leukocytes bearing adhesins and the dynamics of the concentrations of adhesins in response to both exercise training and overtraining.[195–200]

C. THE GLUCOCORTICOSTEROIDS

It has been known for a considerable length of time that the immune system contains cells of varying resistance to cortisol.[17] *In vitro* mitogenic responses to PHA, CON A, and PWM can be significantly suppressed by the addition of cortisol to cultures.[60,201-206] Although, at low concentrations, cortisone has been shown to enhance Ig production in PWM stimulated cultures.[207]

In vivo cortisol is released from the adrenal cortex in reponse to adrenocorticotrophic hormone secreted from the anterior pituitary gland.[57] In low doses, corticosteroids have been shown to induce immune suppression *in vivo* while at greater than normal physiological concentrations, lethal modification to the immune system is possible.[208,209] The administration of hydrocortisone, dexamethasone, or prednisolone has been shown to significantly suppress the ability of leukocytes to respond to mitogens and by Ig production *in vitro*.[177,205,211] An apparent circadian rhythm of T-cell mitogen responses has been shown to coincide with changes in plasma cortisol, suggesting that at physiological levels, cortisol is able to influence lymphocyte metabolism significantly or lead to subpopulation changes in peripheral circulation.[212] Several workers have shown that the number of neutrophils is raised in circulation following exercise.[63,139,213,214] Moorthy and Zimmerman[214] have suggested that this is due to increases in plasma cortisol which finds some support from the work of several other groups. This indicated that corticosteroids can induce a neutrophilia.[215-217] The extent to which cortisol can be influenced by exercise is still not clearly understood, although it is clear that plasma cortisol levels rise during exercise but may not peak until some hours later.[57,151,218-223] While there have been suggestions that plasma cortisol levels may decrease at workloads less than 50% of maximal oxygen uptake and only begin to increase when oxygen uptake is greater than 60% of maximum,[219,220,224] it has been suggested that increase in plasma cortisol in response to exercise may persist for some time and contribute to some of the physiological adaptations associated with training.[56] The levels of other hormones have been shown to be modified by exercise such as insulin, aldosterone, antidiuretic hormone, and the thyroid hormones, as well as sex hormones; all of these have the potential to significantly influence immunological function.[57]

It is also becoming clear that exercise induces significant changes in the hypothalamic-pituitary-adrenal axis, which can lead to immunomodulation. The role of this more central effect to the development of overtraining needs to be fully explored. There is, as yet, a largely unexplored area which may link hormonal, metabolic, and psychic stress to the development, in some elite athletes and others, of the so-called overtraining syndrome.[3] It is well-known that Olympic athletes and other high-performing sports people are under significantly more emotional and psychic stress than recreational athletes.[3,147-150,164,225] It has also been suggested for many years that psychic stress and psychic stress combined with physical stress has immunosuppressive properties,[3,129,164,226–238] and a major component to overtraining in the elite athlete appears to be mental stress.[122,155,157,228–240] It is also clear that the chronic overtraining syndrome is characterized by anxiety, depression, chronic fatigue, loss of appetite, weight loss, decreased libido, anger, lack of self esteem, etc. (Table 3)[166,241–244] These responses, along with major changes in the endocrine and neuroendocrine system as a result of overtraining,[28,129,245] all have the potential to lead to major changes in the immune system. Many of these symptoms are similar to those seen in the chronic fatigue syndrome (post viral syndrome, Yuppie flu, etc.).[246,247] Based on a study of 100 chronic fatigue syndrome sufferers, there appeared to be evidence of impaired immune response in many cases.[248] Some of the symptoms of apparent immune suppression have been atypical lymphocytosis, or lymphopenia in peripheral blood; isolated Ig deficiencies; impaired cellular responses to mitogens *in vitro;* impaired skin delayed type hypersensitivity (DTH) — responses and decreased absolute numbers of T-lymphocytes (CD2 +); T helper/inducer (CD4 +) and T cytotoxic/suppressor (CD8 +) lymphocytes.[247] Lloyd et al.[248] have argued that excessive production of cytokines may also be implicated.

Therefore, in light of the foregoing, it is tempting to speculate that with so many common symptoms between chronic overtraining and the chronic fatigue syndrome, it should not be surprising if depressed immunity is found in many cases of chronic overtraining.[149,150]

The unanswered question now is when does overtraining (and overreaching) begin to significantly and adversely affect immune responsiveness of the individual?

As we have indicated earlier, most of the studies to date which claim to investigate overtraining by our definitions[3] must be redefined as studies of overreached athletes. Very few studies on athletes defined as suffering the overtraining syndrome have been reported to date. The results imply that there is as yet some undefined stage of chronic overtraining where immunological problems will begin to appear in an athlete. This condition is likely to appear well before the most serious outcome of prolonged excessive overload training, the overtraining syndrome. A crucial role, if any, for immune suppression in these areas of long-term training has yet to be defined.

REFERENCES

1. **Bompa, T. O.,** *Theory and Methodology of Training,* Kendall/Hunt, Dubuque, IO, 1983.
2. **Kuipers, H. and Keizer, H. A.,** Overtraining in elite athletes: review and directions for the future, *Sports Med.,* 6, 79, 1988.
3. **Fry, R. W., Morton, A. R., and Keast, D.,** Overtraining in athletes: an update, *Sports Med.,* 12, 32, 1991.
4. **Selye, H.,** *The Stress of Life,* Longmans Green, London, 1957.

5. **Counsilman, J. E.**, *The Science of Swimming,* Prentice Hall, Englewood Cliffs, NJ, 1968.
6. **Matveyev, L.**, *Fundamentals of Sports Training* (Translation of the revised ed.), Progress Publishing, USSR, 1981.
7. **Harre, D.**, *Principles of Sports Training: Introduction to the Theory and Methods of Training* (Translated from German), Sportverlag, Berlin, 1982.
8. **Bompa, T. O.**, Physiological intensity values employed to plan endurance training, *Track Technique (Summer),* 3435, 1989.
9. **Kukushkin, K. I.**, *The System of Physical Education in the USSR,* Readugi Publishing, Moscow, 1983.
10. **Astrand, P. O. and Rodhal, K.**, *Textbook of Work Physiology,* McGraw-Hill, New York, 1977.
11. **Schueler, K. P.**, Untersuchungen des Wiederherstellungsverlauf nacheiner Langzeit-daurbelastung auf dem Fahrradergometer: research on the recovery after an effort of long duration on the bicycle ergometer, *Medizin und Sport,* 21, 10, 1981.
12. **Clijsen, L. P. V. M., Linden, J., Welbergen, E., and Boer, R. W.**, Supercompensation in external power of well-trained cyclists, in *Medical and Scientific Aspects of Cycling,* Burke, E. R. and Newom, M. M., Eds., Human Kinetics, Champaign, IL, 1988.
13. **Adams, W. C.**, The effects of selective pace variations on the O_2 requirements of running a 4:37 mile, National College of Physical Education, Association for Men, 1966.
14. **Costill, D. L., Flynn, M. G., Kirwin, J. P., et al.**, Effects of repeated days of intensified training on muscle glycogen and swimming performance, *Med. Sci. Sports Exercise,* 20, 249, 1988.
15. **Costill, D. L., King, D. S., Thomas, R., and Hargreaves, M.**, Effects of reduced training on muscular power in swimmers, *Physician Sportsmed.,* 13, 94, 1985.
16. **Surkina, I. D.**, Stress and immunity among athletes, *Teoriya i Pratika Fizicheskoi Kultury,* 3, 18, 1981; Translation in *Soviet Sports Review* 17, 198, 1982.
17. **Roitt, I., Brostoff, J., and Male, D.**, *Immunology,* 2nd ed., Gower Publishing, London, 1989.
18. **Ardawi, M. S. M. and Newsholme, E. A.**, Metabolism in lymphocytes and its importance in the immune response, *Essays Biochem.,* 21, 1, 1985.
19. **Ardawi, M. S. and Newsholme, E. A.**, Maximum activities of some enzymes of glycolysis, the tricarboxcylic acid cycle and ketone-body and glutamine utilisation pathways in lymphocytes of the rat, *Biochem. J.,* 208, 743, 1982.
20. **Ardawi, M. S. and Newsholme, E. A.**, Glutamine metabolism in lymphocytes of the rat, *Biochem. J.,* 212, 835, 1983.
21. **Keast, D. and Newsholme, E. A.**, Effects of mitogens on the maximal activities of hexokinase, lactate dehydrogenase, citrate synthase and glutaminase in rat mesenteric lymphnode lymphocytes and splenocytes during the early period in culture, *Int. J. Biochem.,* 22, 133, 1989.
22. **Newsholme, P., Gordens, P., and Newsholme, E. A.**, Rates of utilization and fates of glucose, glutamine, pyruvate, fatty acids and ketone bodies by mouse macrophages, *Biochem. J.,* 292, 632, 1987.
23. **Griffiths, M. and Keast, D.**, The effect of glutamine on murine splenic leukocyte responses to T- and B-cell mitogens, *Immun. Cell Biol.,* 68, 405, 1990.
24. **Hebble, C. and Keast, D.**, Glutamine and macrophage function, *Metabolism,* in press, 1992.
25. **Newsholme, E. A.**, Psychoimmunology and cellular nutrition: an alternative hypothesis, *Biol. Psychiatry,* 27, 1, 1990.
26. **Parry-Billings, M., Evans, J., Calder, P. C., and Newsholme, E. A.**, Does glutamine contribute to immunosuppression after burns? *Lancet,* 336, 523, 1990.
27. **Parry-Billings, M., Blomstrand, E., McAndrew, N., and Newsholme, E.**, A communicational link between skeletal muscle, brain and cells of the immune system, *Int. J. Sports Med.,* (Special Suppl.) 11, 1, 1990.

28. **Keast, D., Cameron, K., and Morton, A. R.,** Exercise and the immune response, *Sports Med.,* 5, 248, 1988.
29. **Green, R. L., Kaplan, S. S., Rabin, B. S., et al.,** Immune function in marathon runners, *Ann. Allergy,* 47, 73, 1981.
30. **Nash, H. L.,** Can exercise make us immune to disease? *Physician Sports Med.,* 14, 250, 1986.
31. **Koch, C.,** Cold protection, *Triathlon Magazine,* p. 16, January 1988.
32. **Anderson, O.,** A run a day keeps the doctor away, *Runners World,* p. 54, January 1989.
33. **Nieman, D. C., Johanssen, L. M., and Lee, J. W.,** Infectious episodes in runners before and after a road race, *J. Sports Med. Phys. Fitness,* 29, 289, 1989.
34. **Fiatarone, M. A., Morley, J. E., Bloom, E. T., et al.,** The effect of exercise on natural killer cell activity in young and old subjects, *J. Gerontol.,* 44, M37, 1989.
35. **Smith, J. A., Telford, R. D., Mason, I. B., and Weidmann, M. J.,** Exercise, training and neutrophil microbial activity, *Int. J. Sports Med.,* 11, 179, 1990.
36. **Pedersen, B. K., Tvede, N., Klarlund, K., et al.,** Indomethacin *in vitro* and *in vivo* abolishes post-exercise suppression of natural killer cell activity in peripheral blood, *Int. J. Sports Med.,* 11, 127, 1990.
37. **Ivanova, N. I. and Talko, V. V.,** The effect of physical loads on the immune systems, *Teorya i Praktika Fizichesko: Kultury* 1, 24, 1981; Translation in *Soviet Sports Rev.,* 16, 208, 1981.
38. **Soman, V. R., Koivisto, V. A., Grantham, P., and Felig, P.,** Increased insulin binding to monocytes after acute exercise in normal man, *J. Clin. Endocrinol. Metab.,* 47, 216, 1978.
39. **Soman, V. R., Koivisto, V. A., Deibert, D., et al.,** Increased insulin sensitivity and insulin binding to monocytes after physical training, *N. Engl. J. Med.,* 29, 1200, 1979.
40. **Koivisto, V. A., Soman, V. R., DeFronzo, R., et al.,** Insulin binding to monocytes in trained athletes: changes in resting state after exercise, *J. Clin. Invest.,* 64, 1011, 1979.
41. **Koivisto, V. A., Soman, V. R., DeFronzo, R., and Felig, P.,** Effects of acute exercise and training on insulin binding to monocytes and insulin sensitivity *in vivo, Acta Paediatr. Scand. Suppl.,* 283, 70, 1980.
42. **Bieger, W. P., Weiss, M., Michel, G., and Weicher, H.,** Exercise induced monocytosis and modulation of monocyte function, *Int. J. Sports Med.,* 1, 30, 1980.
43. **Pedersen, O., Beck-Nielsen, H., and Heding, L.,** Increased insulin receptors after exercise in patients with insulin-dependent diabetes mellitus, *N. Engl. J. Med.,* 302, 886, 1985.
44. **Michel, G., Vocke, T., Fiehn, W., et al.,** Bidirection alteration of insulin receptor affinity by different forms of physical exercise, *Am. J. Physiol.,* 246, E153, 1984.
45. **Pedersen, B. K., Tvede, N., Hansen, F. R., et al.,** Modulation of natural killer cell activity in peripheral blood by physical exercise, *Scand. J. Immunol.,* 27, 673, 1988.
46. **Brahmi, Z., Thomas, J. E., Park, M., et al.,** The effect of acute exercise on natural killer-cell activity of trained and sedentary human subjects, *J. Clin. Immunol.,* 5, 321, 1985.
47. **Mackinnon, L. T.,** Exercise and natural killer cells: what is the relationship? *Sports Med.,* 7, 141, 1989.
48. **Nieman, D. C., Nehlsen-Cannerella, S. L., Donohue, K. M., et al.,** The effects of acute moderate exercise on leukocyte and lymphocyte sub-populations, *Med. Sci. Sports Exercise,* 23, 578, 1991.
49. **Berk, L. S., Nieman, D. C., Youngerberg, W. S., et al.,** The effect of long endurance running on naural killer cells in marathoners, *Med. Sci. Sports Exercise,* 22, 207, 1990.
50. **Simpson, J. R. and Hoffman-Goetz, L.,** Exercise stress and murine natural killer cell function, *Proc. Soc. Exp. Biol. Med.,* 195, 125, 1990.

51. **Good, R. A. and Fernandez, G.,** Enhancement of immunologic function and resistance to tumor growth in BALB/C mice by exercise, *Fed. Proc.,* 40, 1040, 1981.

52. **Keast, D.,** *Stress and Cancer,* Bammer, K. and Newberry, B.H., Eds., Hogrefe, Toronto, 1981, 71.

53. **Crist, D. M., Mackinnon, L. T., Thompson, R. F., et al.,** Physical exercise increases natural cellular-mediated tumor cytotoxicity in elderly women, *Gerontology,* 35, 66, 1989.

54. **Barone, J., Herbert, J. R., and Reddy, M. M.,** Dietary fat and natural-killer-cell activity, *Am. J. Clin. Nutr.,* 50, 861, 1989.

55. **Richter, E. A., Kiens, B., Raben, A., et al.,** Immune parameters in male athletes after a lacto-ovo vegetarian diet and a mixed Western diet, *Med. Sci. Sports Exercise,* 23, 517, 1991.

56. **Galbo, H.,** in *Hormonal and Metabolic Adaptation to Exercise,* Thieme, G., Ed., Springer-Verlag, Stuttgart, Austria, 1983.

57. **Bunt, J. C.,** Hormonal alterations during exercise, *Sports Med.,* 3, 331, 1986.

58. **Hadden, J. W., Hadden, E. M., Middleton, Jr., E., and Good, R. A.,** Lymphocyte blast formation. I. Demonstration of adrenergic receptors in human peripheral lymphocytes, *Cell. Immunol.,* 1, 583, 1970.

59. **Estes, G., Soloman, S., and Norton, W. L.,** Inhibition of lymphocyte stimulation by cyclic and non cyclic nucleotides, *J. Immunol.,* 107, 1489, 1971.

60. **Goodwin, J. S. and Webb, D. R.,** Regulation of the immune response by prostaglandins, *Clin. Immunol. Immunopathol.,* 15, 106, 1980.

61. **Crary, B., Hauser, S. L., Borysenko, M., et al.,** Epinephrine-induced changes in the distribution of lymphocyte subsets in the peripheral blood of humans, *J. Immunol.,* 131, 1178, 1983.

62. **Watson, R. R., Mariguchi, S., Jackson, J. C., et al.,** Modification of cellular immune functions in humans by endurance exercise training during beta-adrenergic blockade with atenolol or proprano, *Med. Sci. Sports Exercise,* 18, 95, 1986.

63. **Eskola, J., Ruuskanen, O., Soppi, E., et al.,** Effect of sport stress on lymphocyte transformation and antibody formation, *Clin. Exp. Immunol.,* 33, 339, 1978.

64. **Cameron, K. R., Morton, A. R., and Keast, D.,** T-cell sub-populations and polyclonal lymphocyte function in continuous and intermittent exercise, *Aust. J. Sci. Med. Sport,* 21, 15, 1989.

65. **Fry, R. W., Morton, A. R., Garcia-Webb, P., Crawford, G. P. M., and Keast, D.,** Acute anaerobic interval training and haematology, *Excel,* 1991, in press.

66. **Shouten, W. J., Verschuur, R., and Kemper, H. C.,** Physical activity and upper respiratory tract infections in a normal population of young men and women: the Amsterdam growth and health study, *Int. J. Sports Med.,* 9, 451, 1988.

67. **Roberts, J. A., Wilson, J. A., and Clements, G. B.,** Virus infections and sports performance: a prospective study, *Br. J. Sports Med.,* 22, 161, 1988.

68. **Midtvedt, T. and Midtvedt, K.,** Sport and infection, *Scand. J. Soc. Med. Suppl.,* 29, 242, 1982.

69. **Peters, E. M. and Bateman, E. D.,** Ultramarathon running and upper respiratory tract infections — an epidemiological survey, *S. Afr. Med. J.,* 64, 582, 1983.

70. **Heath, G. W., Ford, E. S., Craven, T. E., et al.,** Exercise and the incidence of upper respiratory tract infections, *Med. Sci. Sports Exercise,* 23, 152, 1991.

71. **Cabinian, A. E., Kiel, R. J., Smith, F., et al.,** Modification of exercise-aggravated coxsackievirus B3 murine myocarditis by T lymphocyte suppression in an inbred model, *J. Lab. Clin. Med.,* 115, 454, 1990.

72. **Lee, P. S. and Lau, E. Y.,** Risk of acute non-specific upper respiratory tract infections in healthy men taking dapsone-pyrimethamine for prophylaxis against malaria, *Br. Med. J.,* 26, 893, 1988.

73. **Liu, Y. G. and Wang, S. Y.,** The enhancing effect of exercise on the production of antibody to Salmonella tyhi in mice, *Immunol. Lett.,* 14, 117, 1987.

74. **Nehlsen-Cannarella, S. L., Nieman, D. C., Balk-Lamberton, A. J., et al.,** The effects of moderate exercise training on immune response, *Med. Sci. Sports Exercise,* 23, 64, 1990.
75. **Tomasi, T. B., Trudeau, F. B., Czerwinski, D., and Erredge, S.,** Immune parameters in athletes before and after strenuous exercise, *J. Clin. Immunol.,* 2, 173, 1982.
76. **Roitt, I. M. and Lehner, T.,** *Immunology of Oral Disease,* 2nd ed., Blackwell, Oxford, U.K., 1983.
77. **Carmack, M. A.,** Exercise-Induced Modifications in Immune Responsiveness in Rats, unpublished doctoral dissertation, University of Oregon, Corvallis, 1984.
78. **Cross, B. B.,** The Effect of Aerobic Conditioning on Antibody Production in BALB/C Mice, unpublished doctoral disseration, University of Maryland, College Park, 1985.
79. **Douglas, D. J.,** The effects of physical training on the immunological response in mice, *J. Sports Med. Phys. Fitness,* 14, 48, 1974.
80. **Morse, L. J., Bryan, J. A., and Murle, J. P.,** Holy Cross football team hepatitis outbreak, *J. Am. Med. Assoc.,* 219, 706, 1972.
81. **Weinstein, L.,** Poliomyelitis — a persistent problem, *N. Engl. J. Med.,* 288, 370, 1973.
82. **Baron, R. C., Hatch, M. H., Kleeman, K., and MacCormack, J. N.,** Aseptic meningitis among members of a high school football team, *J. Am. Med. Assoc.,* 248, 1724, 1982.
83. **Fox, G. N.,** Revisiting the revisited football team hepatitis outbreak, correspondence, *J. Am. Med. Assoc.,* 254, 317, 1985.
84. **Friedman, L. S., O'Brien, T. F., and Morse, L. J.,** Revisiting the Holy Cross football team outbreak (1969) by serological analysis, *J. Am. Med. Assoc.,* 254, 774, 1985.
85. **Ludlam, H. and Cookson, B.,** Scrum kidney: pyoderma caused by a nephrotogenic streptococcus pyogenes in a rugby team, *Lancet,* 9, 331, 1986.
86. **Becker, T. M., Kodsi, R., Bailey, P., et al.,** Grappling with herpes: herpes gladiatorum, *Am. J. Sports Med.,* 16, 665, 1988.
87. **Rees, J. and Price, J.,** *ABC of Asthma,* British Medical Association, London, 1989, 1.
88. **McCarthy, P.,** Wheezing or breezing through exercise-induced asthma, *Physician Sportsmed.,* 17, 125, 1989.
89. **Barnes, P. J.,** A new approach to the treatment of asthma, *N. Engl. J. Med.,* 321, 1, 1989.
90. **Moscato, G., Rampula, C., Dellabianca, A., et al.,** Increased neutrophil chemotactic activity in exercise- and "fog"—induced asthma, *Allergy,* 41, 581, 1986.
91. **Sly, R. M.,** Evaluation of disodium cromoglycate in asthmatic children, *Ann. Allergy,* 28, 299, 1970.
92. **Fitch, K. D. and Morton, A. R.,,** Sodium Cromoglycate BP in the prevention of exercise induced asthma, *Med. J. Aust.,* 2, 158, 1974.
93. **Sly, R. M.,** Beta-adrenergic drugs in the management of asthma in athletes, *J. Allergy Clin. Immunol.,* 73, 680, 1984.
94. **Konig, P., Hordvik, N. L., and Kreutz, C.,** The preventative effect and duration of action of nedocromil sodium on exercise induced asthma, *J. Allergy Clin. Immunol.,* 79, 64, 1987.
95. **Fitch, K. D., Turner, K. J., and Morton, A. R.,** The relationship between serum IgE levels and exercise induced asthma, *Ann. Allergy,* 30, 497, 1972.
96. **Morton, A. R., Turner, K. J., and Fitch, K. D.,** Protection from exercise induced asthma by pre-exercise cromolyn sodium and its relationship to serum IgE levels, *Ann. Allergy,* 31, 265, 1973.
97. **Smith, J. K., Chi, D. S., Krish, G., et al.,** Effect of exercise on complement activity, *Ann. Allergy,* 65, 304, 1990.
98. **Luric, A., Dessanges, J. F., Delautier, D., et al.,** Exercise- and allergen-induced asthma do not change the production of pap-acethier by neutrophils and platelets, *Bull. Eur. Physiopathol. Respir.,* 23, 347, 1987.

99. **Silverman, M., Konig, P., and Godfrey, S.,** The use of serial exercise tests to assess the efficacy and duration of action of drugs for asthma, *Thorax,* 28, 574, 1973.

100. **Anderson, S. D., Seale, J. P., Ferris, L., et al.,** An evaluation of pharmacotherapy for exercise-induced asthma, *J. Allergy Clin. Immunol.,* 64, 612, 1979.

101. **Anderson, S. D.,** Drugs affecting the respiratory system with particular reference to asthma, *Med. Sci. Sports Exercise,* 13, 259, 1981.

102. **Sly, R. M., Heimlich, E. M., Busser, R. J., and Strick, L.,** Exercise-induced bronchospasm: effect of adrenergic or cholinergic blockade, *J. Allergy,* 40, 93, 1967.

103. **Hahn, A., Anderson, S. D., Morton, A. R., et al.,** A re-interpretation of the effect of temperature and water content of the inspired air in exercise-induced asthma, *Am. Rev. Resp. Dis.,* 130, 575, 1984.

104. **Jones, R. S., Buston, M. H., and Wharton, M. J.,** The effect of exercise on ventilatory function in the child with asthma, *Br. J. Dis. Chest,* 56, 78, 1962.

105. **Fitch, K. D. and Morton, A. R.,** Respiratory disease, in *The Olympic Book of Sports Medicine,* Dirix, A., Knuttgen, H. G., and Tittel, K., Eds., Blackwell, Oxford, U.K., 1988, 531.

106. **Belcher, N. G., O'Hickey, S., Arm, J. P., and Lee, T. H.,** Pathogenic mechanisms of exercise induced asthma and the refractory period, *N. Engl. J. All. Proc.,* 9, 199, 1988.

107. **Lee, T. H., Nagakura, J., and Papageorgiou, N.,** Exercise-induced late asthmatic reactions with neutrophil chemotactic activity, *N. Engl. J. Med.,* 308, 1502, 1983.

108. **Schoffell, R. E., Anderson, S. D., Gillam, I., and Lindsay, D. A.,** Multiple exercise and histamine challenge in asthmatic patients, *Thorax,* 35, 164, 1980.

109. **Blythe, S. A. and Lemanska, Jr., R. F.,** Pulmonary late phase-allergic reactions, *Pediat. Pulmonol.,* 4, 173, 1988.

110. **Zawadski, D. K., Lenner, K. A., and McFadden, Jr., E. R.,** Re-examination of the late asthmatic response to exercise, *Am. Rev. Resp. Dis.,* 137, 837, 1988.

111. **Woolfe, C. R. and Suero, J. T.,** Alterations in lung mechanics and gas exchange following training in chronic obstructive lung disease, *Dis. Chest,* 55, 37, 1969.

112. **Fitch, K. D., Morton, A. R., and Blanksby, B. A.,** Effects of swimming training on children with asthma, *Arch. Dis. Child,* 51, 190, 1976.

113. **Afzelius-Frist, I., Grimby, G., and Lindholm, N.,** Physical training in patients with asthma, *Poumon. Coeur.,* 33, 33, 1977.

114. **Freeman, W., Nute, M. G., Brooks, S., and William, C.,** Responses of the asthmatic and non asthmatic athletes to prolonged treadmill running, *Br. J. Sports Med.,* 24, 183, 1990.

115. **Varray, A. L., Mercier, J. G., Terral, C. M., and Prefaut, C. G.,** Individual aerobic and high intensity training for asthmatic children in an exercise readaptation program. Is training always helpful for better adaptation to exercise? *Chest,* 99, 579, 1991.

116. **Varray, A., Mercier, J., Terral, C., and Prefaut, C.,** Effects of individualized aerobic training in re-adaptation of the asthmatic child to exercise, *Rev. Mal. Respir.,* 7, 581, 1990.

117. **Bungaard, A., Ingemann-Hansen, T., Halkjaer-Kristensen, J., et al.,** Short term physical training in bronchialasthma, *Br. J. Dis. Chest,* 77, 147, 1983.

118. **Weiler, J. M., Metzer, W. J., Donnelly, A. L., et al.,** Prevalence of bronchial hyperresponsiveness in highly trained athletes, *Chest,* 90, 23, 1986.

119. **Pierson, W. E. and Voy, R. O.,** Exercise-induced bronchspasm in the XXIII Summer Olympic Games, *N. Engl. Reg. All. Proc.,* 9, 209, 1988.

120. **Freeman, W., Nute, M. G., and Williams, C.,** The effect of endurance running training on asthmatic adults, *Br. J. Sport Med.,* 23, 115, 1989.

121. **Freeman, W., Williams, C., and Nute, M. G.,** Endurance running performance in athletes with asthma, *J. Sports Sci.,* 8, 103, 1990.

122. **Selye, H.,** *Stress in Health,* Butterworth, Boston, 1976.

115

123. **Keizer, H. A., Kuipers, H., DeHaan, J., et al.,** Multiple hormonal responses to exercise in eumenorrheic trained and untrained women, *Int. J. Sports Med.,* 8, 139, 1987.
124. **Keizer, H. A., Kuipers, H., DeHaan, J., et al.,** Effect of 3 month endurance training program on metabolic and multiple hormonal responses to exercise, *Int. J. Sports Med.,* 8, 154, 1987.
125. **Viru, A.,** Hormonal ensemble in exercise, in *Hormones in Muscular Activity,* CRC Press, Boca Raton, FL, 1985.
126. **Viru, A.,** Adaptive effect of hormones in exercise, in *Hormones in Muscular Activity,* CRC Press, Boca Raton, FL, 1985.
127. **Blalock, J. E., Harbour-McMenamin, E., and Smith, E. M.,** Peptide hormones shared by the neuroendocrine and immunologic systems, *J. Immunol.,* 135, 858s, 1985.
128. **Johnson, H. M. and Torres, B. A.,** Regulation of lymphokine production by arginine vasopressin and oxytocin: modulation of lymphocyte function by neurohypophyseal hormones, *J. Immunol.,* 135, 773s, 1985.
129. **Khansari, D. N., Murgo, A. J., and Faith, R. E.,** Effects of stress on the immune system, *Immunol. Today,* 11, 170, 1990.
130. **Gisler, R. H., Bussard, A. E., Mazie, J. C., and Hess, R.,** Hormonal regulation of the immune response. I. Induction of an immune response *in vitro* with lymphoid cells from mice exposed to systemic stress, *Cell. Immunol.,* 2, 634, 1971.
131. **Monjan, A. A. and Collector, M. I.,** Stress-induced modulation of the immune response, *Science,* 196, 307, 1977.
132. **di Giovine, F. S. and Duff, G. W.,** Interleukin 1: the first interleukin, *Immunol. Today,* 11, 13, 1990.
133. **Simon, H. B.,** The immunology of exercise, *JAMA,* 252, 2735, 1984.
134. **Kishimoto, T.,** The biology of interleukin-6, *Blood,* 74, 1, 1989.
135. **Hirano, T., Akira, S., Taga, T., and Kishimoto, T.,** Biological and clinical aspects of interleukin 6, *Immunol. Today,* 11, 443, 1990.
136. **Hikida, R. S., Staron, R. S., Hagerman, F. C., et al.,** Muscle fiber necrosis associated with human marathon runners, *J. Neurol. Sci.,* 59, 185, 1983.
137. **Friden, J.,** Muscle soreness after exercise: implications of morphological change, *Int. J. Sports Med.,* 4, 170, 1984.
138. **Hagerman, F. C., Hikida, R. S., Staron, R. S., et al.,** Muscle damage in marathon runners, *Physician Sportsmed.,* 12, 39, 1984.
139. **Lewicki, R., Tchorzewski, H., Denys, A., et al.,** Effects of physical exercise on some parameters of immunity in conditioned sportsmen, *Int. J. Sports Med.,* 8, 309, 1987.
140. **Espersen, G. T., ElbÆk, A., Ernst, E., et al.,** Effect of physical exercise on cytokines and lymphocyte subpopulations in human peripheral blood, *APMIS,* 98, 395, 1987.
141. **Gemsa, D., Leser, F. G., Deimann, W., et al.,** Suppression of T lymphocyte proliferation during lymphoma growth in mice: role of PGE_2-producing macrophages, *Immunobiology,* 161, 385, 1982.
142. **Goodwin, J. S., Messner, R., and Peake, G. L.,** Prostaglandin suppression of mitogen-stimulated lymphocytes *in vitro:* changes with mitogen dose and preincubation, *J. Clin. Invest.,* 62, 753, 1978.
143. **Gordon, D., Henderson, D. C., and Westwick, J.,** Effects of prostaglandins E_2 and I_2 on human lymphocyte transformation 144 in the presence and the absence of inhibitors of prostaglandin synthesis, *J. Pharmacol.,* 67, 17, 1979.
144. **Kappel, M., Tvedec, N., Galbo, H., et al.,** Evidence that the effect of physical exercise on NK cell activity is mediated by epineprine, *J. Appl. Physiol.,* 70, 2530, 1991.
145. **Novgrodsky, A., Rubin, A. L., and Steryl, K. H.,** Selective suppression by blastogenesis induced by different mitogens, *J. Immunol.,* 122, 1, 1979.

146. **Thompson, S. P., Jelinek, D. F., and Lipsky, P. E.,** Regulation of human B cell proliferation by prostaglandin E₂, *J. Immunol.*, 133, 2446, 1984.

147. **Jelinek, D. F., Thompson, P. A., and Lipsky, P. E.,** Regulation of human B-cell activation by prostaglandin E₂: suppression of the generation of immunoglobulin-secreting cells, *J. Clin. Invest.*, 75, 1339, 1985.

148. **Fitzgerald, L.,** Exercise and the immune system, *Immunol. Today,* 9, 337, 1988.

149. **Fry, R. W., Morton, A. R., and Keast, D.,** The symptoms of and contributing factors to overtraining and their similarities to the chronic fatigue syndrome. I. Overtraining, *N. Z. J. Sports Med.,* 1991, in press.

150. **Fry, R. W., Morton, A. R., and Keast, D.,** The symptoms of and contributing factors to overtraining and their similarities to the chronic fatigue syndrome. II. Fatigue syndrome, *N. Z. J. Sports Med.,* 1991, in press.

151. **Fry, R. W., Morton, A. R., Garcia-Webb, P., and Keast, D.,** Monitoring exercise stress by changes in metabolic and hormonal responses over a 24 hour period, *Eur. J. Appl. Physiol.,* 1991, in press.

152. **Fry, R. W., Morton, A. R., Garcia-Webb, P., Crawford, G. P. M., and Keast, D.,** The *in vitro* leucocyte responses to acute exercise, what do they mean? submitted for publication, 1991.

153. **Gaudeiri, S., Fry, R. W., Morton, A. R., and Keast, D.,** The effect of exercise on interleukin 1 and 2 production *in vivo* and *in vitro,* unpublished results, 1991.

154. **Karpovitch, P. V.,** *Physiology of Muscular Activity,* Saunders, Philadelphia, 1965.

155. **Costill, D. L.,** *Inside Running — Basics of Sports Physiology,* Benchmark Press, Indianapolis, IN, 1986.

156. **Town, G. P.,** *Science of Triathlon Training and Competition,* Human Kinetics, Champaign, IL, 1985.

157. **O'Brien, T. F.,** Overtraining and sports psychology, in *The Olympic Book of Sports Medicine,* Vol. 1, Dirix, A., et al., Eds., Blackwell, Cambridge, MA, 1988, 635.

158. **Falsetti, H. L.,** Overtraining in athletes — a round table, *Physician Sportsmed.,* 11, 93, 1983.

159. **Stray-Gundersen, J., Videman, T., and Snell, P. G.,** Changes in selected objective parameters during overtraining, *Med. Sci. Sports Exercise,* 18 (Abstr.), 268, 1986.

160. **Noakes, T.,** *Lore of Running,* Oxford University Press, Cape Town, 1989.

161. **Verma, S. K., Mahindroo, S. R., and Kansal, D. K.,** Effect of four weeks of hard physical training on certain physiological and morphological parameters of basketball players, *J. Sports Med.,* 18, 379, 1978.

162. **Heis, F.,** Unfallverhutung Beim Sport, Hoffman, Schorndorf, 1971, 17.

163. **Jokl, E.,** The immunological status of athletes, *J. Sports Med.,* 14, 165, 1984.

164. **Asgeirsson, G. and Bellanti, J. A.,** Exercise, immunology, and infection, *Semin. Adoles. Med.,* 3, 199, 1987.

165. **Salo, D. C.,** Does swimming make you sick? *Swimming World,* 1989, p. 59, October, 1989.

166. **Morgan, W. P., Morgan, D. R., Raglin, J. S., et al.,** Psychological monitoring of overtraining and staleness, *Brit. J. Sports Med.,* 21, 107, 1987.

167. **Douglas, D. J. and Hansen, P. G.,** Upper respiratory infections in the conditioned athlete, *Med. Sci. Sports Exercise,* 10 (Abstr.), 55, 1978.

168. **Johanssen, C.,** Individually programmed training and prevention of injuries in elite orienteers, Abstr. 23rd FIMS World Congr. Sports Med., 1986.

169. **Reilly, T. and Rothwell, J.,** Correlates of injury and illness in female distance runners, *Br. Assoc. Sports Med.,* Congress, Univeristy of Liverpool, 1987.

170. **Matvienko, L. A.,** A study of peripheral blood in track and field athletes, *Teoriyaki Praktika Fizicheskoi Kultury,* 2, 31, 1979; translation in *Soviet Sports Rev.,* 16, 50, 1981.

171. **Umarova, L. S.,** The state of natural immunity in athletes of different ages, *Teoriyaki Praktika Fizicheskoi Kultury,* 26, 8, 1981; translation in *Soviet Sports Rev.,* 17, 104, 1982.

172. **Maianski, D. N. and Voronina, N. P.,** Changes of macrophage function after graded physical loading, *Patol. Fiziol. Eksp.*, 3, 56, 1989.
173. **Petrova, I. V., Kuzmin, S. N., Kurshakova, T. S., et al.,** Neutrophil phagocytic activity and the humoral factors of general and local immunity under intensive physical loading, *Zhurnal. Mikrobiologii. Epidemiologii. i Immunobiologii.*, 12, 53, 1983.
174. **Papa, S., Vitale, M., Mazzotti, G., et al.,** Impaired lymphocyte stimulation induced by long term training, *Immunol. Lett.*, 22, 29, 1989.
175. **Kokot, K., Schaefer, R. M., Teschner, M., et al.,** Activation of leucocytes during prolonged physical exercise, *Adv. Exp. Med. Biol.*, 240, 57, 1988.
176. **Fauci, A. S.,** Mechanisms of corticosteroids on lymphocyte subpopulations. I. Redistribution of circulating T- and B-lymphocytes to the bone marrow, *Immunology*, 28, 669, 1975.
177. **Fauci, A. S.,** Mechanisms of corticosteroids on lymphocyte subpopulations. II. Differential effect of *in vivo* hydrocortisone, prednisone and dexamethasone on *in vitro* expression of lymphocyte function, *Clin. Exp. Immunol.*, 224, 54, 1976.
178. **Male, D., Champion, B., and Cooke, A.,** *Advanced Immunology*, Gower, London, 1987.
179. **Carli, G., Martelli, G., Viti, A., et al.,** Modulation of hormone levels in male swimmers during training, *Biomechanics and Medicine in Swimming; International Series on Sports Sciences*, 14, 33, 1983.
180. **Barron, J. L., Noakes, T. D., Levy, W., et al.,** Hypothalamic dysfunction in overtrained athletes, *J. Clin. Endocrinol. Metab.*, 60, 803, 1985.
181. **Wishnitzer, R., Berribi, A., Hurwitz, N., et al.,** Decreased cellularity and hemosiderin of the bone marrow in healthy overtrained competitive distance runners, *Physician Sportsmed.*, 14, 86, 1986.
182. **Budgett, R., Koutedakis, Y., Walker, R., et al.,** The overtraining syndrome/staleness, *Proc. IOC Conf.*, Colorado Springs, 1989.
183. **Belcastro, A. N., Dallaire, J., McKenzie, D. C., et al.,** CASS overstress study: blood monitoring, *Med. Sci. Sports Exercise*, 22, S131, 1990.
184. **Flynn, M. G., Pizza, F. X., Boone, J. B., et al.,** Indices of overtraining syndrome during a running season, *Med. Sci. Sports Exercise*, 22, 131, 1990.
185. **Strom, T. B., Lundin, A. P., and Carpenter, C. B.,** The role of cyclic nucleotides in lymphocyte activation and function, *Prog. Clin. Immunol.*, 3, 115, 1977.
186. **Watson, J.,** The involvement of cyclic nucleotide metabolism in the initiation of lymphocyte proliferation induced by mitogens, *J. Immunol.*, 117, 1656, 1976.
187. **Sherman, W. M., Costill, V. L., Fink, W. J., et al.,** Effect of a 4.2 km foot race and subsequent rest or exercise on muscle glycogen and enzymes, *J. Appl. Physiol.*, 55, 1219, 1983.
188. **Kindermann, W.,** Overtraining — an expression of faulty regulated development, Translated from *Deutsche Zeitschrift fur Sport-medizin*, 37, 238, 1986.
189. **Gader, A. M. A. and Cash, J. D.** The effect of adrenaline, noradrenaline, isoprenoline and salbutamol on the resting levels of white blood cells in man, *Scand. J. Haematol.*, 14, 5, 1975.
190. **Steel, C. M., French, E. B., and Aitchison, W. R. C.,** Studies on adrenaline-induced leucocytosis in normal man. I. The role of the spleen and the thoracic duct, *Br. J. Haematol.*, 21, 413, 1971.
191. **Mishler, J. M. and Sharp, A. A.,** Adrenaline: further discussion of its role in mobilization of neutrophils, *Scand. J. Haematol.*, 17, 78, 1976.
192. **Muir, A. L., Cruz, M., Martin, B. A., et al.,** Leukocyte kinetics in the human lung: role of exercise and catecholamines, *J. Appl. Physiol.*, 57, 711, 1984.
193. **Sprent, J.,** Circulating T and B lymphocytes in the mouse. I. Migratory properties, *Cell. Immunol.*, 7, 10, 1973.

194. **Hedfors, E., Holm, G., and Ohnell, B.,** Variations of blood lymphocytes during work studied by cell surface markers, DNA synthesis and cytotoxicity, *Clin. Exp. Immunol.,* 24, 328, 1976.
195. **Woodruff, J. G., Clarke, L. M., and Chin, Y. H.,** Specific cell adhesion mechanisms determining migration pathways of recirculating lymphocytes, *Annu. Rev. Immunol.,* 5, 291, 1987.
196. **Hamann, A., Jablonski-Westrich, D., Duijvestyn, N., et al.,** Evidence for an accessary role of LFA-1 in lymphocyte-high epithelium interaction during homing, *J. Immunol.,* 140, 693, 1988.
197. **Springer, T. A.,** Adhesion receptors of the immune system, *Nature (London),* 346, 425, 1990.
198. **Singer, K. H.,** Interactions between epithelial cells and T-lymphocytes: role of adhesion molecules, *J. Leukocyte Biol.,* 48, 367, 1990.
199. **Wardlow, A.,** Leukocyte adhesion to endothelium, *Clin. Exp. Allergy,* 20, 619, 1990.
200. **O'Rourke, A. M. and Mescher, M. F.,** T-cell receptor-activated adhesion systems, *Curr. Opin. Cell. Biol.,* 2, 888, 1990.
201. **Nowell, P. C.,** Inhibition of human leukocyte mitosis by prednisolone *in vitro, Cancer Res.,* 21, 1518, 1961.
202. **Smith, K. A., Crabtree, G. R., Kenned, S. J., and Munck, A. V.,** Glucocorticoid receptors and glucocorticoid sensitivity of mitogen stimulated and unstimulated human lymphocytes, *Nature (London),* 267, 523, 1977.
203. **Webel, M. L. and Ritts, R. E.,** The effects of corticosteroid concentrations on lymphocyte blastogenesis, *Cell. Immunol.,* 32, 287, 1977.
204. **Neifeld, J. P. and Tormey, D. C.,** Effects of steroid hormones on phytohaemagglutinin stimulated human peripheral blood lymphocytes, *Transplantation,* 27, 309, 1979.
205. **Gillis, S., Crabtree, G. R., and Smith, K. A.,** Glucocorticoid-induced inhibition of T cell growth factor production. I. The effect of mitogen-induced lymphocyte proliferation, *J. Immunol.,* 123, 1624, 1979.
206. **Gordon, D. and Nouri, A. M. E.,** Comparison of the inhibition by glucocorticosteroids and cyclosporin A of mitogen-stimulated human lymphocyte proliferation, *Clin. Exp. Immunol.,* 44, 287, 1981.
207. **Cooper, B. T., Douglas, S. A., Firth, L. A., et al.,** Erosive gastritis and gastrointestinal bleeding in a female runner, *Gastroenterology,* 92, 2019, 1987.
208. **Keast, D.,** A simple runting index for the measurement of the runting syndrome and its use in the study of the influence of the gut flora in its production, *Immunology,* 15, 237, 1968.
209. **Keast, D.,** The murine runting syndrome and neoplasia, *Immunology,* 16, 693, 1969.
210. **Fauci, A. S.,** Human B lymphocyte function: cell triggering and immunoregulation, *J. Infec. Dis.,* 145, 602, 1982.
211. **Saxon, A., Stevens, R. H., Ramer, S. J., et al.,** Glucocorticoids administered *in vivo* inhibit human suppressor T-lymphocyte function and diminish B-lymphocyte responsiveness in *in vivo* immunoglobulin synthesis, *J. Clin. Invest.,* 61, 922, 1978.
212. **Tavadia, H. B., Fleming, K. A., Hume, P. D., and Simpson, H. W.,** Circadian rhythmicity of human plasma cortisol and PHA-induced lymphocyte transformation, *Clin. Exp. Immunol.,* 22, 190, 1975.
213. **De Lanne, R., Barnes, J. R., and Broucher, L.,** Haematological changes during muscular activity and recovery, *J. Appl. Physiol.,* 15, 31, 1960.
214. **Moorthy, A. V. and Zimmerman, W.,** Human leucocyte response to an endurance race, *Eur. J. Appl. Physiol.,* 38, 271, 1984.
215. **Bishop, C. R. and Athens, J. W.,** Leukokinetic studies. XIII. A non steady state kinetic evaluation of the mechanism of cortisone-induced granulocytosis, *J. Clin. Invest.,* 47, 249, 1968.
216. **Cream, J. J.,** Prednisolone-induced granulocytosis, *Br. J. Haematol.,* 15, 259, 1968.

217. **Dale, D. C., Fauci, A. S., Guerry, I. V. D., and Wolff, S. M.,** Comparison of agents producing a Neurophilic leucocytosis in man: hydrocortisone, prednisone, endotoxin and eitocholanolone, *J. Clin. Invest.,* 56, 808, 1975.

218. **Sutton, J., Young, J. D., Lazarus, L., et al.,** The hormonal response to physical exercise, *Aust. Ann. Med.,* 18, 84, 1969.

219. **Davies, C. T. M. and Few, J. D.,** Effects of exercise on adrenocorticoid function, *J. Appl. Physiol.,* 35, 877, 1973.

220. **Few, J. D.,** Effect of exercise on the secretion and metabolism of cortisol in man, *J. Endocrinol.,* 2, 342, 1974.

221. **Desspris, A., Kuoppasalmi, K., and Aldercreutz, H.,** Plasma cortisol, testosterone, androstenedione and luteinizing hormone in a non competitive marathon run, *J. Steroid Biochem.,* 7, 33, 1976.

222. **Gawel, M. J., Park, D. M., Alaghband-Zadeh, J., et al.,** Exercise and hormonal secretion, *Postgrad. Med. J.,* 55, 373, 1979.

223. **Kuoppasalmi, K., Naveri, H., Harkonen, M., et al.,** Plasma cortisol, androstenedione, testosterone and luteinizing hormone in running exercise of different intensities, *Scand. J. Clin. Lab. Invest.,* 40, 403, 1980.

224. **Cornil, A., DeCoster, A., Copinski, G., and Franckson, J. R. M.,** The effect of muscular exercise on the plasma cortisol level in man, *Acta Endocrinol.,* 48, 163, 1965.

225. **Simon, H. B.,** The immunology of exercise, *JAMA,* 292, 2735, 1984.

226. **Spitz, R.A.,** Hospitalism, *Psychoanal. Study Child,* 1, 53, 1945.

227. **Spitz, R. A.,** Anaclitic depression, *Psychoanal. Study Child,* 2, 313, 1946.

228. **Solomon, G. F., Amkrant, A. A., and Kasper, P.,** Immunity, emotions and stress, *Ann. Clin. Res.,* 6, 313, 1974.

229. **Bartrop, R. W., Lockhurst, E., Lazarus, L., et al.,** Depressed lymphocyte function after bereavement, *Lancet,* 1, 834, 1977.

230. **Rogers, M. P., Dubey, D., and Reich, P.,** The influence of the psyche and the brain on immunity and disease susceptibility: a critical review, *Psychosom. Med.,* 41, 147, 1979.

231. **Fauman, F. A.,** The central nervous system and the immune system, *Biol. Psychiatry,* 17, 1459, 1982.

232. **Borysenko, M. and Borysenko, J.,** Stress, behavior and immunity: animal models and mediating mechanisms, *Gen. Hosp. Psychiatry,* 4, 69, 1982.

233. **Lake, S. E.,** Stress adaptation and immunity: studies in humans, *Gen. Hosp. Psychiatry,* 4, 49, 1982.

234. **Jemmott, J. B., III, Borysenko, J. Z., Borysenko, M., et al.,** Academic stress, power motivation and decrease in salivary immunoglobulin A secretion rate, *Lancet,* 1, 1400, 1983.

235. **Schleifer, S. J., Keller, S. E., Camerino, M., et al.,** Suppression of lymphocyte stimulation following bereavement, *JAMA,* 250, 377, 1983.

236. **Jemmott, J. B. and Magloire, K.,** Academic stress, social support and secretory immunoglobulin A, *J. Pers. Soc. Psychol.,* 55, 803, 1988.

237. **Kiecolt-Glaser, J. K. and Glasor, R.,** Psychological influences on immunity-implications for AIDS, *Am. Psychol.,* 43, 892, 1988.

238. **Kerezty, A.,** Overtraining, in *Encyclopedia of Sport Sciences and Medicine,* Larson, L. A., Ed., Macmillan, New York, 1971, 218.

239. **Nideffer, R. M.,** Psychological factors associated with overtraining, Second Elite Coaches Seminar, Australian Inst. Sport, 1988.

240. **O'Conner, P. J. and Morgan, W. P.,** Athletic performance following rapid transversal, of multiple time zones, *Sports Med.,* 10, 20, 1990.

241. **Feigley, D. A.,** Psychological burn out in high level athletes, *Physician Sportsmed.,* 12, 109, 1984.

242. **Morgan, W. P.,** Selected psychological factors limiting performance: a mental health model, in *Units of Human Performance,* Clark, D. H. and Eckert, H. M., Eds., Human Kinetics, Champaign, IL, 1985.

243. **Miller, T. W., Vaughn, M. P., and Miller, J. M.,** Clinial issues and treatment strategies in stress-orientated athletes, *Sports Med.,* 9, 370, 1990.

244. **Raglin, J. S.,** Exercise and mental health beneficial and detrimental effects, *Sports Med.,* 9, 323, 1990.

245. **Adner, M. M.,** Haematology, in *Sports Medicine,* Strauss, R. H., Ed., Saunders, Philadelphia, 1984, 120.

246. **Holmes, G. P., Kaplan, J. E., and Gantz, N. M.,** Chronic fatigue syndrome: a working case definition, *Ann. Intern. Med.,* 108, 387, 1988.

247. **Gin, W., Christiansen, F. T., and Peter, J. B.,** Immune function and the chronic fatigue syndrome, *Med. J. Aust.,* 151, 117, 1989.

248. **Lloyd, A. R., Wakefield, D., Boughton, C. R., and Dwyer, J. M.,** Immunological abnormalities in the chronic fatigue syndrome, *Med. J. Aust.,* 151, 122, 1989.

Chapter 8

EXERCISE AND INFECTION

David C. Nieman and Sandra L. Nehlsen-Cannarella

TABLE OF CONTENTS

I. INFECTION IN ATHLETES

Several types of infectious diseases affect athletes, often because they perform in an environment in which certain pathogenic microorganisms are particularly widespread, or, due to the type of sport, abrasions or other tissue injuries are more likely.[1,2] Athletes may be at increased risk for various infections because of cross-infection from other athletes with whom they are in close contact, and potential immunosuppression from both the psychosocial stress and direct physiological effects associated with overtraining and competitive athletic events. In addition, exposure to alien environmental pathogens during foreign travel may result in infection due to lack of specific immunity.[3] We have previously reviewed information on the athlete's risk of acquiring various infections (e.g., impetigo, erysipelas, herpes simplex, tinea pedis, hepatitis B, infectious mononucleosis, and myalgic encephalomyelitis).[4]

In this chapter, emphasis will be placed on the relationship between varying levels of exercise and respiratory tract infections. Much attention has recently been focused on stress, both physical and psychological, as a potential modulating factor in immune function and status, and respiratory tract infections.[4-7] There is a common belief among the general and athletic populations alike that regular exercise training decreases the risk of acquiring a cold or flu, while severe exertion may increase risk. The Center for Disease Control has estimated that the 429 million colds and flus occurring annually in the U.S. result in $2.5 billion in lost school and work days, and medical costs.[8,9] Understanding the relationship between exercise and respiratory tract infections has potential public health implications, and for the athlete, may mean the difference between being able to compete or missing the event due to illness.

II. "J"-SHAPED MODEL RELATIONSHIP BETWEEN EXERCISE AND RESPIRATORY TRACT INFECTION

We have previously proposed that the relationship between exercise and respiratory tract infection may be modeled in the form of a "J" curve[4] (Figure 1). This model suggests that while the risk of respiratory tract infection may decrease below that of a sedentary individual when one engages in moderate exercise training, risk may rise above average during periods of excessive amounts of exercise. The evidence for and against this model will be reviewed starting with the effect of unusually heavy exertion.

A. HEAVY EXERTION AND INFECTION

Many athletes feel that while their regular training programs promote resistance to respiratory tract infections,[10] the actual competitive event increases their risk. Nieman et al.[11] administered a questionnaire to ten experienced marathon runners; nine out of ten felt that their training program during the previous 5 years had helped them to reduce the number of respi-

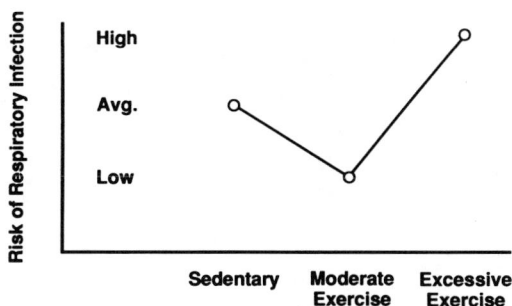

FIGURE 1. "J"-shaped model of relationship between varying amounts of exercise and risk of respiratory tract infections. This model suggests that moderate exercise may lower risk of respiratory infection while excessive amounts may increase the risk.

ratory tract infections, while one felt that the incidence was increased. However, seven of the ten marathoners felt that, following marathon race events, their risk of infection was increased, while three felt that their risk was the same as normal.

There is considerable anecdotal information from coaches and physicians of athletic teams in support of the belief that severe exertion, especially when coupled with mental stress, places them at increased risk for respiratory tract infection.[12,13] It has been reported that at the 1988 Olympic Games, some of the world's best athletes were unable to compete due to infectious illness.[12] The respiratory tract infection that afflicted U.K. Olympic gold medalist Sebastian Coe, for example, during the U.K. Olympic trials in August, so affected his running that he failed to qualify for the Olympic team.

1. Epidemiological Evidence

Several epidemiological reports suggest that athletes engaging in marathon type events and/or very heavy training are at increased risk of respiratory tract infections.[14-16] Nieman et al.[15] researched the incidence of such infections in a group of 2,311 marathon runners who varied widely in running ability and training habits. Using a pilot-tested questionnaire, runners self-reported demographic, training, and respiratory tract infection episodes and symptom data for the 2-month period (January, February) prior to, and the 1-week period immediately following the race.

An important finding was that 12.9% of Los Angeles Marathon (LAM) participants reported an infectious episode during the week following the race in comparison to only 2.2% of similarly experienced runners who had applied but did not participate (for reasons other than sickness). Controlling for important demographic and training data by using logistic regression, it was determined that the odds were 6 to 1 in favor of sickness for the LAM participants vs. the nonparticipating runners (Figure 2).

Forty percent of the runners reported at least one respiratory tract infectious episode during the 2-month winter period prior to the LAM. Controlling

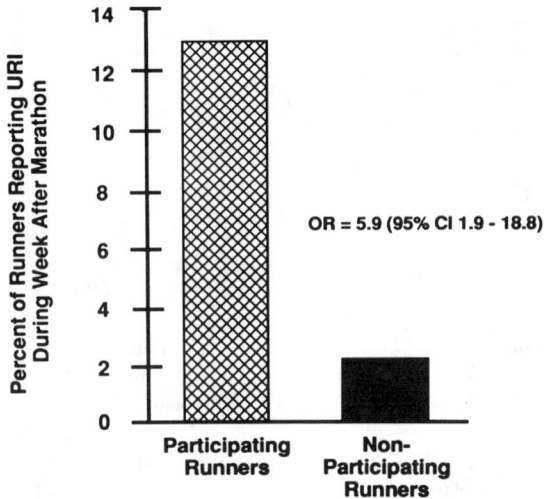

FIGURE 2.   Self-reported respiratory tract infection in 2,300 Los Angeles Marathon runners during the week following the 1987 Los Angeles Marathon. After controlling for confounding variables using logistic regression, the odds for experiencing a respiratory tract infection by runners who ran the marathon were nearly sixfold greater than for equally experienced runners who applied for the race but did not run (for reasons other than sickness). (Data from Nieman, D. C., Johanssen, I. M., Lee, J. W., and Arabatzis, K., *J. Sports Med. Phys. Fitness,* 30, 316, 1990.)

for important confounders, it was determined that runners training more than 60 mi/week (96 km/week) doubled their odds for sickness compared to those training less than 20 mi/week (32 km/week). Although the lowest odds of sickness were in the less than 20 mi/week group, the odds ratio did not increase significantly until 60 mi/week was exceeded (Figure 3). The researchers concluded that runners may experience increased risk for respiratory tract infection during heavy training or following a marathon race event.

Other epidemiological data support these findings. Peters and Bateman[16] studied the incidence of respiratory tract infections in 150 randomly selected runners who took part in a 56-km race in comparison to matched controls who did not run. Symptoms of respiratory tract infections occurred in 33.3% of runners compared with 15.3% of controls during the 2-week period following the race, and were most common in those who achieved the faster race times, (Figure 4). The most prevalent symptoms reported after the race were sore throats and nasal symptoms. Of the total number of symptoms reported by the runners, 80% lasted for longer than 3 d, suggesting an infective origin.

Linde[14] studied respiratory tract infections in a group of 44 elite orienteers and 44 nonathletes of the same age, sex, and occupational distribution during a 1-year period. The orienteers experienced significantly more infectious episodes during the year in comparison to the control group (2.5 vs. 1.7

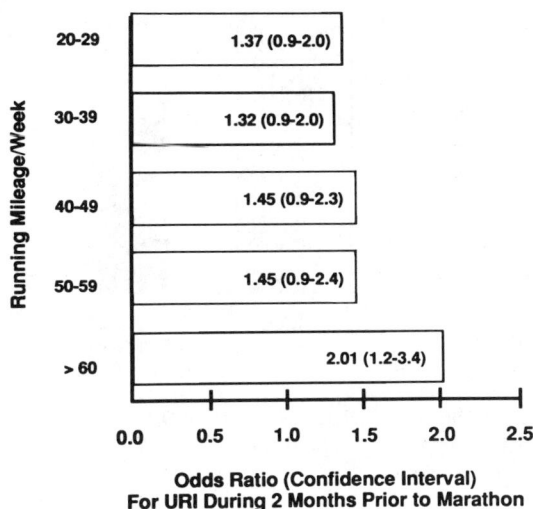

FIGURE 3. Self-reported respiratory tract infection in 2,300 Los Angeles Marathon runners during the two month period (January, February) prior to the 1987 Los Angeles Marathon. After controlling for confounding variables using logistic regression, the odds for experiencing a respiratory tract infection by runners who trained more than 60 miles/week were twofold greater than for those training less than 20 miles/week. (Data from Nieman, D. C., Johanssen, I. M., Lee, J. W., and Arabatzis, K., *J. Sports Med. Phys. Fitness,* 30, 316, 1990.)

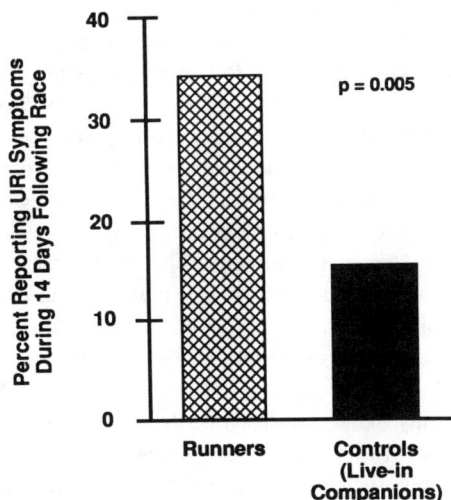

FIGURE 4. Upper respiratory tract infections (URI) in runners vs. controls during a 2-week period following a 56-km race in South Africa. (Data from Peters, E. M. and Bateman, E. D., *S. Afr. Med. J.,* 64, 582, 1983.)

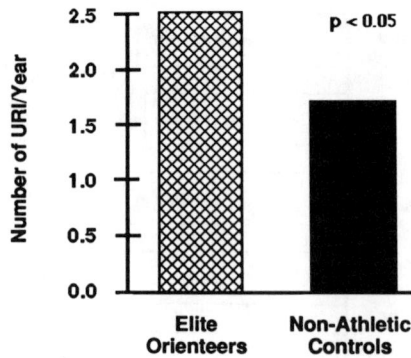

FIGURE 5.   Upper respiratory tract infections (URI) in Danish elite orienteers vs. nonathletic controls during a 1-year period. (Data from Linde, F., *Scand. J. Sports Sci.*, 9, 21, 1987.)

episodes, respectively) (Figure 5). While one-third of the controls reported no respiratory tract infections during the year-long study period, this applied to only 10% of the orienteers. The average duration of symptoms in the group of orienteers was 7.9 d compared to 6.4 d in the control group (NS). The control group had the expected seasonal variation with the peak incidence in winter and relatively few cases in summer, while the orienteers tended to show a more even distribution.

Heath et al.[17] followed a cohort of 530 runners who self-reported any symptoms of respiratory infections daily for 1 year. The average runner in the study was about 40 years of age, ran 20 mi/week (32 kms/week), and experienced a rate of 1.2 respiratory infections per year. Controlling for various confounding variables using logistic regression, the lowest odds ratio for respiratory infection was found in those running less than 10 mi/week (16 km/week). The odds ratio more than doubled for those running more than 17 mi/week (27 km/week). This study is somewhat difficult to interpret for several reasons. In contrast to other studies,[15] living alone and a low body mass index (kg/m^2) were found to be risk factors for developing a respiratory infection within this group of runners. These two factors, when included within the logistic regression model, may have altered the running distance threshold at which the odds ratio for respiratory infection became significant. Nonetheless, this study demonstrated that total running distance for a year is a significant risk factor for upper respiratory tract infections, with risk increasing as the running distance rises. The threshold at which running distance becomes a risk factor awaits further investigation.

In a 1-year prospective study of respiratory tract infections in 137 children (average age 12.7 years), participation in sports (gymnastics, swimming, or ice hockey) did not have an effect on the occurrence of illness.[18] This study is difficult to interpret, however, in that duration and intensity of exercise was not quantified. The control students (those not engaging in supervised sports training) were enrolled in physical education classes, and were allowed to take part in extracurricular physical activities. Thus, although sports participation by children appears to have no effect on occurrence of respiratory tract infections, data from this study cannot be used to answer the question as to whether or not varying levels of physical activity have an effect.

Although there have been other published reports on the relationship between exercise or sports participation and respiratory tract infections, the methods used in these investigations make it difficult to draw conclusions or make comparisons with other studies.[19-22] For example, Schouten et al.[19] conducted a 6-month retrospective study of 199 young adults, and concluded that the incidence and duration of respiratory tract infections was not significantly related to physical activity and fitness levels. However, in this study, no attempt was made to control for potential confounding factors, and the accuracy with which young adults are able to recall the incidence and duration of respiratory tract infections from the previous 6 months is questionable.

2. Clinical Evidence and Possible Mechanisms

The epidemiological studies reviewed thus far suggest that heavy acute or chronic exercise is associated with increased risk of respiratory infection. This interpretation is consistent with both human and animal experimental evidence.[23]

a. Changes in Immunity from Physiological Stress

Nieman et al.[11,24] ran ten seasoned marathoners at their fastest marathon pace on treadmills for 3 h. Subjects averaged just under 13 km/h at an average intensity of 70% VO_2 max. Blood samples were collected before, at 1 h of running, and 5 min, 1.5 6, and 21 h following the 3-h exercise bout. The samples were analyzed for cortisol and catecholamines, and a wide variety of tests for immune status and function were performed.

Cortisol rose 59% above baseline levels after the 3-h run, remaining elevated for 1.5 h of recovery before falling to normal daytime levels. This increase in cortisol correlated strongly ($r = 0.80$) with the three- to fourfold increase in both total leukocytes and granulocytes which peaked at 1.5 h of recovery. Cortisol levels after exercise correlated inversely with the 25 to 46% decrease in natural killer (NK) cell activity at 1.5 h of recovery, which persisted for nearly 6 h (Figure 6). The decrease in NK cell activity was coincident with a 50% decrease in lymphocytes bearing the antigen CD16. No decrease, however, was measured in number of lymphocytes bearing the antigen CD56 that identifies those cells most effective in exhibiting NK cell activity.[5] Thus, the decrease in NK cell activity was probably not entirely due to a redistribution of NK cells to the periphery. Rather, a true suppression in the activity of circulating NK cells appeared to occur for several hours after the 3-h running bout, which we have interpreted as a temporary suppression of immunosurveillance.[25]

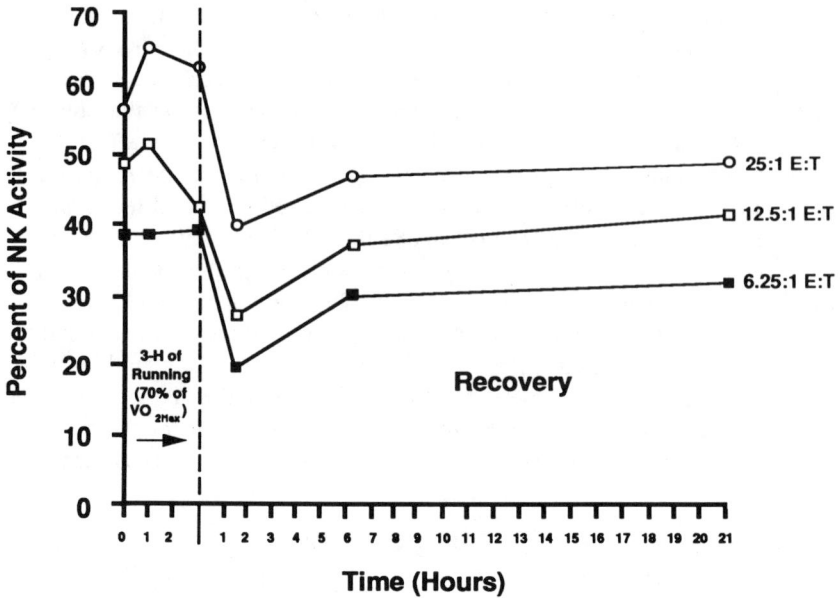

FIGURE 6. Changes in percent natural killer cell activity in 10 male marathon runners at three E:T ratios in response to a 3-h run at 70% VO_2 max. E:T, effector:target ratios; effector cells, peripheral blood mononuclear cells; target cells, K562 cells derived from patient with myelogenous leukemia; *, $p < 0.05$, contrast with baseline. (Data from Berk, L. S., Nieman, D. C., and Youngberg, W. S., *Med. Sci. Sports Exercise,* 22, 207, 1990.)

This interpretation is consistent with the findings of Pedersen et al.[26,27] who have carefully demonstrated that the post-exercise suppression of NK cell activity is due to increased levels of prostaglandins released from monocytes and neutrophils.

Our interpretation that both heavy acute and chronic exertion adversely effects immune status and function is consistent with the findings of many other researchers. Eskola et al.[28] and Gmünder et al.[29] have reported a significant decrease in lymphocyte proliferative response for several hours after a marathon (Figure 7). Following 1 h of cycling at 80% VO_2 max by untrained individuals, Tvede et al.[30] found suppression of B-lymphocyte function for at least 2 h because of an inhibitory effect of activated monocytes. Smith et al.[31] have determined that neutrophil killing capacity is decreased in elite athletes engaging in prolonged periods of intensive training in comparison to untrained controls. Nieman et al.[32] and Smith et al.[33] have reported significantly lower serum complement in long distance runners relative to sedentary controls. A significant decrease in salivary immunoglobulin concentrations following 2 h of intense cycling or 50 km of cross-country ski racing has been described by two groups of investigators[34,35] (Figure 8). Israel et al.[36]

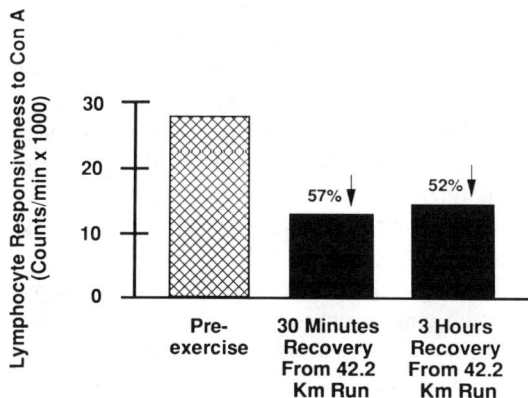

FIGURE 7. Effect of running 42.2 km on the lymphocyte proliferative response to the mitogen concanavalin A (Con A) in four elite Finnish marathon runners. (Data from Eskola, J., Ruuskanen, O., and Soppi, E., et al., *Clin. Exp. Immunol.*, 32, 339, 1978.)

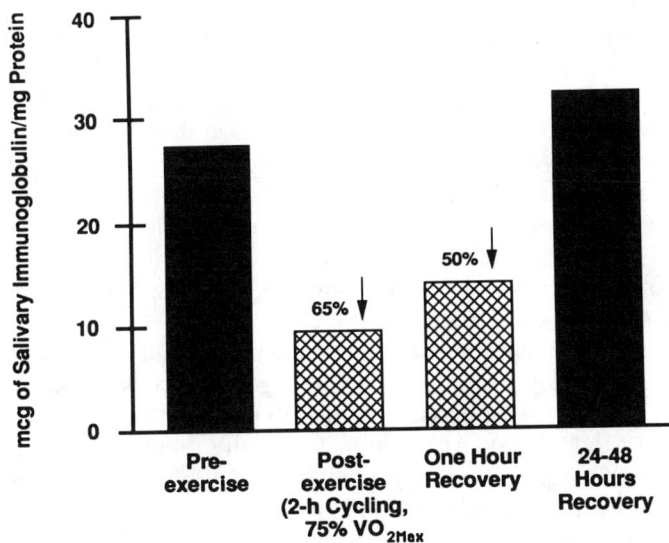

FIGURE 8. Effect of 2 h of cycle ergometer exercise (75% VO$_2$ max) on salivary IgA levels in eight well-trained male competitive bicyclists (expressed as mcg salivary IgA/mg protein). (Data from Mackinnon, L. T., Chick, T. W., Van As, A., and Tomasi, T. B., *Adv. Exp. Med. Biol.*, 216A, 869, 1987.)

have reported that serum immunoglobulins fall 10 to 28% for at least 1 d after athletes run 45 or 75 km at high intensity.

Russian investigators have reported that exhaustion of immune reserves can be observed during periods of important competitions, manifested by lowered immunoglobulin levels and suppression of phagocytic activity of neutrophils.[37-39] Under such conditions of physical and emotional stress, both interferon[40] and immunoglobulin[41] preparations have been shown to exert a protective antiviral effect, and may prove useful for athletes in competitive environments.

Results from animal studies have rather consistently supported the viewpoint that heavy acute and chronic exertion are related to negative changes in immune function. Several researchers have reported that exhaustive single bouts of exercise by both trained and untrained animals, or 6 d to 4.5 months of heavy exercise training, are linked to increased splenic epinephrine and cortisol levels and decreased splenic natural killer and T-cell lymphocyte function.[42-45] Thus, both circulating immune cells and those found in secondary lymphoid tissues may have their function suppressed because of the increase in cortisol and catecholamine levels that occur following heavy exertion.

These data, however, must be balanced against the findings of other researchers who have come to alternate conclusions. Pedersen et al.[46] has reported significantly higher basal NK cell activity in 27 elite Danish cyclers relative to untrained subjects, suggesting that as a result, their resistance to infection was improved. Fehr et al.[47] have related that the enzyme content and phagocytic activity of connective tissue macrophages increase when competitors run 15 km at high intensity. Macrophages from the lung, however, may respond differently than those from connective tissue areas following exercise. For example, Wong et al.[48] have established that the antimicrobial function of alveolar macrophages is strongly suppressed for 3 d in horses following single bouts of strenuous exercise.

MacNeil et al.[49] have reported that lymphocyte proliferative response is decreased for at least 2 h following cycle ergometer exercise, regardless of intensity (30 to 75% VO_2 max), duration (30 to 120 min), or subject fitness level (low-fit to high-fit). Although high-intensity exercise and high-fitness status tended to impair lymphocyte proliferation to the greatest extent, differences with other subgroups were not marked.

Further research is warranted to better elucidate the clinical significance of exercise-induced changes in immune status and function (many of which are transient in nature), and which variables best predict potential changes in host protection. The data at present are not consistent enough between studies to even suggest thresholds for various immune system markers that may indicate increased risk of respiratory infection. For example, although serum and salivary immunoglobulins have been shown to be low in some elite athletes during the competitive season, data to link these low levels of immunoglobulins to increased acute respiratory infection are unconvincing.[36,50]

b. Possible Synergism from Psychological Stress

Psychological factors may also play an important role in the relationship between exercise and respiratory infection. Exercise is a form of physiological stress, varying according to the intensity and duration of the training program. In particular, exercise-induced elevations in plasma catecholamines and glucocorticoids are of interest, because these hormones have been shown to effect immune function. The acute response of the immune system to psychological stressors is, in many ways, similar to those that occur in response to acute exercise.[51]

If the exercise training program is deemed stressful by the athlete, the combined psychological and physiological impact may overwhelm the ability of the immune system to protect the host.[4] Mental stress alone has been related to a wide variety of negative changes in immunity. Bereavement, major depression, loneliness, schizophrenia, marital discord, and other forms of mental stress have all been associated with suppression of immune function.[52-55]

A biochemical basis for bidirectional communication between the immune system and neuroendocrine system has been established.[56-59] These systems produce and use many of the same signal molecules in the form of hormones, lymphokines, and monokines for inter- and intrasystem communication and regulation. Lymphoid organs are innervated by the autonomic nervous system, and lymphocytes have receptors for the various stress hormones. In the other direction, for example, products of leukocytes have been shown to alter neuronal activity in certain areas of the brain.

Thus, stress of any form may decrease host protection from infection through both autonomic nervous system and hormonal mechanisms. Research by Graham and associates,[6] for example, has demonstrated that during a given 6-month period of time, highly stressed individuals have twice as many days with respiratory infection symptoms as compared with low-stressed people. Although specific research in this area has not yet been conducted, it would seem logical to assume that athletes, around the time of competition when both physiological and psychological stress are high, would be most vulnerable to respiratory infections. It would be of interest to study the confounding effect that competition outcome may have on the relationship between competitive exertion and infection. For example, could the jubilation associated with performing well partially neutralize some of the negative physiological effects?

c. The Acute-Phase Response

Another factor that may prove to be important with respect to risk of respiratory infection in athletes is the involvement of the immune system in the tissue repair process that occurs following strenuous exercise. It has been well established that both heavy acute and chronic exertion are associated with muscle cell damage, local inflammation, and the stereotyped sequence of host defense reactions known as the acute-phase response.[60-62]

The acute-phase response following long endurance exercise involves the complement system, neutrophils, macrophages, various cytokines, and acute-phase proteins, and can last for several days, promoting clearance of damaged tissue and setting the stage for repair and growth.[60,61,63] Lymphocytes, neutrophils, and macrophages are attracted to the injured muscle cells, and invade the area to aid in the process. Neutrophils phagocytize tissue debris and release a wide variety of factors that aid in the digestion of adjacent dead tissue cells.[62] Macrophages have surface receptors which allow them to react nonspecifically to a variety of substances, a process enhanced by the presence of opsonins (primarily complement and antibody). Macrophages also are a prime source of cytokines that mediate most of the physiological and inflammatory reactions accompanying muscle cell injury.[61] Dufaux and Order[64] have shown that plasma elastase-alpha 1-antitrypsin, neopterin, tumor necrosis factor, and soluble interleukin-2 receptor increase during recovery from a 2.5-h running test, supporting the concept of a functional involvement of polymorphonuclear neutrophils and an activation of macrophages and T-lymphocytes.

We have demonstrated that serum complement levels are lower in athletes relative to controls, and also decrease during recovery from an exhaustive 3-h run.[25,32] Dufaux and Order[65] have provided evidence for complement activation after 2.5 h of running. Together, these data suggest that serum complement may contribute to extravascular pools during recovery from marathon running, assisting macrophages and leukocytes in the resolution and repair process of injured muscle cells.

Could the active enmeshment of the immune system in the muscle-tissue repair and inflammation process mean that protection from respiratory infection is compromised? Research to answer this question is certainly warranted, and may greatly increase our understanding as to how and why athletes appear to be more susceptible to respiratory tract infections during periods of heavy training.

III. MANAGEMENT OF THE ATHLETE DURING INFECTION

At present, insufficient evidence exists to recommend precisely what laboratory tests of immune function should be conducted to ascertain when an athlete is at increased risk of an infectious episode due to overtraining and/ or psychosocial stress. Although some evidence would suggest that low immunoglobulin and complement levels, decreased lymphocyte proliferative response, diminished neutrophil phagocytic activity, depressed NK cell activity, low total lymphocyte count, and low helper/suppressor T-cell ratio are each important markers of increased risk, the exact level at which one or a combination of some or all of these immune components becomes predictive is unknown.[4] In most clinical situations, the trend in laboratory values established over a length of time is much more useful than absolute numbers at single points. In other words, athletes should be monitored at intervals with each new value compared to those previously obtained. However, at this time there is no single test or small battery of tests that can be recommended as being the best or even sufficient monitor of depressed immune function in athletes. It is doubtful that tests for immune function or status will be used in the immediate future because of various practical considerations, including time and cost.

If an athlete experiences sudden and unexplained deterioration in performance during training or competition, viral infection should be suspected.[66,67] It is well established that various measures of physical performance capability are reduced during an infectious episode.[68-74] Several case histories have been published demonstrating that sudden and unexplained deterioration in athletic performance can, in some individuals, be traced to either recent respiratory tract infections or subclinical viral infections that run a protracted course.[67] Daniels et al.,[68] for example, concluded that during a mild fever state, there is a marked effect upon the ability and/or willingness of some individuals to perform both cardiorespiratory and musculoskeletal exercise. Other researchers have reported decrements in measurements of muscle strength, including Friman et al.,[69,70] who have shown that isometric muscle strength in both the upper and lower extremities is reduced to 85 to 95% of late convalescent values in patients who were hospitalized with various acute infectious diseases. While studies consistently show decrements in measurements of exercise performance, the mechanism for these decreases is not completely known. Friman et al.[73] have suggested that infection-induced degradation of various performance-related muscle enzymes may be one important factor.

Should athletes exercise when they have a viral infection? Most clinical authorities in this area recommend that if the athlete has symptoms of a common cold with no constitutional involvement, then regular training may be safely resumed a few days after the resolution of symptoms.[67,75] Mild exercise during sickness with the common cold does not appear to be contraindicated but there is insufficient evidence at present to say one way or the other. However, if there are symptoms or signs of systemic involvement (fever, extreme tiredness, muscle aches, swollen lymph glands, etc.), then 2 to 4 weeks should probably be allowed before resumption of intensive training. These precautions are advised because of the well documented relationship between intensive exercise and risk of developing viral cardiomyopathy and other severe forms of viral infection.[76]

Clinicians since the 1940s have observed that certain patients with paralytic poliomyelitis give a history of severe exertion immediately preceding or during the onset of paralysis.[77] Levinson et al.[78] found that the incidence and severity of paralysis was greater in monkeys subjected to exhausting exercise than in control animals. Weinstein[79] concluded that participation in strenuous sport late in the incubation period increased the risk of extensive and severe paralysis in school boys during an epidemic of poliomyelitis in Greenwich, CT.

Several studies have demonstrated that exhaustive exercise after contracting an infection may be detrimental. In particular, the virulence of the Coxsackie virus, which has a predilection for the heart muscle, has been shown to be increased by intense exercise. Reyes and Lerner,[80] for example, showed that when weanling Swiss Albino mice are inoculated with the Coxsackie virus and subsequently forced to swim vigorously daily, a dramatic increase in virus multiplication occurred in the hearts, as compared to that observed in the inactive control mice.

It has been known for several decades that many types of viral infections can produce myocarditis and/or pericarditis.[81] Respiratory infections, including the "common cold" and "flu" syndromes are all potentially serious; the patient may be prone to develop cardiac damage and sudden death through acute arrhythmias. Patients who develop viral cardiomyopathy are usually previously healthy, young people who have stressed themselves with vigorous, prolonged physical exercise during the height of a viral infection, or soon thereafter. Furthermore, these subjects usually have continued with stressful exercise, while ignoring the early onset of dyspnea, palpitation, weakness, fatigability, and general ill feeling — all symptoms and signs also observed in persons suffering cardiac damage. It is recommended that strenuous physical stress be avoided for at least two weeks post-infection.[81]

There are numerous case reports of death in young healthy people who engaged in vigorous exercise during an acute viral illness.[66,67,76,82,83] Phillips et al.[84] reviewed the clinical and autopsy records of the 19 sudden cardiac deaths that occurred among 1.6 million Air Force recruits during basic training. Strenuous physical exertion was associated with sudden death in 17 of 19 cases, and the most frequent underlying etiology was myocarditis. In view of the fact that viral illness is endemic in barrack-residing recruits, the authors conjectured that exertion may have exacerbated subclinical cases of myocarditis, leading to sudden death in seven of eight recruits that had myocarditis. Drory et al.[85], in their study of 20 male soldiers in the Israel Defense Forces (1974 to 1986) who had died suddenly and unexpectedly within 24 h of strenuous exertion, also concluded that febrile disease may have been a cause of death in some of the subjects.

IV. MODERATE EXERCISE TRAINING AND INFECTION

What about the common belief that moderate physical activity is beneficial in decreasing risk of respiratory tract infections and improving immune function? Very few studies have been carried out in this area, and more research is certainly warranted to investigate this interesting question.

A. EPIDEMIOLOGICAL EVIDENCE

As mentioned earlier, in the study by Nieman et al.,[15] the odds ratio for respiratory tract infection did not become significant until runners trained

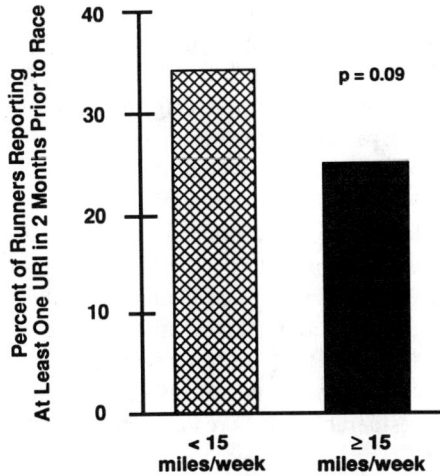

FIGURE 9. Percentage of runners reporting at least one respiratory infectious episode during a 2-month period prior to a 5-, 10-K or half-marathon road race. Twenty-five percent of runners training more than 15 miles/week (average of 26 miles/week) reported at least one infectious episode in comparison to 34% of runners training less than 15 miles/week (average of 7.5 miles or 12 kilometers/week). (Data from Nieman, D. C., Johanssen, I. M., and Lee, J. W., *J. Sports Med. Phys. Fit.,* 29, 289, 1989.)

more than 60 miles/week (96 kilometers/week) when using less than 20 miles/week as a reference point. In another study by Nieman et al.,[86] 25% of runners training more than 15 miles/week (24 kilometers/week) (average of 26 miles or 42 kilometers/week) reported at least one infectious episode during a 2-month winter period in comparison to 34% of runners training less than 15 miles/week (average of 7.5 miles or 12 kilometers/week) (Figure 9). The higher mileage runners trained more frequently than the lower mileage runners (4.6 vs. 2.7 sessions/week), suggesting that frequent but moderate amounts of exercise training may improve immunosurveillance. These two studies suggest that moderate amounts of training are associated with a lower risk of respiratory infection than high-distance training. However, these two studies did not address the question as to whether or not individuals who exercise moderately have different rates of respiratory infection when compared to sedentary controls.

B. CLINICAL EVIDENCE AND POSSIBLE MECHANISMS

The influence of exercise training on resistance to infection has been investigated using animal models since the turn of the century. Cannon and Kluger[87] have reviewed the animal literature and concluded that moderate exercise prior to infection may increase resistance to infection, but that exhaustive exercise after contracting an infection may be detrimental. In accordance with this viewpoint, Slubik et al.[88] have reported that moderate physical exercise preceding irradiation diminishes radiation injury in animals while intensive exercise and stress may aggravate the damage.

Smith et al.[31] have shown that 1 h of cycling at 60% VO_2 max may increase resistance to infection by improving the "killing capacity" of neutrophils, an effect which persists for at least 6 h of recovery. In that neutrophils are the body's best phagocyte, these findings suggest that regular episodes of moderate exercise may increase resistance to infection.

We recently conducted the first randomized controlled study on the effects walking had on immune response and acute respiratory infection tract symptomatology.[89,90] We chose a group of sedentary, mildly obese women from the community, and randomly divided them into walking and sedentary control groups. This type of subject was chosen because women of this age have been reported to have the highest rates of respiratory infection among adults, and to experience considerable cardiorespiratory benefits from regimens of brisk walking.

The 15-week research project extended from the last week in January to mid-May 1989. The exercise subjects walked 45 min/session, 5 times/week, for 15 continuous weeks on a measured course under supervision. Based on graded exercise test results, the exercise heart rates were kept at 60% of heart rate reserve, and recorded every half mile by an exercise supervisor. Subjects averaged slightly more than 3 mi per session at a heart rate of 138 beats per minute. Testing was conducted at three time periods — baseline, 6, and 15 weeks. Blood samples were collected 36 h after the last exercise session and analyzed in our immunology laboratory for a wide variety of indicators of immune system status and function. Subjects recorded health problems in a daily log book using 10 codes supplied to us by the Centers for Disease Control. A respiratory tract infectious episode was defined if symptoms persisted for at least 48 h and was separated by at least one week from a previous episode.

Our most important finding was that exercise subjects experienced one-half the days with respiratory infection symptoms during the 15-week period compared to that of the sedentary control group (5.1 ± 1.2 vs. 10.8 ± 2.3 d, respectively; p = 0.039). The number of separate infectious episodes did not vary between groups (1.0 ± 0.2 vs. 1.1 ± 0.2 for exercise and sedentary groups, respectively; p = 0.693) but the number of symptom days per infectious episode was significantly lower in the exercise group (p = 0.049) (Figure 10).

Moderate exercise training led to a 20% net increase in each of the three serum immunoglobulins, and was significantly correlated with fewer respiratory infection symptoms days, as was improvement in cardiorespiratory fitness (Figure 11). Improvement in fitness was also correlated significantly with increases in each of the three classes of serum immunoglobulins.[50] These results are similar to those of Liu and Wang[91] who have reported that in mice, 13 weeks of exercising 20 min/d led to significantly higher antibody levels following immunization.

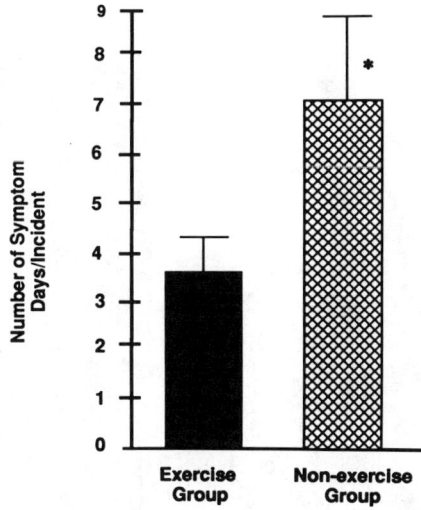

FIGURE 10. Moderate exercise training effects on the duration of symptoms from respiratory tract infection during a 15-week period in 18 walkers vs. 18 sedentary controls. The number of symptom days per infectious incident in the exercise group was approximately half that of the nonexercise group. *, $p < 0.05$. (Data from Nieman, D. C., Nehlsen-Cannarella, S. L., and Markoff, P. A., et al., *Int. J. Sports Med.*, 11, 467, 1987.)

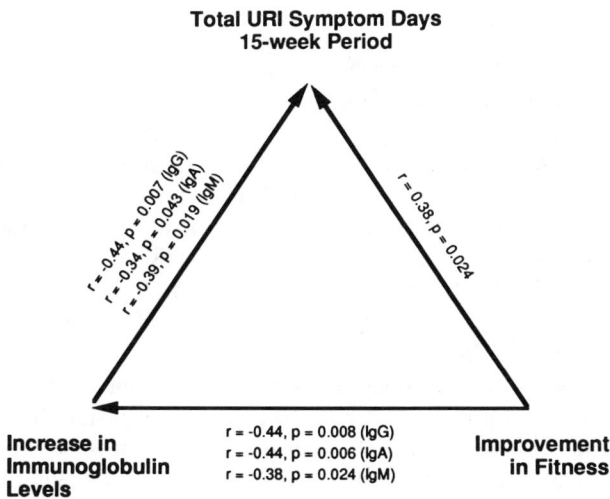

FIGURE 11. Correlations between improvement in cardiorespiratory fitness, increase in serum immunoglobulins, and total upper respiratory tract infection (URI) symptom days during a 15-week moderate exercise training study. (Data from Nehlsen-Cannarella, S. L., Nieman, D. C., and Balk-Lamberton, A. J., et al., *Med. Sci. Sports Exercise*, 23, 64, 1991.)

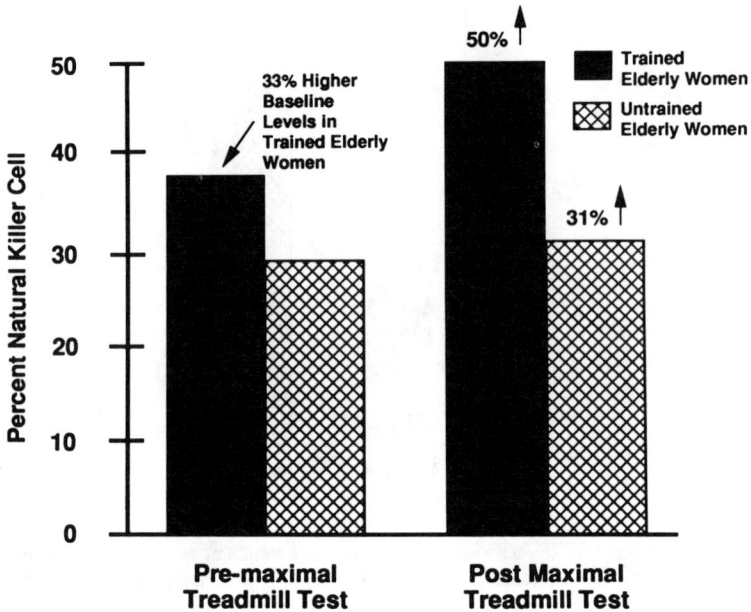

FIGURE 12. Percent natural killer cell activity in seven trained (age, 73 years) and seven untrained (age, 71 years) elderly women before and after a graded-maximal treadmill test. (Data from Crist, D. M., Mackinnon, L. T., Thompson, R. R., Atterbom, H. A., and Egan, P. A., *Gerontology*, 35, 66, 1989.)

Exercise training also led to a significant 57% increase in NK cell activity after 6 weeks of training, which preceded a seasonal improvement in NK cell activity in the sedentary group by mid-May.[89] The increase in NK cell activity occurred despite no change in NK cell number in either group, meaning that the activity of each NK cell was improved in response to walking. NK cell activity at 6 weeks was significantly correlated with a decrease in the duration of respiratory infection symptoms per episode. These results are similar to those of Crist et al.,[92] who moderately exercised elderly women for 16 weeks and measured a 33% higher NK cell activity at rest and a heightened increase following maximal testing (Figure 12).

As a follow-up to this prospective study, we brought into our Human Performance Lab the same basic group of women to measure the acute 24-h response of the immune system to a single 45-min bout of walking at 60% VO_2 max.[93,94] We were interested to see if acute effects would differ from those of more intense exercise bouts. Treatment order between walking or seated rest in the same environment was counterbalanced on two testing occasions with the women acting as their own controls. The 45-min walk increased heart rates to 138 bpm, which corresponded to just under 5 METS and a perceived exertion between "fairly light" and "somewhat hard".

Our most important finding was that serum immunoglobulins increased moderately and transiently immediately after the 45-min walk, relative to the rest condition, for IgG, IgA, and IgM.[94] Additionally, a moderate, transient lymphocytosis occurred, with NK cells representing two-thirds of the increase and T-cells representing the other third.[93] The increase in T-cells was primarily CD8 cells. Closer inspection revealed, however, that nearly all of the increase in CD8 cells were of the dim-CD8 variety, a subset of cells that are thought to be NK cells. In other words, walking recruits lymphocytes from peripheral lymphoid tissues that are, or act as, NK cells, cells that are vitally important in the first-line defense actions of the immune system. Interestingly, these changes in the immune system in response to walking are exactly opposed to what occurs after intense marathon running. Repeated walking bouts may then lead to (based on data from our 15-week training study[89,90]) a chronic increase in natural killer cell activity and serum immunoglobulin levels.

The acute response of the immune system to exercise may have much to do with the degree of intensity and total exertion load, and corresponding changes in concentrations of cortisol and epinephrine. Both of these hormones have been associated with many negative effects on immune function.[95-97] Lymphocytes have β-adrenergic receptors, and the presence of epinephrine during exercise increases receptor number on T-suppressor/cytotoxic and natural killer cells, which are the major lymphocyte subsets that increase in response to an exercise challenge.[58,59] The degree to which these lymphocyte subsets increase in the peripheral blood as they are recruited from lymphoid tissue pools is highly dependent on the magnitude of change in epinephrine. Additionally, the effect on lymphocyte function is also dependent on the change in both epinephrine and cortisol. Moderate exercise, such as walking, does not increase the concentration of these two hormones in the blood, resulting in a small lymphocytosis in contrast to intense exercise in which levels of both hormones increase.[93] (Figure 13). Thus, it may be argued that moderate exercise induces a small increase in NK and CD8 T cells without the potential suppressive effect of epinephrine or cortisol, which may be favorable for host protection. There are only a finite number of lymphocytes that are specific to any particular antigen. Theoretically, by recruiting lymphocytes from the periphery, exercise may increase the rate of lymphocyte circulation through the body, improving the potential for interaction of lymphocyte and antigen without the attending negative effects of stress hormones.[4]

V. EXERCISE BY AIDS PATIENTS

Acquired Immune Deficiency Syndrome (AIDS) is a major public health problem of this generation.[98] People who are sexually active with multiple partners or who use IV drugs are at significant risk for contracting AIDS.

Within several weeks to several months after infection with the human immunodeficiency virus (HIV), many individuals develop an acute self-limited mononucleosis-like illness lasting for a week or two.[99] Most persons

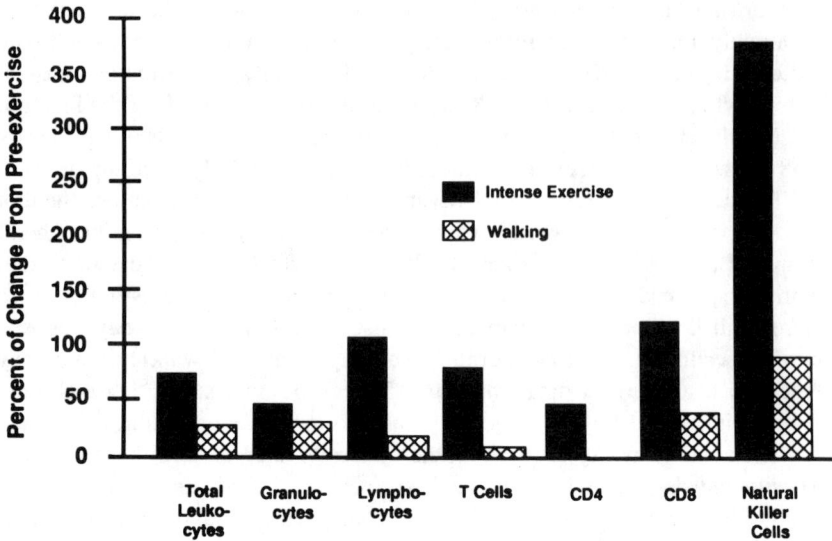

FIGURE 13.   Review of literature on walking-induced vs. intense exercise-induced acute changes in circulating immune system variables. Data expressed as percent change in mean circulating numbers of cells before and immediately post-exercise.

infected with HIV develop detectable antibodies within 1 to 3 months, al-though occasionally, there may be a more prolonged interval. HIV-infected persons may be free then of clinical signs or symptoms for many months to years before onset of clinical illness which starts with a constellation of nonspecific symptoms (AIDS-related complex or ARC) and then proceeds to AIDS. Fully developed AIDS infection also includes more than a dozen additional opportunistic infections and several cancers. The proportion of HIV-infected persons who will ultimately develop AIDS is not precisely known. Although the vast majority of HIV-infected persons is projected to develop AIDS within 15 to 20 years, with modern therapy the incubation period is expected to be considerably longer. Without specific therapy, the case fatality rate of AIDS has been very high, with 80 to 90% of patients dying within 3 to 5 years after diagnosis.

The primary target of this virus is the T-helper/inducer cell because it binds directly to the CD4 surface membrane receptor, and kills the cell as replication proceeds. As a result, AIDS patients have a marked reduction in the number of CD4 cells, the most evident hallmark of disease progression, with symptoms usually rare until the count falls below 400 to 500 cells/mm^3. When CD4 cell counts fall below 50 cells/mm^3, most patients develop the most serious of the opportunistic infections associated with AIDS. Other immunologic abnormalities develop in these patients, including a deficiency in ability to mount an appropriate antibody response, defects in monocyte function, a reduction in NK cell activity, and a marked decrease in T-cell proliferative response to mitogens.[100]

Pertinent questions have been raised regarding HIV transmission during sports that require close physical contact. Most patients diagnosed with active AIDS are acutely and chronically ill and are not likely to participate in athletic endeavors. For each patient with clinically apparent AIDS, however, there are many more who are HIV-infected, but are free of clinical manifestations or present with nonspecific symptoms (ARC), who may be capable of normal participation in sports.

Routine social or community contact with an HIV-infected person carries no risk of transmission; only sexual exposure and exposure to blood or tissues carries a risk.[99] While the HIV has been found in saliva, tears, urine, and bronchial secretions, there is no evidence that the virus can be transmitted after contact with these secretions. There are several situations, however, in which the transmission of HIV is of concern in athletic settings. In sports in which athletes can be cut, such as in boxing or wrestling, or in other contact sports such as football, basketball, and baseball, risk of HIV transmission exists when the mucous membranes of a healthy athlete are exposed to the blood of an infected athlete. At present, the feeling is that testing all athletes prior to sports participation is impractical, unethical, and unrealistic.[98] Therefore, the team physician and athletic trainer are urged to provide information about the transmission of HIV, recommended behavior to reduce risks, and referral for follow-up care or diagnosis.[101]

These concerns and concepts have been summarized by the World Health Organization and International Federation of Sports Medicine in their consensus report "AIDS and Sports". Included in this report are the following:

1. No evidence exists for a risk of transmission of HIV when infected persons, without bleeding wounds or skin lesions, engage in sports. There is a potential, very low risk of HIV transmission, however, during combative sports when an infected athlete with a bleeding wound or a skin lesion with exudate comes in contract with another athlete who has a skin lesion or an exposed mucous membrane. It should be the responsibility of any athlete participating in a combative sport who has a wound or other skin lesion to report it immediately to a responsible official and seek medical attention. Athletes who know they are HIV-infected should seek medical counseling about further participation in sports.

2. Sports organizations, clubs, and groups have special opportunities to educate athletes and ancillary personnel about AIDS, and should ensure that each are aware of the major issues involved.

3. There is no medical or public health justification for testing or screening for HIV infection prior to participation in sports activities.

Can exercise training be used as a method to delay the progression from HIV infection to AIDS? At present, only a handful of investigators have published results in this area.[102-105] Rigsby et al.[102] studied the effect of an exercise program (three 1-h sessions per week of strength training and aerobic exercise) on 37 HIV-infected subjects who spanned the range of HIV disease progression from asymptomatic to a diagnosis of AIDS (CD4 counts ranged from 9 to 804 cells/mm^3). Subjects were randomly assigned to either a 12-week exercise training or a counseling control group. Although exercise training had the expected effect in improving both strength and cardiorespiratory fitness in exercise subjects, no significant change in CD4 cell counts or the CD4/CD8 ratio was found for either condition. The exercise group experienced an average increase of 58 CD4 cells/mm^3 during the study compared to no change in the counseling group, but the heterogenous nature of the relatively small study group weakened the likelihood of the change being statistically significant. The increase in strength with weight training, which has also been reported by Spence et al.[106] in AIDS subjects, is noteworthy in that muscle atrophy and nervous system disorders are common among ARC and AIDS patients. Weight training may provide one means of retarding the wasting syndrome which accompanies AIDS and improve the quality of life for these individuals.

LaPerriere et al.[103-105] randomly assigned 50 asymptomatic, healthy homosexual males to 10 weeks of either an aerobic exercise training or a measurement-only control group. The subjects included 12 seronegative exercisers, 10 seropositive exercisers, 11 seronegative controls, and 6 seropositive controls. The aerobic exercise training involved 45 min of stationary bicycle ergometry exercise three times per week, at an intensity of 70 to 80% of age-predicted maximum heart rate, and resulted in significant improvement in cardiorespiratory endurance. Both HIV seronegative and seropositive subjects in the exercise group showed an increase in CD4 cells, with the magnitude greater in the seronegative group (220 vs. 115 cells/mm^3, respectively). Seropositive exercisers experienced a smaller decrease in NK cells than seropositive control subjects (38 vs. 170 cells/mm^3, respectively). Results of this study suggest that exercise training in asymptomatic HIV positive subjects (with CD4 counts in the normal range) may attenuate the usual decrements seen in immune status and function. However, long-term studies with greater numbers of subjects are needed before any definitive conclusions can be drawn.

One tentative conclusion that can be made from these studies is that appropriately supervised exercise training does not appear to adversely affect HIV-infected individuals.[105] Several potential benefits of both aerobic and strength training by HIV-infected individuals, especially when initiated early in the disease state, include improvement in psychological coping, maintenance of health and physical function for a longer period, and attenuation of negative immune system changes. LaPerriere et al.[105] have recommended that exercise prescriptions for all HIV-infected individuals should be made on an individual basis, with appropriate initial screening. The exercise prescription should emphasize both cardiorespiratory and musculoskeletal training components.

VI. SUMMARY

In general, the data reviewed in this chapter suggest that unusually heavy training and/or intense exercise bouts lead to several negative changes in immunosurveillance, many of which are probably related to the effects of cortisol and epinephrine. These changes may lead to an infectious illness, especially when psychological stress is a contributing factor. Regular moderate exercise training, on the other hand, may decrease the individual's risk of acquiring an infection. There are several immune system changes that occur during moderate exercise that may improve host protection.

There is an interesting similarity in the metabolic and immunologic responses to intense endurance exercise and to an infectious challenge.[4,107-109] In both conditions, the number of circulating leukocytes increases, lymphopenia occurs (especially T-cells with cells trafficking to peripheral tissues), the lymphocyte responses to PHA and Con-A decrease, body core temperature rises, plasma levels of acute-phase proteins increase, and degranulation of neutrophils develops. Since endurance exercise is associated with muscle cell damage and an increased intake of potential pathogens through heightened ventilation, it is logical that in preparation for such a challenge, the immune system receives a signal from the neuroendocrine network that activates the immune system.

Why, then, do epidemiological data and clinical experience point toward an increased risk of respiratory infection in some athletes? The mass of evidence favors the view that psychosocial variables play an important role in affecting immunologic competence. The net effect of combined psychological and physiological stress from unusually heavy endurance exercise, especially during times of competition, may lead to suppression or downregulation of the immune system.

For those athletes who must exercise intensely for competitive reasons, several precautions can help decrease the risk of sickness. These include spacing vigorous workouts and race events as far apart as possible, eating a well-balanced diet, keeping other life stresses to a minimum, avoiding overtraining and chronic fatigue, and obtaining adequate sleep. Before and following intense race events, the athlete should try to avoid contact with sick people, if at all possible.

REFERENCES

1. **Midvedt, T. and Midtvedt, K.,** Sport and infection, *Scand. J. Soc. Med. Suppl.,* 29, 241, 1982.
2. **Conklin, R. J.,** Common cutaneous disorders in athletes, *Sports Med.,* 9, 100, 1990.
3. **Girdwood, R. W. A.,** Infections associated with sport, *Brit. J. Sports Med.,* 22, 117, 1988.
4. **Nieman, D. C.,** Physical activity, fitness and infection, in *Exercise and Health: A Consensus of Current Knowledge,* Bouchard, C., Ed., Human Kinetics Publishers, Champaign, IL, 1993, in press.
5. **Graham, H. M. H., Douglas, R. M., and Ryan, P.,** Stress and acute respiratory infection, *Am. J. Epidemiol.,* 124, 389, 1986.
6. **Landmann, R. M. A., Muller, F. B., Perini, C. H., et al.,** Changes in immunoregulatory cells induced by psychological and physical stress: relationship to plasma catecholamines, *Clin. Exp. Immunol.,* 58, 127, 1984.
7. **Mackinnon, L. T. and Tomasi, T. B.,** Immunology of exercise, *Ann. Sports Med.,* 3, 1, 1986.
8. **Schoenborn, C. A. and Marano, M.,** Current estimates from the National Health Interview Survey, Vital and Health Statistics, Series 10, No. 166, National Center for Health Statistics, Public Health Service, Washington, D.C., United States Government Printing Office, 1988.
9. The Office of Disease Prevention and Health Promotion, *Disease Prevention/Health Promotion: The Facts,* U.S. Public Health Service, U.S. Department of Health and Human Services, Bull Publishing, Palo Alto, CA, 1988.
10. **Green, R. L., Kaplan, S. S., Rabin, B. S., Stanitski, C. L., Zdziarski, U.,** Immune function in marathon runners, *Ann. Allergy,* 47, 73, 1981.
11. **Nieman, D. C., Berk, L. S., Simpson-Westerberg, M., et al.,** Effects of long endurance running on immune system parameters and lymphocyte function in experienced marathoners, *Int. J. Sports Med.,* 10, 317, 1989.
12. **Fitzgerald, L.,** Exercise and the immune system, *Immunol. Today,* 9(11), 337, 1988.
13. **Jokl, E.,** The immunological status of athletes, *J. Sports Med.,* 14, 165, 1974.
14. **Linde, F.,** Running and upper respiratory tract infections, *Scand. J. Sport Sci.,* 9, 21, 1987.
15. **Nieman, D. C., Johanssen, I. M., Lee, J. W., and Arabatzis, K.,** Infectious episodes in runners before and after the Los Angeles Marathon, *J. Sports Med. Phys. Fitness,* 30, 316, 1990.
16. **Peters, E. M. and Bateman, E. D.,** Respiratory tract infections: an epidemiological survey, *S. Afr. Med. J.,* 64, 582, 1983.
17. **Heath, G. W., Ford, E. S., Craven, T. E., et al.,** Exercise and the incidence of upper respiratory tract infections, *Med. Sci. Sports Exercise,* 23, 152, 1991.
18. **Osterback, L. and Qvarnberg, Y.,** A prospective study of respiratory infections in 12-year old children actively engaged in sport, *Acta Paediatr. Scand.,* 76, 944, 1987.
19. **Schouten, W. J., Verschuur, R., and Kempter, H. C. G.,** Physical activity and upper respiratory tract infections in a normal population of young men and women: the Amsterdam Growth and Health Study, *Int. J. Sports Med.,* 9, 451, 1988.
20. **Budgett, R. G. M. and Fuller, G. N.,** Illness and injury in international oarsmen, *Clin. Sports Med.,* 1, 57, 1989.
21. **Strauss, R. H., Lanese, R. R., and Leizman, D. J.,** Illness and absence among wrestlers, swimmers, and gymnasts at a large university, *Am. J. Sports Med.,* 16, 653, 1988.
22. **Seyfried, P. L., Toibin, R. S., Brown, N. E., and Ness, P. F.,** A prospective study of swimming-related illness. I. Swimming-associated health risk, *Am. J. Public Health,* 75, 1068, 1985.

23. **Shubik, V. M.**, Immunity in sportsmen, *J. Hyg. Epidemiol. Microbiol. Immunol.*, 34, 107, 1990.
24. **Berk, L. S., Nieman, D. C., Youngberg, W. S., et al.**, The effect of long endurance running on natural killer cells in marathoners, *Med. Sci. Sports Exercise*, 22, 207, 1990.
25. **Nieman, D. C. and Nehlsen-Cannarella, S. L.**, Effects of endurance exercise on immune response, in *Endurance in Sport*, Shephard, R. J. and Astrand, P. O., Eds., Blackwell Scientific Publications, Oxford, 1991.
26. **Pedersen, B. K., Tvede, N., Klarlund, K., et al.**, Indomethacin *in vitro* and *in vivo* abolishes post-exercise suppression of natural killer cell activity in peripheral blood, *Int. J. Sports Med.*, 11, 127, 1990.
27. **Pedersen, B. K., Tvede, N., Hansen, F. R., et al.**, Modulation of natural killer cell activity in peripheral blood by physical exercise, *Scand. J. Immunol.*, 27, 673, 1988.
28. **Eskola, J., Ruuskanen, O., Soppi, E., et al.**, Effect of sport stress on lymphocyte transformation and antibody formation, *Clin. Exp. Immunol.*, 32, 339, 1978.
29. **Gmunder, F. K., Lorenzi, G., Bechler, B., et al.**, Effect of long-term physical exercise on lymphocyte reactivity: similarity to spaceflight reactions, *Aviat. Space Env. Med.*, 59, 146, 1988.
30. **Tvede, N., Heilmann, C., Halkjaer-Kristensen, J., and Pedersen, B. K.**, Mechanisms of B-lymphocyte suppression induced by acute physical exercise, *J. Clin. Lab. Immunol.*, 30, 169, 1989.
31. **Smith, J. A., Telford, R. D., Mason, I. B., and Weidemann, M. J.**, Exercise, training and neutrophil microbicidal activity, *Int. J. Sports Med.*, 11, 179, 1990.
32. **Nieman, D. C., Tan, S. A., Lee, J. W., and Berk, L. S.**, Complement and immunoglobulin levels in athletes and sedentary controls, *Int. J. Sports Med.*, 10, 124, 1989.
33. **Smith, J. K., Chi, D. S., Krish, G., Reynolds, S., Cambron, G.**, Effect of exercise on complement activity, *Ann. Allergy*, 65, 304, 1990.
34. **Mackinnon, L. T., Chick, T. W., Van As, A., and Tomasi, T. B.**, The effect of exercise on secretory and natural immunity, *Adv. Exp. Med. Biol.*, 216A, 869, 1987.
35. **Tomasi, T. B., Trudeau, F. B., Czerwinski, D., and Erredge, S.**, Immune parameters in athletes before and after strenuous exercise, *J. Clin. Immunol.*, 2, 173, 1982.
36. **Israel, S., Buhl, B., Drause, M., and Neumann, G.**, Die konzentration der immunglobuline A, G und M im serum bei trainierten und untrainierten sowie nach verschiedenen sportlicken ausdauerleistungen, *Medizin und Sport*, 22, 225, 1982.
37. **Pershin, B. B., Kus'min, S. N., Suzdal'nitskii, R. S., and Levando, V. A.**, Reserve potentials of immunity, *Zh. Mikrobiol. Epidemiol. Immunobiol.*, 6, 59, 1985.
38. **Petrova, I. V., Kuz'mion, S. N., Durshakova, T. S., Suzdail'nitskii, R. S., and Levando, V. A.**, The phenomenon of the formation of universal rosette-forming cells under superextreme loads, *Zh. Mikrobiol. Epidemiol. Immunobiol.*, 2, 72, 1985.
39. **Petrova, I. V., Kuz'min, S. N., Durshakova, T. S., Suzdail'nitskii, R. S., and Pershin, B. B.**, Neutrophil phagocytic activity and the humoral factors of general and local immunity under intensive physical loading, *Zh. Mikrobiol. Epidemiol. Immunobiol.*, 12, 53, 1983.
40. **Ershov, F. I., Gotovtseva, E. P., and Surkina, I. D.**, Use of recombinant alpha 2-interferon in athletes, *Vopr. Virusol.*, 33, 693, 1988.
41. **Ricken, K. H. and Kindermann, W.**, Behandlungsmoglichkeiten der infedktanfalligkeit des leistungssportiers, *Deutche Zeitschrft fur Sporsmedizin*, 37, 146, 1986.
42. **Simpson, J. R. and Hoffman-Goetz, L.**, Exercise stress and murine natural killer cell function, *Proc. Soc. Exp. Bio. Med.*, 195, 129, 1990.
43. **Ferry, A., Weill, B. L., and Rieu, M.**, Immunomodulations induced in rats by exercise on a treadmill, *J. Appl. Physiol.*, 69, 1912, 1990.
44. **Hoffman-Goetz, L., Keir, R., Thorne, R., Houston, M. E., and Young, C.**, Chronic exercise stress in mice depresses splenic T lymphocyte mitogenesis *in vitro*, *Clin. Exp. Immunol.*, 66, 551, 1986.

45. **Mahan, M. P. and Yound, M. R.,** Immune parameters of untrained or exercise-trained rats after exhaustive exercise, *J. Appl. Physiol.,* 66, 282, 1989.

46. **Pedersen, B. K., Tvede, N., Christensen, L. D., et al.,** Natural killer cell activity in peripheral blood of highly trained and untrained persons, *Int. J. Sports Med.,* 10, 129, 1989.

47. **Fehr, H. G., Lotzerich, H., and Michna, H.,** Human macrophage function and physical exercise: phagocytic and histochemical studies, *Eur. J. Appl. Physiol.,* 58, 613, 1989.

48. **Wong, C. W., Thompson, H. L., Thong, Y. H., and Thornton, J. R.** Effect of strenuous exercise stress on chemiluminescence response of equine alveolar macrophages, *Equine. Vet. J.,* 22, 33, 1990.

49. **MacNeil, B., Hoffman-Goetz, L., Kendall, A., Houston, M. and Arumugam, Y.,** Lymphocyte proliferation response after exercise in men: fitness, intensity, and duration effects, *J. Appl. Physiol.,* 70, 179, 1991.

50. **Nieman, D. C. and Nehlsen-Cannarella, S. L.,** The effects of acute and chronic exercise on immunoglobulins, *Sports Med.,* 11, 183, 1991.

51. **Naliboff, B. D., Benton, D., Solomon, G. F., et al.,** Immunological changes in young and old adults during brief laboratory stress, *Psychosom. Med.,* 53, 121, 1991.

52. **Jemmott, J. B. and Locke, S. E.,** Psychosocial factors, immunologic mediation, and human susceptibility to infectious diseases: how much do we know? *Psychol. Bull.,* 95, 78, 1984.

53. **Stein, M., Keller, S. E., and Schleifer, S. J.,** Stress and immunomodulation: the role of depression and neuroendocrine function, *J. Immunol.,* 135, 827s, 1985.

54. **Khansari, D. N., Murgo, A. J., and Faith, R. E.,** Effects of stress on the immune system, *Immunol. Today,* 11(5), 170, 1990.

55. **Kronfol, Z. and House, J. D.,** Lymphocyte mitogenesis, immunoglobulin and complement levels in depressed patients and normal controls, *Acta Psychiatr. Scand.,* 80, 142, 1989.

56. **Blalock, J. E.,** A molecular basis for bidirectional communication between the immune and neuroendocrine systems, *Physiol. Rev.,* 69, 1, 1989.

57. **Maki, T., Leinonen, H., Naveri, H., et al.,** Response of the beta-adrenergic system to maximal dynamic exercises in congestive heart failure secondary to idiopathic dilated cardiomyopathy, *Am. J. Cardio.,* 63, 1348, 1989.

58. **Van Tits, L. J., Michel, M. C., Grosse-Wilde, H., et al.,** Catecholamines increase lymphocyte beta 2-adrenergic receptors via a veta 2-adrenergic, spleen-dependent process, *Am. J. Cardio.,* 63, 1348, 1989.

59. **Maisel, A. S., Harris, T., Rearden, C. A., and Michel, M. C.,** β-Adrenergic receptors in lymphocyte subsets after exercise: alteration in normal individuals and patients with congestive heart failure, *Circulation,* 82, 2003, 1990.

60. **Armstron, R. B.,** Muscle damage and endurance events, *Sports Med.,* 3, 370, 1986.

61. **Evans, W. J. and Cannon, J. G.,** The metabolic effects of exercise-induced muscle damage, *Ex. Sport Sci. Rev.,* 19, 125, 1991.

62. **Smith, L. L.,** Acute inflammation: the underlying mechanism in delayed onset muscle soreness? *Med. Sci. Sports Exer.,* 23, 542, 1991.

63. **Irintchev, A. and Wernig, A.,** Muscle damage and repair in voluntarily running mice: strain and muscle difference, *Cell Tissue Res.,* 249, 509, 1987.

64. **Dufaux, B. and Order, U.,** Plasma elastase-alpha 1-antitrypsin, neopterin, tumor necrosis factor, and soluble interleukin-2 receptor after prolonged exercise, *Int. J. Sports Med.,* 10, 434, 1989.

65. **Dufaux, B. and Order, U.,** Complement activation after prolonged exercise, *Clin. Chim. Acta,* 179, 45, 1989.

66. **Roberts, J. A.,** Loss of form in young athletes due to viral infection, *Br. J. Med.,* 290, 357, 1985.

67. **Roberts, J. A.,** Viral illnesses and sports performance, *Sports Med.,* 3, 296, 1986.

68. **Daniels, W. L., Sharp, D. S., Wright, J. E., et al.,** Effects of virus infection on physical performance in man, *Milit. Med.,* 150, 8, 1985.
69. **Friman, G.,** Effect of acute infectious disease on isometric muscle strength, *Scand. J. Clin. Lab. Invest.,* 37, 303, 1977.
70. **Friman, G., Wright, J. E., Ilback, N. G., et al.,** Does fever or myalgia indicate reduced physical performance capacity in viral infections? *Acta Med. Scand.,* 217, 353, 1985.
71. **Friman, G.,** Effects of acute infectious disease on circulatory function, *Acta Med. Scand. Suppl.,* 592, 5, 1976.
72. **Friman, G., Ilback, N. G., and Beisel, W. R.,** Effects of *Streptococcus pneumoniae, Salmonella typhimurium* and *Francisella tularensis* infections on oxidative, glycolytic and lysosomal enzyme activity in red and white skeletal muscle in the rat, *Scand. J. Infect. Dis.,* 16, 111, 1984.
73. **Friman, G., Ilback, N. G., Crawford, D. J., and Neufeld, H. A.,** Metabolic responses to swimming exercise in *Streptococcus pneumoniae* infected rats, *Med. Sci. Sports Exercise,* 23, 415, 1991.
74. **Ilback, N. G., Friman, G., Crawford, D. J., and Neufeld, H. A.,** Effects of training on metabolic responses and performance capacity in *Streptococcus pneumoniae* infected rats, *Med. Sci. Sports Exercise,* 23, 422, 1991.
75. **Simon, H. B.,** Exercise and infection, *Physician Sportsmed.,* 15(10), 135, 1987.
76. **Sharp, J. C. M.,** Viruses and the athlete, *Br. J. Sports Med.,* 23, 47, 1989.
77. **Horstmann, D. M.,** Acute poliomyelitis: relation of physical activity at the time of onset to the course of the disease, *JAMA,* 142, 236, 1950.
78. **Levinson, S. O., Milzer, A., and Lewin, P.,** Effect of fatigue, chilling and mechanical trauma on resistance to experimental poliomyelitis, *Am. J. Hygiene,* 42, 204, 1945.
79. **Weinstein, L.,** Poliomyelitis: a persistent problem, *N. Engl. J. Med.,* 288, 370, 1973.
80. **Reyes, M. P. and Lerner, A. M.,** Interferon and neutralizing antibody in sera of exercised mice with Coxsackie virus B-3 myocarditis, *Proc. Soc. Exp. Bio. Med.,* 151, 333, 1976.
81. **Burch, G. E.,** Viral diseases of the heart, *Acta Cardiologica.,* 34(1), 5, 1979.
82. **Baron, R. C., Hatch, M. H., Kleeman, K., and MacCormack, J. N.,** Aseptic meningitis among members of a high school football team, *JAMA,* 248, 1724, 1982.
83. **Krikler, D. N. and Zilberg, B.,** Activity and hepatitis, *Lancet,* 2, 1046, 1966.
84. **Phillips, M., Robinowitz, M., Higgins, J. R., et al.,** Sudden cardiac death in Air Force recruits: a 20-year review, *JAMA,* 256, 2696, 1986.
85. **Drory, Y., Kramer, M. R., and Lev, B.,** Exertional sudden death in soldiers, *Med. Sci. Sports Exercise,* 23, 147, 1991.
86. **Nieman, D. C., Johanssen, I. M., and Lee, J. W.,** Infectious episodes in runners before and after a roadrace, *J. Sports Med. Phys. Fit.,* 29, 289, 1989.
87. **Cannon, J. G. and Kugler, J. J.,** Exercise enhances survival rate in mice infected with *Salmonella typhimurium, Proc. Soc. Exp. Bio. Med.,* 175, 518, 1984.
88. **Slubik, V. M., Levin, M. I., Mashneva, N. I., and Pulkov, V. M.,** The combined effect of ionizing radiation and physical exercises on some indices of nonspecific protection and immunity, *Radiobiologiia,* 27, 548, 1987.
89. **Nieman, D. C., Nehlsen-Cannarella, S. L., Markoff, P. A., et al.,** The effects of moderate exercise training on natural killer cells and acute upper respiratory tract infections, *Int. J. Sports Med.,* 11, 467, 1987.
90. **Nehlsen-Cannarella, S. L., Nieman, D. C., Balk-Lamberton, A. J., et al.,** The effects of moderate exercise training on immune response, *Med. Sci. Sports Exercise,* 23, 64, 1991.
91. **Liu, Y. G. and Wang, S. Y.,** The enhancing effect of exercise on the production of antibody to *Salmonella typhi* in mice, *Immunol. Lett.,* 14, 117, 1987.
92. **Crist, D. M., Mackinnon, L. T., Thompson, R. R., Atterbom, H. A., and Egan, P. A.,** Physical exercise increases natural cellular-mediated tumor cytotoxicity in elderly women, *Gerontology,* 35, 66, 1989.

93. **Nieman, D. C., Nehlsen-Cannarella, S. L., Donohue, K. M., et al.,** The effects of acute moderate exercise on leukocyte and lymphocyte subpopulations, *Med. Sci. Sports Exercise,* 23, 578, 1991.

94. **Nehlsen-Cannarella, S. L., Nieman, D. C., Jessen, J., et al.,** The effects of acute moderate exercise on lymphocyte function and serum immunoglobulins, *Int. J. Sports Med.,* 12, 391, 1991.

95. **Cavallo, R., Dartori, M. L., Gatti, G., and Angeli, A.,** Cortisol and immune interferon can interact in the modulation of human natural killer cell activity, *Experientia,* 42, 177, 1986.

96. **Crary, B., Hauser, S. L., Borysenko, M., et al.,** Epinephirine-induced changes in the distribution of lymphocyte subsets in peripheral blood of humans, *J. Immunol.,* 131, 1178, 1983.

97. **Cupps, T. R. and Fauci, A. S.,** Corticosteroid-mediated immunoregulation in man, *Immunological Rec.,* 65, 133, 1982.

98. **Calabrese, L. H. and Kelley, D.,** AIDS and athletes, *Physician Sportsmed.,* 17(1), 127, 1989.

99. **Benenson, A. S.,** *Control of Communicable Diseases in Man,* American Public Health Association, Washington, D.C., 1990.

100. **Antoni, M. H., Schneiderman, N., Fletcher, M. A., et al.,** Psychoneurommunology and HIV-1, *J. Consul. Clin. Psych.,* 58, 38, 1990.

101. **Walker, E.,** Herpes simplex, hepatitis B and the acquired immune deficiency syndrome, *Br. J. Sports Med.,* 22, 118, 1988.

102. **Rigsby, L. W., Dishman, R. K., Jackson, A. W., Maclean, G. S., and Raven, P. B.,** Effects of exercise training on men seropositive for the Human Immunodeficiency Virus-1, *Med. Sci. Sports Exercise,* 23, 00, 1991.

103. **LaPerriere, A. R., Fletcher, M. A., Antoni, M. H., Klimas, N. G., and Schneiderman, N.,** Aerobic exercise training in an AIDS risk group, *Int J. Sports Med.,* 12 (Suppl. 1), S53, 1991.

104. **LaPerriere, A. R., Antoni, M. H., Schneiderman, N., et al.,** Exercise intervention attenuates emotional distress and natural killer cell decrements following notification of positive serologic status for HIV-1, *Biofeedback Self-Regulation,* 15, 229, 1990.

105. **LaPerriere, A., Antoni, M., Fletcher, M. A., and Schneiderman, N.,** Exercise and health maintenance in AIDS, in *Clinical Assessment and Treatment in HIV: Rehabilitation of a Chronic Illness,* Galantino, M. L., Ed., Slack Inc., Thorofare, New Jersey, 1991, in press.

106. **Spence, D. W., Galantino, M. L. A., Mossberg, K. A., et al.,** Progressive resistance exercise: effect on muscle function and anthropometry of a select AIDS population, *Arch. Phys. Med. Rehabil.,* 71, 644, 1990.

107. **Cannon, J. G. and Kluger, M. J.,** Endogenous pyrogen activity in human plasma after exercise, *Science,* 220, 617, 1983.

108. **Lewis, D. E., Gilbert, B. E., and Knight, V.,** Influenza virus infection induces functional alterations in peripheral blood lymphocytes, *J. Immunol.,* 137, 3777, 1986.

109. **Schaefer, R. M., Kokot, K., Heidland, A., and Plass, R.,** Jogger's leukocytes, *N. Engl. J. Med.,* 316, 223, 1987.

Chapter 9

IMMUNE FUNCTION IN EXERCISE-INDUCED INJURIES

Louis C. Almekinders and Sally V. Almekinders

TABLE OF CONTENTS

I. INTRODUCTION

Medical and epidemiologic research in the past two decades have clearly shown that regular exercise is associated with many health benefits. Both preventive as well as therapeutic effects of exercise have been found in physical and mental illness. Only a relatively few negative health effects from exercise have been reported. These negative effects are predominantly associated with musculoskeletal injuries. Musculoskeletal injury rates have been reported in a variety of sports and age groups[1-3] and appear to be relatively high. However, no studies that compare these overall rates to the incidence of musculoskeletal problems in sedentary individuals are available. The overall importance of exercise-induced injuries relative to the health benefits remains unclear. A clear understanding of the nature of the injury can possibly lead to injury prevention while enabling the individual to enjoy the other health benefits.

Data on effective injury prevention are still emerging, but many studies have addressed the diagnosis, treatment, and rehabilitation of these exercise-induced injuries, since these injuries are thought to be a major impediment to an exercise-oriented lifestyle. Consequently, numerous books and articles[4-6] in the past decade have described modes of treatment for many injuries. In particular, research on surgical treatment of major injuries has been the center of attention. Basic science data on the exact pathophysiology of these and minor injuries are often lacking. Only recently has some of the research taken a step back and focused again on the understanding of basic processes that follow an exercise-induced injury. This chapter will review this basic research as it pertains to the role of the immune system in these injuries. It will also focus on the local immune response at the site of injury.

II. TYPES OF INJURY

Exercise-induced injuries can be classified in many ways. Traditionally, this has been done according to type of tissue and anatomic site involved. The resulting descriptions, such as medial collateral ligament injury of the knee, may be helpful for the clinician, but less so for the basic scientist, since most soft tissue injuries of muscle, tendon, or ligament appear to elicit a similar response from the body and its immune system. Therefore, it may be more appropriate to classify injuries according to the type of insult that caused the injury. This could be a classification based on acute and chronic injuries.[7] Acute injuries are those injuries that are caused by a single traumatic force. This force exceeds the strength of a previously healthy structure and, therefore, results in a macroscopic injury. The typical response to this injury is an inflammatory reaction with subsequent healing. The definition of a chronic injury may be more complicated. A chronic exercise-induced injury should not be equated with a chronic inflammatory reaction. An acute injury often shows a classic, acute, inflammatory reaction, but a chronic injury does not appear to result in a chronic, granulomatous reaction. It is not clear whether inflammation is an important part of most chronic injuries.

In general, a chronic injury is caused by repetitive motion. The force of each cycle by itself does not exceed the strength of the involved structure. However, the cumulative effect of repetitive cycles somehow results in an injury that may only be detectable on a microscopic or even subcellular level. On the other hand, repetitive and submaximal cycles have been shown to stimulate the involved structure to strengthen itself (a training effect). A specific physiological adaptation occurs in response to the imposed demands. For instance, tendons and ligaments become mechanically stronger when exercised repeatedly.[8,9] It is often unclear where a physiologic response to repetitive motion stops and a chronic exercise-induced injury begins. This issue will be discussed in more depth later in this chapter.

III. ACUTE EXERCISE-INDUCED INJURIES

Examples of acute exercise-induced injuries are often easy to find. Ligament tears or sprains and muscle tears or strains are prime examples of such injuries. In most cases, they appear to result from a simple mechanical overload of the involved structure. The macroscopic disruption is associated with tearing of the vascular, neural, and connective tissue elements. This results in local hemorrhage and cell death. The response to such an injury appears to be a "classical", acute, inflammatory response. There are many pathways through which this inflammatory response is mediated.[10-12] It is thought that the initial disruption of cell membranes, collagen fibers, and hemorrhages result in the generation of vasoactive mediators, chemotactic factors, and activation of the complement system. At the same time, neutrophils, macrophages, platelets and a coagulation system are recruited to participate in this response. Apart from activation of this response through inflammatory mediators, it is possible that some breakdown products of the injury are directly responsible for activation. Collagen breakdown products have been shown to result in direct chemotaxis of cells from the immune system.[13] The entire process, the acute-phase response, has been extensively studied in bacterial endotoxin response, but appears to be very similar in an acute exercise-induced injury.

One of the first systems to be activated is the complement system. This cascade of twenty plasma proteins can be activated through the "classical" or "alternative" pathways.[14] The classical pathway can be activated by several inflammatory mediators such as proteases, immune complexes, and polyanions. This pathway requires proteins C1, C2, and C4 before activating C3. The alternative pathway can be stimulated by damaged host cells and results in a direct binding of C3. The final common pathway is the formation of active anaphylatoxins and a membrane attack complex that can induce cell lysis. The functions of the anaphylatoxins are multiple and include increased vascular permeability directly or through basophil and mastcell degranulation.

They also modulate immune function by acting as chemotactic factors for leukocytes. Finally, they can activate arachidonic acid metabolite formation which can further enhance the increase in vascular permeability.

Arachidonic acid can be released from injured and intact phospholipid cell membranes during an acute inflammatory response.[15,16] Activated phospholipases liberate arachidonic acid, which can be metabolized through lipoxygenase and cyclooxygenase pathways. Lipid peroxidation results in the formation of leukotrienes and oxygen radicals. Leukotrienes have been shown to have strong pro-inflammatory action and some of the leukotrienes have been called collectively the slow-reacting substances of anaphylaxis (SRS-A). They can bring about smooth muscle contraction and increased microvascular permeability. The cyclooxygenase pathway results in the formation of prostaglandins and thromboxane. The function of the prostaglandins is more controversial. Several prostaglandins have been shown to have pro-inflammatory effects. However, others appear to function as a negative feedback mechanism on some parts of the developing inflammation and modulate immune functions. For instance, PGE2 is capable of inhibition of interleukin-1 (IL-1), a potent inflammatory cytokine.[17] Some prostaglandins may also have an anabolic effect following an injury, as evidenced by delayed wound[18] and bone healing[19] in the presence of nonsteroidal anti-inflammatory medication which inhibits prostaglandin production.

Following the initial generation of vasoactive, pro-inflammatory mediators, cellular elements are recruited to the area of injury. Both neutrophils, monocytes/macrophages, as well as lymphocytes, are recruited to the area. Chemotactic factors, such as complement-derived C5a and leukotriene B4, result in margination of inflammatory cells along vascular walls at the site of injury. After adherence and migration through the vascular wall, the inflammatory cells can be activated to perform their phagocytic function. The activation or stimulus-response coupling within the neutrophil appears to be regulated through changes in intracellular calcium, activation of phospholipase and protein kinase.[20,21] After activation, clearance of injured and necrotic tissues can commence. Initial engulfment by the neutrophil cell membrane of the necrotic debris results in the formation of a phagosome. After fusion with lysosomes, the proteolytic enzymes can complete the degradation in the phagolysosome.

It is likely that in a later phase of the body response to the injury, a cell-mediated hypersensitivity reaction occurs. For instance, experimentally induced muscle strains develop an extensive macrophage and lymphocyte infiltration several days following the injury.[22] If macrophages continue to be stimulated with an appropriate antigen at the site of injury, they can activate antigen-specific T-lymphocytes. This can occur after binding with the antigen, but also through cytokines such as IL-1 and tumor necrosis factor (TNF) produced by the macrophages. The activated T-lymphocytes release lymphokines which results in additional recruitment of activated inflammatory cells. Lymphocytes and macrophages are responsible for clearing residual cellular and matrix debris.

In addition to phagocytosis, the cellular immune response also appears to play a critical role in the induction of the fibroblast healing response. IL-1 and TNF can be produced by macrophages, and appear to stimulate the subsequent fibroblast proliferation and synthetic activity.[23,24] These cytokines may be responsible in part for modulating the fibroblastic scarring response that occurs at the site of injury. Fibronectin (a glycoprotein), derived from the initial clot, and macrophages attract fibroblasts and allow adherence of matrix and cellular elements.[25] Transforming growth factor-beta (TGF-β) is another macrophage-derived cytokine with profound effects on matrix proliferation.[26] TNF and TGF also influence the ingrowth of new capillaries into the injured area.[27] Besides macrophages and lymphocytes, platelets in the clot that forms in the injured area can induce a healing response. Platelet-derived growth factor may be responsible for some of these effects.[28] Finally, prostaglandins may also modulate the fibroblast response, directly or through other cytokines. The fibroblasts, through their collagen production, are responsible for the eventual recovery of mechanical strength. Modulation of their activity can result in a change in strength. Dahners et al.[29] found an early increase in strength in healing rat ligaments treated with NSAIDs.

Through a complex process with multiple pathways, the body first appears to increase the injury by inducing increased vascular permeability, generating mediators that result in increased pain, and recruiting additional inflammatory cells from the immune system elsewhere in the body (see Figure 1). Although this appears to be detrimental at first glance, it finally results in the resolution of the injury. The pain will force the body to limit the use of the injured structure and thereby contain the injury. The inflammatory cells are, in fact, the only way in which the body can clear necrotic cells and injured extracellular matrix. Only then is ingrowth of new cellular elements possible, which results in a mechanical healing of the injury. A clear example of this principle is the tears of the meniscal cartilage of the knee. Isolated tears have little propensity to heal. However, when the outer vascularized rim is mechanically roughened to stimulate an inflammatory response, the tears can often heal.[30] This process can be augmented by placing a bloodclot within the tear.[31]

An important issue for clinicians dealing with acute exercise-induced injuries is the question of whether the initial response of the body overshoots its goal. Is all the swelling, hemorrhage, and pain necessary before healing can take place? Traditionally, it is felt that the early inflammation should be contained as best as possible through intervention with anti-inflammatory medication and/or physical modalities. Although little is known about this issue, it appears that the available treatment options may have only a limited impact on this post-injury response.[32]

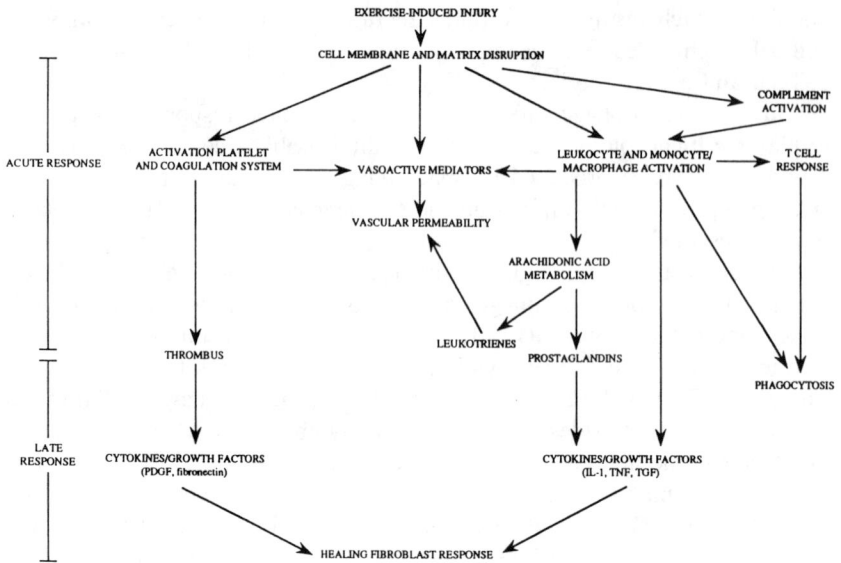

FIGURE 1. Summary of some mechanisms involved in the response of an exercise-induced injury.

IV. CHRONIC EXERCISE-INDUCED INJURIES

As mentioned before, one of the difficulties in studying chronic injuries lies in the close resemblance to changes that occur as a physiologic response to training. For instance, a twofold increase in plasma complement levels has been found following a 2.5-h running protocol.[33] Such a manifestation of the acute-phase response suggests an exercise-induced injury. However, many runners are able to tolerate such a protocol without clinical evidence of injury. Similarly, increases in numbers of circulating neutrophils can be found during and after exercise.[34] Again, this does not necessarily signify a pathologic situation.

At the cellular level, the most studied situation is that of exercise-induced muscle damage. It has been long known that vigorous eccentric exercise results in a delayed onset muscle soreness which usually peaks at about 48 h. Eccentric exercise involves contractions of the muscles as they are lengthened. Exercises, such as running, involve many eccentric contractions since the muscles are often used to absorb the shock of landing on the leg. The muscles contract to dampen the shock, but are still forcibly lengthened by the force of the impact. Investigations in delayed-onset muscle soreness (DOMS) have shown evidence of ultrastructural damage of the muscle, with partial necrotic muscle fibers[35] and loss of striations.[36] Evidence of an immune response was also found by Jones et al.[37] They have shown mononuclear cell infiltration several days following the exercise. Finally, increases in serum levels of myocellular enzymes, such as creatinekinase, have been found. Although this is evidence that the exercise caused a loss of cell membrane integrity, the levels do not correlate well with the ultrastructural damage and loss of function that is seen following the exercise. Again, many of the cellular changes seen after eccentric exercise resemble elements of an inflammatory reaction. However, subsequent bouts of eccentric exercise usually result in a decrease of the DOMS and its cellular changes, suggesting the initial response was merely an adaptation of the body to increased demands. It is possible that weak and inadequate muscle fibers were eliminated during the initial bout of exercise.[38] On the other hand, cellular destruction does appear to take place and it could be an example of a mild injury. Possible explanations of this type of chronic exercise-induced injury could be the mechanical shearing between fibers during exercise, disturbances in cell volume or energy state, and transient ischemia. Reperfusion after ischemia has been shown to result in oxygen radical production by neutrophils and mitochondria.[39,40]

Chronic exercise-induced injuries are often described as repetitive motion or overuse injuries. It is thought that repetitive tensile, compressive, or shear forces eventually exceed the adaptive capabilities of the involved structure. However, each cycle of tensile, compressive, or shear force by itself is not sufficient to cause an acute exercise-induced injury. Many of these injuries are often described as tendonitis, bursitis, or fasciitis, suggesting an inflammatory component to these injuries. This as an assumption that remains to be proven. To date, relatively little is known about the exact pathophysiology of chronic exercise-induced injuries. Some histological studies suggest mainly a degenerative process with very little evidence of inflammatory cell infiltration.[41,42,43] Occasionally, a small lymphocytic infiltration is seen in the synovial tendon sheath.[44] These studies may be biased since they rely on surgical specimens from end-stage injuries. On the other hand, these findings are supported by the fact that treatment of these injuries with anti-inflammatory modalities does not appear very efficacious.[45] The diagnosis of tendonitis may, therefore, not be appropriate and may have to be replaced by tendinosis with secondary paratendonitis.

Early *in vitro* studies are being carried out to study the effect of repetitive motion on cells in cell culture. Low levels of mechanical stimulation have been shown to stimulate cell metabolism towards increased synthesis.[46] These findings probably correlate with the adaptive response of cells to increased demands. Higher and longer levels of mechanical stimulation result in an increased production of prostaglandin E_2 and leukotrienes, suggesting that the arachidonic acid metabolism is activated. After cultured tendon fibroblasts are repetitively stretched at 10 cycles per minute for 3 h or more, they produced markedly increased levels of PGE2.[47] Whether this indicates that the adaptive capabilities of the cells are exceeded is still not clear. However, prostaglandins such as PGE2 have been associated with catabolic responses and its production may still be evidence of cell injury.[48]

It is likely that future research will better define the levels of exercise where an adaptive response is not adequate and more permanent injury occurs. It is currently not clear whether such a chronic and often small injury is capable of invoking a complete immune response from the body. Both collagen and proteoglycan fragments have been shown to be able to be immunoreactive.[49,50] Theoretically, they are capable of eliciting a cellular immune response. Since most of the data thus far have shown little or no inflammatory changes, it is possible that only a limited number of the inflammatory pathways are activated. Once those pathways are identified, treatment can possibly be made more rational. Thus far, most forms of treatment are based on anecdotal and empirical findings rather than truly scientific data.

REFERENCES

1. **Dehaven, K. E. and Lintner, D. M.,** Athletic injuries: comparison by age, sport and gender, *Am. J. Sports Med.,* 14, 218, 1986.
2. **James, S. L., Bates, B. T., and Osternig, L. R.,** Injuries to runners, *Am. J. Sports Med.,* 6, 40, 1978.
3. **Keller, C. S., Noyes, F. R., and Buncher, C. R.,** The medical aspects of soccer injury epidemiology, *Am. J. Sports Med.,* 15, 230, 1987.
4. **Kellett, J.,** Acute soft tissue injuries: a review of the literature, *Med. Sci. Sports Exerc.,* 18, 489, 1986.
5. **O'Donoghue, D. H.,** *Treatment of Injuries to Athletes,* W.B. Saunders, Philadelphia, 1976.
6. **Peterson, L. and Renstrom, P.,** Sports injuries: their prevention and treatment, Yearbook Publishers, Chicago, 1986.
7. **Leadbetter, W. B., Buckwalter, J. A., and Gordon, S. L., Eds.,** *Sports Induced Inflammation,* American Academy of Orthopedic Surgeons, Park Ridge, IL, 1989.
8. **Cabaud, H. E., Chatty, A., Gildengorin, V., et al.,** Exercise effects on the strength of the rat anterior cruciate ligament, *Am. J. Sports Med.,* 8, 79, 1980.
9. **Tipton, C. M., James, S. L., Mergner, W., et al.,** Influence of exercise on strength of medial collateral ligaments in dogs, *Am. J. Physiol.,* 218, 894, 1970.
10. **Houck, J. C., Ed.,** *Chemical Messengers of the Inflammatory Process,* Elsevier/North Holland Biomedical Press, Amsterdam, 1979.
11. **Movat, H. Z.,** *The Inflammatory Reaction,* Elsevier Science Publishers, Amsterdam, 1985.
12. **Weissman, G., Ed.,** *The Cell Biology of Inflammation,* Elsevier/North Holland Biomedical Press, Amsterdam, 1980.
13. **Postlethwaite, A. E. and Kang, A. H.,** Collagen- and collagen peptide-induced chemotaxis of human blood monocytes, *J. Exp. Med.,* 143, 1299, 1976.
14. **Bellanti, J. A., Ed.,** *Immunology III,* 3rd ed., W.B. Saunders, Philadelphia, 1985.
15. **Marcus, A. J.,** The eicosanoids in biology and medicine, *J. Lipid Res.,* 25, 1511, 1984.
16. **Samuelsson, B.,** Leukotrienes: mediators of immediate hypersensitivity reaction and inflammation, *Science,* 220, 568, 1983.
17. **Kunkel, S. L., Chensue, S. W., and Phan, S. M.,** Prostaglandins as endogenous mediators of interleukin-1 production, *J. Immunol.,* 136, 186, 1986.

18. **Proper, S. A., Frenske, N. A., Burnett, S. M., et al.,** Compromised wound repair caused by perioperative use of ibuprofen, *J. Am. Acad. Dermatol.,* 18, 1173, 1988.
19. **Tornkvist, H., Lindholm, S., Netz, P., et al.,** Effect of ibuprofen and indomethacin on bone metabolism reflected in bone strength, *Clin. Orthop. Rel. Res.,* 187, 255, 1984.
20. **Becker, E. L.,** Leucocyte stimulation: receptor, membrane and metabolic events, *Fed. Proc.,* 45, 2148, 1986.
21. **Synderman, R. and Pike, M. C.,** Chemoattractant receptors on phagocytic cells, *Annu. Rev. Immunol.,* 2, 257, 1984.
22. **Almekinders, L. C. and Gilbert, J. A.,** Healing of experimental muscle strains and the effects of non-steroidal anti-inflammatory medication, *Am. J. Sports Med.,* 14, 303, 1986.
23. **Bartold, P. M.,** The effect of interleukin 1 beta on proteoglycans synthesized by gingival fibroblasts in vitro, *Connect. Tissue Res.,* 17, 287, 1988.
24. **Vilcek, J., Palombella, V. J., Henriksen-DiStefano, D., et al.,** Fibroblast growth enhancing activity of tumor necrosis factor and its relationship to other polypeptide growth factors, *J. Exp. Med.,* 163, 632, 1986.
25. **Nathan, C. F.,** Secretory products of macrophages, *J. Clin. Invest.,* 79, 319, 1987.
26. **Roberts, A. B., Sporn, M. B., Assoian, R. K., et al.,** Transforming growth factor type beta: rapid induction of fibrosis and angiogenesis *in vivo* and stimulation of collagen formation *in vitro, Proc. Natl. Acad. Aci. U.S.A.,* 83, 4167, 1986.
27. **Folkman, J. and Klagsbrun, M.,** A family of angiogenic peptides, *Science,* 329, 671, 1987.
28. **Ross, R., Raines, E. W., and Bowen-Pope, D. F.,** The biology of platelet derived growth factor, *Cell,* 46, 155, 1986.
29. **Dahners, L. E., Phillips, H. O., and Almekinders, L. C.,** The effect of piroxicam on ligament healing in rats, *Transact. 32nd Ann. ORS,* 1986; 11, 77, 1986.
30. **Henning, C. E., Lynch, M. A., Clark, J. R.,** Vascularity for healing of meniscus repairs, *Arthroscopy,* 3, 13, 1987.
31. **Arnoczky, S. P., Warref, R. F., and Spivak, J. M.,** Meniscal repair using an exogenous fibrin clot: an experimental study in dogs, *J. Bone Joint Surg.,* 70A, 1209, 1988.
32. **Almekinders, L. C.,** The efficacy on non-steroidal anti-inflammatory medication in ligament injuries, *Sports Med.,* 9, 137, 1990.
33. **Dufaux, B., Muller, R., and Hollmann, W.,** Assessment of circulating immune complexes by a solid-phase Clq-binding assay during the first hours and days after prolonged exercise, *Clin. Chim. Acta,* 145, 313, 1985.
34. **Steel, C. M., Evans, J., and Smith, M. A.,** Physiological variations in circulating B cell:T cell ratio in man, *Nature (London),* 247, 387, 1974.
35. **Hikida, R. S., Staron, R. S., Hagerman, F. C., et al.,** Muscle fiber necrosis associated with human marathon runners, *J. Neuro. Sci.,* 59, 185, 1983.
36. **Friden, J., Seger, J., Sjostrom, M., et al.,** Adaptive response in human skeletal muscle subjected to prolonged eccentric training, *Int. J. Sports Med.,* 4, 177, 1983.
37. **Jones, D. A., Newham, D. J., Round, J. M., et al.,** Experimental human muscle damage: morphological changes in relation to other indices of damage, *J. Physiol. (London),* 375, 435, 1986.
38. **Newham, D. J., Jones, D. A., and Clarlison, D. M.,** Repeated high force eccentric exercise: effects on muscle pain and damage, *J. Appl. Physiol.,* 63, 1381, 1987.
39. **Parker, L.,** Vitamin E, physical exercise and tissue damage in animals, *Med. Biol.,* 62, 105, 1984.
40. **Smith, F. K., Grisham, M. B., Granger, D. N., et al.,** Free radical defense mechanism and neutrophil infiltration in postischemic skeletal muscle, *Am. J. Physiol.,* 256, H789, 1989.
41. **Ferretti, A., Ippolito, E., Mariano, P., et al.,** Jumper's knee, *Am. J. Sports Med.,* 11, 58, 1983.

42. **Jozsa, L., Balint, B. J., Reffy, A., et al.,** Hypoxic alterations of tenocytes in degenerative tendinopathy, *Acta Orthop., Trauma Surg.,* 99, 243, 1982.
43. **Martens, M., Wouters, P., and Burssens, A.,** Patellar tendinitis: pathology and results of treatment, *Acta Orthop. Scand.,* 53, 445, 1982.
44. **Kvist, M., Josza, L., Jarvinen, M., et al.,** Chronic achilles paratendonitis in athletes: a histological and histochemical study, *Pathology,* 19, 11, 1987.
45. **Almekinders, L. C. and Almekinders, S. V.,** Outcome and compliance in treatment of overuse injuries, in press.
46. **Sutker, B. D., Lester, G. E., Banes, A. J., et al.,** Cyclic strain stimulates DNA and collagen synthesis in fibroblasts cultured from rat medial collateral ligaments, *Transact. 36th Annu. Orthop. Res. Soc.,* 15, 130, 1990.
47. **Almekinders, L. C., Banes, A. J., and Ballinger, C. A.,** Unpublished data.
48. **Baracos, V., Rodemann, P., Dinarello, C. A., et al.,** Stimulation of muscle protein degradation and prostaglandin E_2 release by leucocyte pyrogen (interleukin-1), *N. Engl. J. Med.,* 3008, 553, 1983.
49. **Garbrecht, F. C., Ragsdale, C. G., Schultz, J. S., et al.,** Autoimmunity to articular collagen in patients with osteoarticular syndromes, *J. Rheumatol.,* 13, 517, 1986.
50. **Golds, E. E. and Poole, A. R.,** Connective tissue antigens stimulate collagenase production in arthritic diseases, *Cell. Immunol.,* 86, 190, 1984.

Chapter 10

EXERCISE AND AGE-RELATED DECLINE IN IMMUNE FUNCTIONS

Robert S. Mazzeo and Imran Nasrullah

TABLE OF CONTENTS

I. INTRODUCTION

The decline in the responsiveness of the immune system with advancing age is well documented.[43,65,72,77,95] This immunosenescence can result in an increased incidence of tumorgenesis, infectious diseases, and auto-immune disorders in the elderly. While many of the components which make up the immune system are affected by age, the T-cell compartment appears to be most adversely affected (secondary to thymic involution). Both quantitative as well as qualitative changes in several factors associated with cell-mediated immunity, including recognition of antigen/mitogen, cell activation and pro-liferation, total cell numbers and subset distributions, lymphokine production, and receptor expression, have been reported to be altered with age. A few interventions have been employed in an attempt to offset, delay, or restore the age-related decline in immune function. Thymic and bone marrow cell grafts into old mice have been shown to partially restore immune function, suggesting that the involution of the thymus with age plays a major role in immunosenescence.[48,49,106] This is further supported by the observation that administration of thymic hormones can restore T-cell-dependent antibody response in old animals.[23,26,32,111] Most impressive are the results from dietary restriction studies in which the increased longevity and reduction of disease has been attributed, in part, to an enhanced immune function.[22,104,109]

A program of regular aerobic exercise has been shown to elicit beneficial outcomes in both the prevention and rehabilitation of many disease states, including heart disease, stroke, hypertension, diabetes, and cancer. However, the extent to which such an exercise training program can influence immuno-responsiveness is not as clear. Evidence for a positive relationship has been suggested by the observations that a lack of exercise (bedrest, immobilization) has been associated with a depression in immune function,[16,20,36] while in-creased physical activity contributes to both a reduction in tumor growth and the incidence of certain types of cancer.[33,51,107] Thus, the prospect of exercise as an immunoenhancing therapy is beginning to receive more attention; un-fortunately, the information on exercise and immunity is confounding due to differences in species, exercise intensity, and duration, as well as differences between acute and chronic responses. Further, information concerning the role of exercise in offsetting or restoring immune function in elderly popu-lations, as well as any potential deleterious effects, is extremely limited. Our own laboratory has tried to address this issue by looking at key components of the aging immune system in the Fischer 344 rat. Much of our efforts have been to examine cell-mediated immune function, particularly T-cell blasto-genesis, IL-2 production, and natural cytotoxicity.

II. AGE-ASSOCIATED CHANGES IN CELL-MEDIATED IMMUNITY

Among the decline in immune responsiveness with advancing age, T-cell-dependent functions are the most prominent. This has been attributed primarily to the involution of the thymus documented to occur with age.[2,47,50,106] As maturation, as well as differentiation, of T-cells occurs in the thymus, both age-related reductions in functional T-cell number and alterations in the ratios of T-cell subsets have been reported.[40,46,59] In addition, while the exact mechanisms remain uncertain, loss of thymic hormonal activity also contributes to immunosenescence of cell-mediated immunity.[23,26,32,111]

Successful induction of cell-mediated immunity is dependent upon the interaction of many components. Defects in a number of critical variables occur with advancing age. These alterations are briefly summarized below. (For more comprehensive reviews, see References 19, 65, and 72.)

A. MACROPHAGE FUNCTION

Fundamental to an effective immune response is proper function of macrophages. Macrophages attack and process antigens before presentation to T-cells for recognition. Further, macrophages also release interleukin 1 (IL-1) which stimulates activation and proliferation of T-cells. Thus, any malfunctions inherent in macrophage function would result in a blunted immune response independent of antigen-specific T- and B-cell integrity. In general, the capacity of macrophages for phagocytosis and IL-1 production may decrease slightly with age; however, this does not appear to be physiologically significant.[13,45,85,93] Reduced IL-1 synthesis in response to antigen/mitogen occurs in macrophages of aged mice; however, these deficiencies may be compensated by augmented macrophage numbers, at least in the peritoneum.[12] The release of "suppressor molecules" by aged macrophages may contribute to reduced T-cell mediated immunity such as plaque-forming cell (PFC) responses. This is evidenced by the observation that removal of culture supernatant after 24 h followed with the reintroduction of fresh media along with aged B- and T-cells results in PFC reconstitution.[1] Further, the ability of macrophages from aged mice to facilitate cytolytic T-lymphocyte (CTL) reactions to murine tumor lines is attenuated when compared to young mice.[12]

Any decline in T-cell dependent immunity seems more a function of age-related defects inherent in T-cells rather than in monocytes, as will be discussed later. However, decreases in T-cell mediated immunity are in part due to deterioration of accessory cell/T cell interaction, since young accessory cells mixed with aged T-cells showed marked improvement ($p < 0.05$) to mitogen responsiveness, while aged accessory cells do not.[7] Others, however, have found that age-related attenuation of IL-2 receptor expression is similar, independent of accessory cell donor age.[12]

B. T-CELLS

Despite the age-associated involution of the thymus, T-cell numbers appear to be maintained with age in peripheral blood and in lymphoid organs (with the exception of the thymus in which T-cell numbers decline).[56,92,111] However, the percentage of T-cells capable of entering mitosis/replication cycle, necessary for complete immune responsiveness, has been reported to decline with advancing age.[43,71] This is supported by the observation that the proliferative capacity of aged T-cells exposed to mitogens (e.g., conconvalin A, Con-A) is markedly reduced. The proliferative capacity of aged lymphocytes decreases in both rats[38,82,98] and in humans.[21,34,37,66,74] Cheung et al.[15] showed that proliferation in rats peaks at 4 months of age, but declines linearly to the age of 20 months, such that proliferation of the aged animals is 36% that of the young. Protein synthesis also followed the same trend, peaking at 4 months and declining steadily to 20 months; the most radical reductions occurring from 12 to 20 months. Mixed lymphocyte reactions and mitogen stimulation[37,38,74] also show reduced proliferation among aged lymphocytes. In humans, the reduced proliferative capacity, as well as reduced frequency of T-cell responses are evident.[74] Similar results have also been found by Froelich et al.,[34] who showed significant reductions in thymidine uptake by aged peripheral blood lymphocytes. Mechanisms explaining poor proliferation by aged lymphocytes have identified deficiencies in IL-2 production, IL-2 receptors and expression, and calcium kinetics.[31,37,38,41,71,87]

Reports on changes or shifts in the distribution of T-cell subsets with age have been inconsistent. Several studies examining peripheral blood lymphocytes in humans have found no changes in the ratios of T-cell subsets.[61,76] Others have reported both increases and decreases in various subsets particularly in T-helper as well as suppressor/cytolytic cells.[8,59,67,75,91] Data from animal studies on lymphoid tissue have been more definitive in their reports of alterations in T-cell subsets with age.[2,3,13,39,46,105,106]

Cytotoxic T-cells *in vivo* cytotoxicity with BM-2 primed splenocytes show significant activity at all effector:target cell ratios among aged rats.[38] *In vitro* studies show that among young rats, cytotoxic activity is mediated primarily via the cytotoxic T-cells (CTC), and with age the proportion of CTC involved diminishes.[38,67] The functional activity, affinity for target cells, and total number of allogenic T-cytotoxic cells was found to decline with age in senescent mice.[3,6,39,113] Primary and secondary responses to influenza viral infection are also significantly reduced.[20] Cytotoxicity is also reduced significantly against both NK resistant and NK target cell lines over a range of E:T ratios.[66] The reduction in CTC activity that is seen during aging can be alleviated to some extent by the addition of exogenous IL-2.[14,97,99] For example, the primary cytolytic responses increase to near youthful levels, while

TABLE 1
Age-Related Changes on Two Variables of Cell-Mediated Immunity

IL-2 synthesis	T-cell blastogenesis	Ref.
N.A.	CD8+ decrease	66
Decrease	T-cell decrease	98
N.A.	T-cell decrease	12
N.A.	T-cell decrease	7
N.A.	T-cell decrease	74
Decrease	N.A.	97
Decrease	T-cell decrease	38
N.A.	CD8+ decrease	41
Decrease	T-cell decrease	82
Decrease	T-cell decrease	53
Decrease	T-cell decrease	34
Decrease	T-cell decrease	14

Note: N.A., not applicable.

secondary cytolytic responses return to full activity upon addition of exogenous IL-2.[97] This phenomenon may be tissue specific since the addition of exogenous IL-2 to splenic T-cells was found to have no beneficial effect.[38]

C. NATURAL KILLER CELLS

Information pertaining to natural killer (NK) function and aging are somewhat inconclusive. Generally, the majority of studies examining peripheral blood lymphocytes in humans have found no major changes in NK number and activity with age.[27,74,101] Murasko et al.[74] reported no change in percent mean cytotoxicity (E:T of 50:1) between subjects greater than 70 when compared with young adult controls. However, others have documented age-related declines in NK activity in their subjects.[84,89] Data from animal studies (mice, rats) examining splenic cells are more consistent in reporting decreases in both NK number and their ability to lyse susceptible target cells.[5,11,88,90,110] The conflicting data reported in the literature may be related to species or tissue differences.

D. IL-2 PRODUCTION AND RECEPTOR FUNCTION

A primary concern for the aging organism is related to the ability of generation T-cells and their responsiveness to activating stimuli.[3,6,39,113] IL-2 plays a major role in the proliferation and differentiation of helper, cytolytic, and suppressor T-cells. Thus, any reductions in IL-2 activity and function can have rather a significant impact on overall immune responsiveness. As shown in Table 1, this aging effect may be related to deficiencies in IL-2 synthesis and receptor function. In addition, as mentioned earlier, defects in calcium kinetics can also significantly affect cell activation and may contribute to the reduction in cytokine secretion and receptor expression.

A consistent finding in both human and animal models is that aging is associated with a diminished capacity for IL-2 synthesis.[21,37,54,97,98] Aging is associated with a significant decline in IL-2 production when compared to young controls.[21,34,37,82] Thoman and Weigle[98] demonstrated that "young" murine splenocytes produce a tenfold greater amount of IL-2 at peak mitogen doses than do aged donors, over a varied concentration of cells. Mixed lymphocyte reactions (MLTC) using allogeneic BM-2 cells results in decreased IL-2 production by aged rat splenocytes.[38] The decline in IL-2 production may be attributed to a three-fold reduction in the number of cells actively synthesizing IL-2 mRNA, especially intermediate to high levels.[31,112] These findings are further supported by the observation that *in vitro* addition of purified exogenous IL-2 can partially restore functional defects and proliferative capabilities in lymphocytes from elderly subjects.[14,97,99]

The reduction in IL-2 synthesis with advancing age is further complicated by the findings that the number, affinity, and expression of IL-2 receptors is also adversely affected with age.[37,77,91,100,108] Advancing age among humans has been shown to reduce the number of cells which bear IL-2 receptors by 50 to 70% of young controls, while the remainder produce amounts typical of young donor cells.[97] Aging is associated with a reduction of IL-2 receptors and appearance rate of new receptors,[61] as well as a loss in signal transduction due to dysfunction of high affinity IL-2 receptors (alpha beta). Further, there is a concomitant increase in low affinity IL-2 receptors (alpha alpha).[87] These results are similar to Froelich et al.,[34] who showed that aging among humans was associated with a significant reduction in IL-2R, while low affinity (alpha alpha) receptors remained similar. However, no change was reported in the Kd of IL-2R between the two age groups.[34,53]

Finally, defects at the level of calcium influx have routinely been observed in aging T-cells.[41,70,86] Calcium plays a key role in the antigen-induced activation cycle of lymphocytes, including IL-2 secretion and the expression of IL-2 receptors. In this regard, the use of a calcium ionophore (ionomycin) has been documented to partially restore the proliferative response of T-cells from aged mice.[69,100]

E. HUMORAL RESPONSE

Much of the aging process that affects T-cell membrane and intracellular mechanisms can also affect B-cells since both utilize the same scheme in activation events. Calcium mobilization, cyclic nucleotide fluxes, and membrane transmission through surface receptors have reduced fidelity in their functioning. The decline in B-cell function can also be attributed to the decline in lymphokine secretion associated with age-related T-cell function.[19] Gahring and Weigle[35] have shown that antibody production to human gamma globulin (HGG) in aged CBA/CaJ (24 to 27 months) and C57BL/6JNNia (24 to 25

TABLE 2

Influence of Exercise on Various Components of the Immune System

Type of exercise	Proliferation or activity	Secretory product	Population	Ref.
Acute exercise	↓ T-cell	N.A.	↓ T cell	29
Post-marathon	↓ T-cell	↑ anti-tetanus toxoid	N.A.	24
Post-exercise (50 km)	N.A.	↓ IgA	↑ B cell no ΔT cell	102
Post-exercise (8 mi, 75% VO₂ max)	↑ NK activity and B-cell	no Δ IgG, IgA IgM	no ΔT cell	42
6-month swim training	↓ T-cells	↓ IL-2	N.A.	82
8 weeks training + exhaustive exercise	↓ T-cell, suppressor	N.A.	N.A.	94
Post 3-h marathon	↓ NK activity	N.A.	↓ NK cells	9
10 weeks swim training	↓ T-cells	N.A.	N.A.	64
GXT-cycle ergometer	N.A.	N.A.	↑ lymphocytes ↓ OKT4+	68
15-week walking	↑ NK activity	N.A.	no Δ NK	80
Acute cycling; 75% VO₂ max	↑ NK activity	N.A.	↑ NK	55
Acute cycling; various intensities	↓ T-cells	N.A.	N.A.	63
Maximal cycling	N.A.	↓ IL-2	↑ CD4,CD8,NK ↓ CD4:CD8	58
5 km race; trained subjects	N.A.	↓ IL-2, ↑ TNFα	↑ NK and CD4:CD8	25

Note: N.A., not applicable.

months) decreases significantly when compared to young mice (6 to 8 weeks) of respective strains. Although CBA/CaJ mice have better antibody responses to HGG than C57BL/6JNNia at each age, both groups showed large decreases in antibody production with age.

III. THE EFFECT OF EXERCISE ON IMMUNITY

Exercise has been shown to influence immune function (Table 2). The extent to which an acute bout of exercise can modulate immune function is dependent upon a number of variables, including the intensity and duration of exercise as well as training status of the individual. In an attempt to respond to the stress imposed from a single bout of exercise, a number of neuroendocrine responses are elicited. These responses help the individual to adjust, both physiologically and metabolically, to the disruptions in homeostasis imposed by exercise. These neuroendocrine responses can make a significant contribution to the alterations in immune responsiveness documented to occur during exercise.

Endurance training is well known to elicit significant improvements in many cardiovascular and musculoskeletal variables including maximal oxygen consumption, stroke volume, local blood flow, and proliferation of mitochondrial enzymes. The effect of endurance training on immune function is not as well defined; however, recent investigations in young healthy populations have begun to generate interesting findings. As these results have been discussed in other chapters, we will briefly summarize some of these observations below. (See References 57, 62, 81 for extensive reviews.)

A. SEDENTARY POPULATION

In sedentary individuals, exhaustive cycling produces significant but transient increases in the number of leukocytes and lymphocytes, while mononuclear cells remain constant, and neutrophils markedly decrease. This leukocytosis and lymphocytosis induced by exercise can persist for several hours into the recovery period. A number of studies have implicated hormonal mechanisms as a primary regulator, specifically catecholamines and corticosteroids.[10,17,29,68,73,103] A high correlation ($r = 0.939$) exists between percent increase in lymphocyte count and both relative workload, as well as circulating epinephrine content ($r = 0.942$).[68] Further, the combination of moderate exercise with epinephrine infusions significantly enhanced NK cell activity in sedentary males.[55]

However, it is frequently reported that a single bout of heavy exercise can have an immunosuppressive effect on a number of variables associated with cell-mediated immunity, including T-cell blastogenesis, IL-2 production, and populations of subsets.[24,28,44,52,58,64,82] T-cell proliferation decreases in proportion to exercise intensity where the greater the intensity, the greater the reduction in proliferation.[63] Hormonal factors, once again, are thought to be involved in this exercise-induced phenomenon. Generally, values return to baseline levels 3 to 24 h post-exercise.

B. TRAINED POPULATION

Chronic endurance training has been reported to produce both beneficial and derogatory effects on the functioning of the immune system.[24,42,52,64,82,96] Discrepancies may stem from differences in species, tissue, or magnitude of training. Splenocytes isolated from Wistar rats that underwent 10 weeks of swim training demonstrated a protective effect on T-lymphocyte blastogenesis.[64] This was evidenced by a reduced suppressive effect of an exhaustive bout of exercise on T-cell blastogenesis in trained rats compared to controls. Hanson and Flaherty[42] showed that moderate exercise in highly trained runners results in increased NK activity 10 min post-exercise, with these increases still observed 24 h post-exercise. Recently, Tharp and Preuss[96] revealed that rats trained by 8 weeks of treadmill running demonstrated a significantly greater mitogenic responsiveness of spleen lymphocytes than did the sedentary controls. However, other investigators have found either no change or a reduction in a number of immunological variables associated with training in both animals and human models, including mitogen-induced lymphocyte proliferation and IL-2 production.[52,82,83] Pahlavani et al.[82] found that 6 months of swim training was associated with a 23 to 32% reduction in both mitogen-induced lymphocyte proliferation and IL-2 production in isolated splenocytes. In humans, Papa et al.[83] demonstrated a 28% decline in peripheral blood lymphocyte responsiveness to mitogen as well as a reduction in IL-2 receptor expression in athletes involved in long-term training compared to healthy controls.

C. HUMORAL IMMUNITY

Moderate exercise training (15 weeks at 60% VO_2 max) in mildly obese women did not result in significant increases in lymphocyte spontaneous blastogenesis; however, the levels of IgG, IgA and IgM increased significantly (20%) after 15 weeks of training.[78] Hanson and Flaherty[42] showed that moderate intensity exercise (72% VO_2 max) in highly trained runners did not elicit any significant increase in either B- or T-cells after 10 min or 24 h of exercise. Further, IgG, IgM, IgA, and IgE did not increase significantly after exercise. Tomasi et al.,[102] examined B-cell population, IgA and IgG levels in trained nordic skiers after a 50-km (males) and 20-km (female) race. Athletes had significantly less salivary IgA content at rest compared to controls and concentrations decreased to a greater extent following exercise. Results showed significant reductions in IgA 1 h post-exercise, while IgG levels did not change significantly. Percentage of B-lymphocytes was significantly elevated in the athletes after the race when compared with age-matched controls. Others have reported no differences in IgG, IgA, and IgM content at rest or during a graded maximal exercise test between trained marathon runners and sedentary controls.[79] Finally, Eskola et al.[24] showed that after a marathon, runners show normal IgG anti-toxin responsiveness to inoculation with tetanus toxoid after the race.

IV. THE EFFECTS OF EXERCISE ON AGE-RELATED IMMUNOSENESCENCE

Very little is known about the interaction between aging, exercise, and immunity. In this section we will discuss what is currently known, as well as some recent observations from our laboratory.

A. HUMAN STUDIES

Fiatarone et al.[30] examined the effect of a single maximal exercise test on peripheral blood lymphocyte NK cell activity in young (30 $\pm$ 1 year) and old (71 $\pm$ 1 year) women. Baseline function and numbers of NK cells did not differ between the two groups. In response to an acute bout of maximal exercise, NK activity increased significantly in both groups, but again, no difference was observed across age groups. Thus, while the exercise stimulus had an enhancing effect on NK activity, the effect was similar in both age groups. Similar findings were observed with regard to NK responsiveness to IL-2 stimulation.

A study involving 16 weeks of aerobic training with elderly women (72 ± 1 year) determined that the group engaged in regular exercise demonstrated elevated resting values of NK activity (↑ 33%) in peripheral blood lymphocytes when compared with an age-matched sedentary control group.[18] Further, while both groups experienced an increase in NK activity in response to an acute bout of incremental treadmill exercise, the group participating in regular exercise achieved significantly greater values of NK activity compared to controls (50.3 vs. 31.1%, respectively).

B. ANIMAL STUDIES

Animal studies investigating the relationship between exercise, aging, and the immune system have been just as scarce as human studies.

Pahlivani et al.[82] looked at age-related immunosenescence and the role of exercise in male F344 rats. These investigators examined rats of four different age groups (1, 6, 12, and 18 months of age, initially) after a 6-month training program. Rats were swim-trained for 60 min, twice daily, 5 d per week for six months. Age-matched controls were kept sedentary for the duration of the study. Interleukin-2 production and lymphocyte proliferation (both with Con-A and lipopolysaccharide stimulation) were measured in isolated splenocytes. At each age, the swim-trained rats had lower body weights than controls while adrenal hypertrophy was observed to occur in the young swim-trained animals only. Unstimulated, as well as mitogen-induced proliferation of lymphocytes in both trained (↓ 41%) and untrained (↓ 52%) rats declined significantly with increasing age. Consequently, the 24-month-old trained and untrained rats had lower (p < 0.001) proliferative responses as compared to their respective 7-month-old counterparts. Training resulted in a significant reduction in Con-A stimulated lymphocyte proliferation of splenocytes among 7- and 12-month-old rats (32 and 23%, respectively) when compared to their age-matched control groups. Among the 18- and 24-month-old rats, no significant differences were observed between trained and untrained groups. An age-related decline in IL-2 synthesis was observed in both the trained and the untrained rats. Twenty-four-month-old trained and untrained rats exhibited significantly less IL-2 production than their younger counterparts. Swim training was associated with significantly lower levels of IL-2 production when compared to sedentary control groups, but only for the 7-month-old (young) rats.

The authors concluded that exercise training could not prevent the age-related decline in both lymphocyte proliferation as well as IL-2 production. Further, training actually reduced the proliferative response and the ability for IL-2 production in the younger animals.

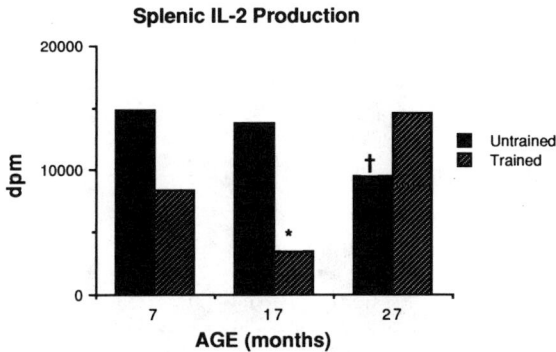

Splenic IL-2 Production

FIGURE 1. Production of IL-2 in isolated splenocytes from young, middle, and old Fischer 344 rats. Trained animals engaged in 15 weeks of treadmill running at 75% maximum capacity. † Significantly different from young animals ($p < 0.05$). * Significantly different from untrained animals ($p < 0.05$).

Data from our laboratory have examined the effect of chronic endurance training on IL-2 synthesis, T-cell proliferation and cytotoxicity in Fischer 344 rats of 7, 17, and 27 months of age. The animals underwent 15 weeks of treadmill running at 75% maximal capacity, 5 days/week for 60 min. Controls remained sedentary throughout the period of the study, but were exposed to 5 min of running once per week. After the 15-week period, animals were sacrificed at least 24 h after their last exercise session. The spleens were removed aseptically, and splenocytes were collected, put into suspension, and used as stock for the various assays. Interleukin-2 was produced by exposing splenocytes to 5 μg/ml Con-A for 24 h; thereafter, supernatants were collected and passed through 0.22 μ filters. IL-2 produced was measured by the IL-2 dependent cell line CTLL-2 as an indicator population. T-cell proliferation was assessed by thymidine uptake upon exposure to varied doses of Con-A over a 48-h period. Natural cytotoxicity was measured using a chromium release assay with YAC-1 cell line serving as the target cell population for splenic effectors.

Splenic IL-2 synthesis declined with age in the sedentary control animals (Figure 1). This significant aging effect was seen at each concentration of IL-2 examined, where the young had significantly greater ($p < 0.05$) levels of IL-2 than the aged. After 15 weeks of endurance training, a trend existed among the young and middle-aged rats indicating a suppression in the ability for IL-2 production in isolated splenocytes. These findings are in agreement with those of Pahlavani et al.[82] cited previously. However, unlike their findings, we found that training caused a dramatic increase in IL-2 production among 27-month-old rats such that levels equivalent to that witnessed in 7-month-old untrained rats were observed. Mitogen-induced splenic lymphocyte proliferation in response to Con-A revealed a pattern similar to that observed for IL-2 (Figure 2). There was a clear and significant decline in T-cell pro-

Splenic T cell Proliferation

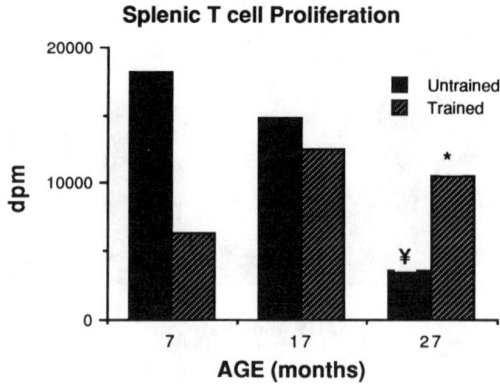

FIGURE 2. Con-A induced proliferation of splenic lymphocytes in trained and untrained rats across various ages. ¥ Significantly different from young and middle-aged animals ($p < 0.05$). * Significantly different from untrained animals ($p < 0.05$).

Thymic T cell proliferation

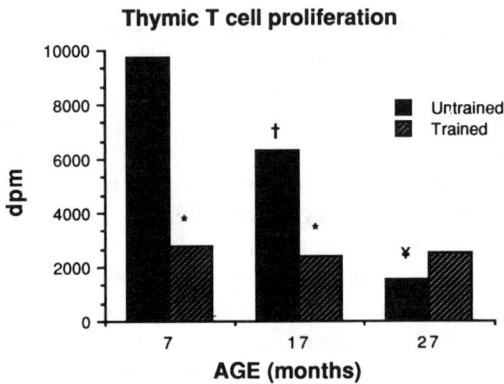

FIGURE 3. Con-A induced proliferation of thymic lymphocytes in trained and untrained animals across various ages. † Significantly different from young animals ($p < 0.05$). ¥ Significantly different from young and middle-aged animals ($p < 0.05$). * Significantly different from untrained animals ($p < 0.05$).

liferation with age such that the young rats demonstrated greater responses than middle-aged rats, while middle-aged rats were greater than aged rats. Once again, as with IL-2 production, blastogenesis was reduced with training among young and middle-aged trained rats compared to their untrained counterparts, similar to the results reported by Pahlavani et al.[82] However, among the aged animals, training was associated with significant increases in T-cell proliferation ($p < 0.05$), as was observed with IL-2 production. A dramatic decline in mitogen-induced proliferation of thymocytes was also demonstrated with advancing age (Figure 3). This was anticipated, based on the well doc-

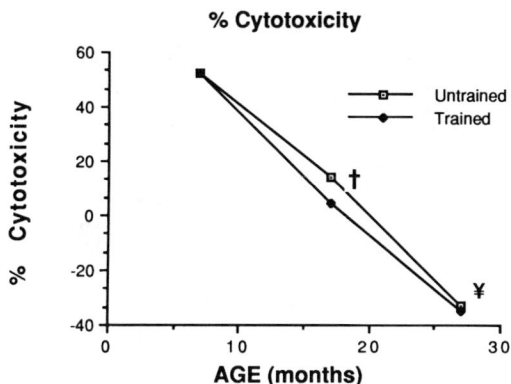

FIGURE 4. Ability of effector cytotoxic cells to lyse target cells (200:1) in trained and untrained Fischer 344 rats across age. † Significantly different from young animals for both trained and untrained rats (*p* < 0.05). ¥ Significantly different from young and middle-aged animals for both trained and untrained rats (*p* < 0.05).

umented involution of the thymus known to occur with age. As was the case for splenic lymphocyte proliferation, endurance training markedly reduced the proliferative capacity of thymocytes in both the young and middle-aged animals, while the opposite effect was observed in the old animals.

As can be seen in Figure 4, the capacity of aged splenocytes to lyse the target YAC-1 cells was greatly reduced. The % cytotoxicity at all effector/target cell ratios tested (200:1, 100:1, 50:1 and 25:1) declined significantly with advancing age. At 27 months, all the E:T ratios were shown to have negative values suggesting a possible protective effect offered to the target cells. This phenomenon has been seen by other laboratories as well, and may be associated with the increase in the release of prostaglandins known to occur with age.[43,72] Endurance training had no effect in offsetting the age-related decline in cytotoxic function at all E:T ratios tested.

Finally, we have also examined the influence of endurance training on humoral immunity in aging Fischer 344 rats.[4] This was assessed *in vivo* with the administration of keyhole limpet hemocyanin (KLH), a T-cell dependent antigen. The humoral immunity response was determined by measurement of serum levels of anti-KLH specific IgG. Figure 5 demonstrates that in response to KLH, IgG antibody production was severely blunted in the old (27 months) when compared to young animals. Further, 10 weeks of endurance training did not improve this antibody response in the old animals.

V. CONCLUSION

As a result of the paucity of investigations examining the role of exercise in modulating the aging immune system, it is difficult at this time to form any definitive conclusions. Longitudinal studies examining the response of

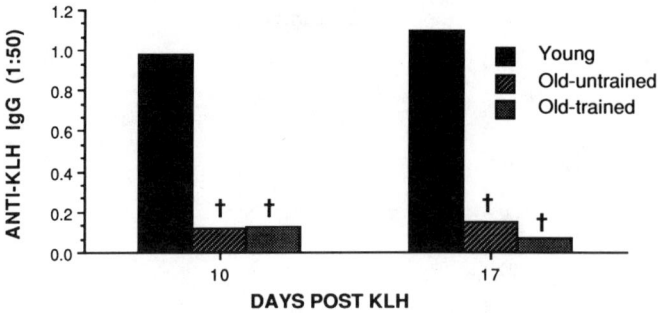

FIGURE 5. The *in vivo* antibody response (IgG) to keyhole limpet hemocyanin (KLH) administration in young vs. old Fischer 344 rats. † Significantly different from young animals (*p* < 0.05). (Modified from Barnes, C. A., Forster, M. J., Fleshner, M., et al., *Neurobiol. Aging,* 12, 47, 1991.)

variables which make up both cell-mediated as well as humoral immunity need to be completed in order to assess to what extent a lifetime of regular exercise can prevent or offset the age-related decline in immune function. Further, more research is required to document the degree to which a single bout of exercise (dependent upon intensity and duration) can influence immune function in aged populations both during as well as into the post-exercise recovery period. Generally, the studies to date suggest that both acute and chronic exercise does alter several components of the immune systems while others remain unaffected. From a mechanistic viewpoint, it is attractive to speculate that neuroendocrine pathways may play a prominent role in regulation of the immune system. Given that the neuroendocrine response is significantly altered with both the aging process and during the stress imposed by physical exercise, coupled with the observation that neuroendocrine activity directly impacts immune function, it is likely that this pathway contributes to aging and exercise immunity. Clearly, further research into this area of immunology is required in order to elucidate cellular interactions involved with immunity, exercise, and aging. Finally, the clinical applications of exercise and immunity must be examined in order to determine potential therapeutic modes for benefiting the elderly population.

ACKNOWLEDGMENTS

The research presented in Figures 1 through 5 was supported by NIH-NIA Grant #AGO7180.

REFERENCES

1. **Antonaci, S., Jirillo, E., Munno, I., et al.**, Monocyte- and cytokine-mediated effects on T immunoregulatory activity in the elderly, *Cytobios.*, 58, 155, 1989.
2. **Asano, Y., Komuro, T., Kubo, M., et al.**, Age-related degeneracy of T cell repertoire: influence of the age environment on T cell allorecognition, *Gerontology*, 36, 3, 1990.
3. **Bach, M.**, Influence of aging on T cell subpopulation involved in the in vitro generation of allogeneic cytotoxicity, *Clin. Immunol. Immunopath.*, 13, 220, 1979.
4. **Barnes, C. A., Forster, M. J., Fleshner, M., et al.**, Exercise does not modify spatial memory, brain autoimmunity, or antibody response in aged F-344 rats, *Neurobiol. Aging*, 12, 47, 1991.
5. **Bash, J. A. and Vogel, D.**, Cellular immunosenescence on F344 rats: decreased natural killer activity involves changes in regulatory interactions between NK cells, interferon, prostaglandin and macrophages, *Mech. Ageing Dev.*, 24, 49, 1984.
6. **Becker, M. J., Farkas, R., Schneider, M., et al.**, Cell-mediated cytotoxicity in humans; age related decline as measured by a xenogeneic assay, *Clin. Immunol. Immunopathol.*, 14, 204, 1979.
7. **Beckman, I., Dimopoulos, K., Xu, X. N., et al.**, T cell activation in the elderly: evidence for specific deficiencies in T-cell/accessory cell interactions, *Mech. Ageing Dev.*, 51, 265, 1990.
8. **Bender, B. S., Chrest, F. J., Nagel, J. A., et al.**, Peripheral blood CD8+ subsets in young and elderly adults; enumeration by two-color immunofluorescence and flow cytometry, *Aging Immunol. Infect. Dis.*, 1, 23, 1988.
9. **Berk, L. S., Nieman, D. C., Youngberg, K. A., et al.**, The effect of long endurance running on natural killer cells in marathoners, *Med. Sci. Sports Exercise*, 22, 207, 1990.
10. **Besedovsky, H. O., Del Rey, A., Sorkin, E., et al.**, Immunoregulation mediated by the sympathetic nervous system, *Cell. Immunol.*, 48, 346, 1979.
11. **Blair, P. B., Staskawicz, M. O., and Sam, J. S.**, Suppression of natural killer cell activity in young and old mice, *Mech. Ageing Dev.*, 40, 57, 1987.
12. **Bruley-Rosset, M. and Vergnon, I.**, Interleukin-1 synthesis and activity in aged mice, *Mech. Ageing Dev.*, 24, 247, 1984.
13. **Callard, R. E.**, Immune function in aged mice. III, *Eur. J. Immunol.*, 8, 697, 1978.
14. **Chang, M., Makinodan, T., Peterson, W. J., et al.**, Role of T cells and adherent cells in age-related decline in murine interleukin 2 production, *J. Immunol.*, 129, 2426, 1982.
15. **Cheung, H. T., Shin, Jr., T. W. U., and Richardson, A.**, Mechanism of the age related decline in lymphocyte proliferation: role of IL-2 production and protein synthesis, *Exp. Gerontol.*, 18, 451, 1983.
16. **Chukhlovin, B. A. and Burov, S. A.**, Resistance to infection under conditions of hypodynamia, *Probl. Kosm. Biol.*, 113, 116, 1969.
17. **Crary, B., Hauser, S. L., Borysenko, M., et al.**, Epinephrine-induced changes in the distribution of lymphocyte subsets in peripheral blood of humans, *J. Immunol.*, 131, 1178, 1983.
18. **Crist, D. M., Mackinnon, L. T., Thompson, R. F., et al.**, Physical exercise increases natural cellular-mediated tumor cytoxicity in elderly women, *Gerontology*, 35, 66, 1989.
19. **Dixon, F. J.**, The cellular and subcellular bases of immunosenescence, *Adv. Immunol.*, 46, 221, 1989.
20. **Durnova, G. N., Kaplansky, A. S., and Portugalov, V. V.**, Effect of a 22-day space flight on the lymphoid organs of rats, *Aviat. Space Environ. Med.*, 37, 588, 1976.
21. **Effros, R. B. and Walford, R. W.**, The immune response of aged mice to influenza: diminished T-cell proliferation, interleukin-2 production and cytotoxicity, *Cell. Immunol.*, 81, 298, 1983.

22. **Effros, R. B., Walford, R. L., Weindruch, R., et al.,** Influences of dietary restriction on immunity to influenza in aged mice, *J. Gerontol.,* 46, B142, 1991.
23. **Ershler, W. B., Coe, C. L., Laughlin, N., et al.,** Aging and immunity in non-human primates. II. Lymphocyte response in thymosin treated middle-aged monkeys, *J. Gerontol.,* 43, B142, 1988.
24. **Eskola, J., Ruuskanen, E., Soppi, E., et al.,** Effect of sport stress on lymphocyte transformation and antibody production, *Clin. Exp. Immunol.,* 32, 339, 1978.
25. **Espersen, G. T., Elbelaek, A., Ernest, E., et al.,** Effect of physical exercise on cytokines and lymphocyte subpopulations in human peripheral blood, *APMIS,* 98, 395, 1990.
26. **Fagiolo, U., Amadori, A., Borghesan, F., et al.,** Immune dysfunction in the elderly: effect of thymic hormone administration on several *in vivo* and *in vitro* immune function parameters, *Aging,* 2, 347, 1990.
27. **Fernandes, G. and Gupta, S.,** Natural killing and antibody dependent cytotoxicity by lymphocyte subpopulations in young and aging humans, *J. Clin. Immunol.,* 1, 141, 1981.
28. **Ferry, A., Picard, F., Duvallet, A., et al.,** Changes in blood leucocyte populations induced by acute maximal and chronic submaximal exercise, *Eur. J. Apply. Physiol.,* 59, 435, 1990.
29. **Ferry, A., Weill, B. L., and Rieu, M.,** Immunomodulations induced in rats by exercise on a treadmill, *J. Appl. Physiol.,* 69, 1912, 1990.
30. **Fiatarone, M. A., Morley, J. E., Bloom, E. T., et al.,** The effect of exercise on natural killer cell activity in young and old subjects, *J. Gerontol.,* 44, m37, 1989.
31. **Fong, T. C. and Makinodan, T.,** *In situ* hybridization analysis of the age associated decline of IL-2 mRNA expressing murine T cells, *Cell. Immunol.,* 118, 199, 1989.
32. **Frasca, D., Adorini, L., Mancini, C., et al.,** Reconstruction of T-cell functions in aging mice by thymosin alpha one, *Immunopharmacology,* 11, 155, 1986.
33. **Frisch, R. E., Wyshak, G., Albright, N. L., et al.,** Lower prevalence of breast cancer and cancer of the reproductive system among former college athletes compared to non-athletes, *Br. J. Cancer,* 52, 885, 1985.
34. **Froelich, C. J., Burkett, J. S., Guiffaut, S., et al.,** Phytohemagglutinin induced proliferation by aged lymphocytes: reduced expression of high affinity interleukin-2 receptors and interleukin-2 secretion, *Life Sci.,* 43, 1583, 1988.
35. **Gahring, L. C. and Weigle, W. O.,** The effect of aging on the induction of humoral and cellular immunity and tolerance in two long-lived mouse strains, *Cell. Immunol.,* 128, 142, 1990.
36. **Galaktionov, V. G. and Ushakov, A. S.,** Effect of hypokinesia on cellular and humoral indices of antibody formation in rats, *Kosm. Biol. Aviakosm. Med.,* 3, 43, 1969.
37. **Gillis, S., Kozak, R., Durante, M., et al.,** Decreased production of and response to T-cell growth factor by lymphocytes from aged humans, *J. Clin. Invest.,* 67, 937, 1981.
38. **Gilman, S. C., Rosenburg, J. S., and Feldman, J. D.,** T lymphocytes of young and aged rats. II. Functional defects and the role of interleukin-2, *J. Immunol.,* 128, 644, 1982.
39. **Goodman, S. A. and Makinodan, T.,** Effect of age on cell-mediated immunity in long-lived mice, *Clin. Exp. Immunol.,* 19, 533, 1975.
40. **Gottesman, S. R., Edington, J. M., and Thorbecke, G. J.,** Proliferative and cytotoxic immune functions in aging mice. IV. Effects of suppressor cell populations from aged and young mice, *J. Immunol.,* 140, 1783, 1988.
41. **Grossman, A., Ledmetter, J. A., and Rabinovitch, P. S.,** Reduced proliferation in T-lymphocytes in aged humans is predominantly in the CD8+ subset, and is unrelated to defects in transmembrane signaling which are predominantly in the CD4+ subset, *Exp. Cell. Res.,* 180, 367, 1989.
42. **Hanson, P. G. and Flaherty, D. K.,** Immunological responses to training in conditioned runners, *Clin. Sci. London,* 60, 225, 1981.

43. **Hausman, P. B. and Weksler, M. E.,** Changes in the immune response with age, in *Handbook Biology of Aging,* Finch, C. E. and Schneider, E. L., Eds., Van Nostrand Reinhold Company, New York, 1985, 414.
44. **Hedfors, E., Holm, G., and Öhnell, B.,** Variations of blood lymphocytes during work studied by cell surface markers, DNA synthesis and cytotoxicity, *Clin. Exp. Immunol.,* 24, 328, 1976.
45. **Heidrich, M. L. and Makinodan, T.,** Presence of impairment of humoral immunity in non-adherent spleen cells of old mice, *J. Immunol.,* 111, 1502, 1973.
46. **Helfrich, B. A., Segre, M., and Segre, D.,** Age-related changes in the degeneracy of the mouse T-cell repertoire, *Cell. Immunol.,* 118, 1, 1989.
47. **Hirokawa, K. and Makinodan, T.,** Thymic involution: effect on T cell differentiation, *J. Immunol.,* 114, 1659, 1975.
48. **Hirokawa, K., Sato, K., and Makinodan, T.,** Influence of age of thymic grafts on the differentation of T cells in nude mice, *Clin. Immunol. Immunopathol.,* 24, 251, 1982.
49. **Hirokawa, K. and Utsuyama, M.,** Combined grafting of bone marrow and thymus, and sequential multiple thymus graftings in various strains of mice. The effect on immune functions and life span, *Mech. Ageing Dev.,* 49, 49, 1989.
50. **Hirokawa, K., Utsuyama, M., and Kasai, M.,** Role of the thymus in aging of the immune system, in *Biomedical Advances in Aging,* Goldstein, A. L., Ed., Plenum Press, New York, 1990, 375.
51. **Hoffman, S. A., Paschkis, K. E., DeBias, D. A., et al.,** The influence of exercise on the growth on the growth of transplanted rat tumors, *Cancer Res.,* 22, 597, 1962.
52. **Hoffman-Goetz, L., Keir, R., Thorne, R., et al.,** Chronic exercise stress in mice depresses splenic T lymphocyte mitogenesis *in vitro, Clin. Exp. Immunol.,* 66, 551, 1986.
53. **Holbrook, N. J., Chopra, R. K., McCoy, M. T., et al.,** Expression of interleukin-2 receptor in aging rats, *Cell. Immunol.,* 120, 1, 1989.
54. **Iwashima, M., Nakayama, T., Kubo, M., et al.,** Analysis of the age-related degeneracy of T cells from aged and chimeric mice, *Int. Archs. Allergy Appl. Immun.,* 83, 129, 1987.
55. **Kappel M., Tvede, N., Galbo, H., et al.,** Evidence that the effect of physical exercise on NK cell activity is mediated by epinephrine, *J. Appl. Physiol.,* 70, 2530, 1991.
56. **Kay, M. M. B.,** Parainfluenza infection of aged mice results in autoimmune disease, *Clin. Immunol. Immunopathol.,* 12, 301, 1979.
57. **Keast, D., Cameron, K., and Morton, A. R.,** Exercise and the immune response, *Sports Med.,* 5, 248, 1988.
58. **Lewicki, R., Tchorzewski, H., Majewska, E., et al.,** Effect of maximal physical exercise on T lymphocyte subpopulations and on interleukin 1(IL-1) and interleukin 2 (IL-2) production *in vitro, Int. J. Sports Med.,* 9, 114, 1988.
59. **Lighthart, G. J., Schuit, H. R. E., and Hijmans, W.,** Subpopulations of mononuclear cells in aging; expansion of the number of T and B cells in human blood, *Immunol.,* 55, 15, 1985.
60. **Lighthart, G. J., Schuit, H. R. E., and Hijmans, W.,** Natural killer cell function is not diminished in the healthy aged and is proportional to the number of NK cells in the peripheral blood, *Immunol.,* 68, 396, 1989.
61. **Lustyik, G. Y. and O'Leary, J. J.,** Aging and intracellular free calcium response in human T cell after stimulation by phytohemagglutinin. *J. Gerontol.,* 44, 1330, 1989.
62. **Mackinnon, L. T. and Tomasi, T. B.,** Immunology of exercise, in *Sports Medicine, Fitness, Training, Injuries,* Urban and Schwarzenberg, Baltimore, MD, 1988, 273.
63. **MacNeil, B., Hoffman-Goetz, L., Kendall, A., et al.,** Lymphocyte proliferation responses after exercise in men: fitness, intensity, and duration, *J. Appl. Physiol.,* 70, 179, 1991.
64. **Mahan, M. P. and Young, R. Y.,** Immune parameters of untrained or exercised-trained rats after exhaustive exercise, *J. Appl. Physiol.,* 66, 282, 1989.

65. **Makinodan, T. and Kay, M. M. B.**, Age influence on the immune system, *Adv. Immunol.*, 29, 287, 1980.

66. **Mariani, E., Rhoda, P., Mariani, A. R., et al.**, Age-associated changes in CD8 + and CD16 + cell reactivity: clonal analysis, *Clin. Exp. Immunol.*, 81, 479, 1990.

67. **Mascart-Lemone, F., Delespesse, G., Servais, G., et al.**, Characterization of immunoregulatory T lymphocytes during aging by monoclonal antibodies, *Clin. Exp. Immunol.*, 48, 148, 1982.

68. **Masuhara, M., Kami, K., Umebayasi, K., et al.**, Influences of exercise on leukocyte count and size, *J. Sports Med.*, 27, 285, 1987.

69. **Miller, R. A.**, Immunodeficiency of aging: restorative effects of phorbol ester combined with calcium ionophore, *J. Immunol.*, 137, 805, 1986.

70. **Miller, R. A., Jacobson, B., Weil, G., et al.**, Diminished calcium influx in lectin-stimulated T cells from old mice, *J. Cell. Physiol.*, 132, 337, 1987.

71. **Miller, R. A.**, The cell biology of aging: immunological models, *J. Gerontol.*, 44, B4, 1989.

72. **Miller, R. A.**, Aging and the immune response, in *Handbook Biology of Aging*, Van Nostrand Reinhold Company, New York, 1990, 157.

73. **Muir, A. L., Cruz, M., Martin, B. A., et al.**, Leukocyte kinetics in the human lung: role of exercise and catecholamines, *J. Appl. Physiol.*, 57, 711, 1984.

74. **Murasko, D. M., Nelson, B. J., Silver, R., et al.**, Immunologic response in an elderly population with a mean age of 85, *Am. J. Med.*, 81, 612, 1986.

75. **Nagel, J. E., Chrest, F. J., and Adler, W. H.**, Enumeration of T lymphocyte subsets by monoclonal antibodies in young and aged humans, *J. Immunol.*, 127, 2086, 1981.

76. **Nagel, J. E., Chrest, F. J., Pyle, R. S., et al.**, Monoclonal antibody analysis of T-lymphocyte subsets in young and aged adults, *Immunol. Commun.*, 12, 223, 1983.

77. **Nagel, J. E. and Adler, W. H.**, Immunology, in *Human Aging Research: Concepts and Techniques*, Kent, B. and Butler, R. N., Eds., Raven Press, New York, 1988, 299.

78. **Nehlsen-Cannarella, S. L., Nieman, D. C., and Balk-Lamberton, A. J.**, The effects of moderate exercise training on immune response, *Med. Sci. Sports Exercise*, 23, 64, 1991.

79. **Nieman, D. C., Tan, S. A., Lee, J. W., et al.**, Complement and immunoglobulin levels in athletes and sedentary controls, *Int. J. Sports Med.*, 10, 124, 1989.

80. **Nieman, D. C., Nehlson-Cannarella, S. L., Markoff, P. A., et al.**, The effects of moderate exercise training on natural killer cells and acute upper respiratory tract infections, *Int. J. Sports Med.*, 11, 467, 1990.

81. **Nieman, D. C. and Nehlson-Cannarella, S. L.**, The effects of acute and chronic exercise on immunoglobulins, *Sports Med.*, 11, 183, 1991.

82. **Pahlavani, M. A., Cheung, T. H., Chesky, J. A., et al.**, Influence of exercise on the immune function of rats at various ages, *J. Appl. Physiol.*, 64, 1997, 1988.

83. **Papa, S., Vitale, M., Mazzotti, G., et al.**, Impaired lymphocyte stimulation induced by long-term training, *Immunol. Lett.*, 22, 29, 1989.

84. **Penschow, J. and Mackay, I. R.**, NK and K cell activity of human blood: differences according to sex, age, and disease, *Ann. Rheum. Dis.*, 39, 82, 1980.

85. **Perkins, E. H.**, Phagocyte activity of aged mice, *J. Reticuloendothel. Soc.*, 9, 642, 1971.

86. **Proust, J. J., Filburn, C. R., Harrison, S. A., et al.**, Age-related defect in signal transduction during lectin activation of murine T lymphocytes, *J. Immunol.*, 139, 1472, 1987.

87. **Proust, J. J., Kittur, D. S., Buchholz, M. A., et al.**, Restricted expression of mitogen induced high affinity IL-2 receptors in aging mice, *J. Immunol.*, 141, 4209, 1988.

88. **Roder, J. C.**, Target-effector interaction in the natural killer (NK) system. VI. The influence of age and genotype on NK binding characteristics, *Immunology*, 41, 483, 1975.

177

89. **Sato, T., Fuse, A., and Kuwata, T.,** Enhancement by interferon of natural cytotoxic activities of lymphocytes from human cord blood and peripheral blood of aged persons, *Cell. Immunol.,* 45, 458, 1979.

90. **Saxena, R. K., Saxena, Q. B., and Adler, W. H.,** Interleukin-2-induced activation of natural killer activity in spleen cells from old and young mice, *Immunology,* 51, 719, 1984.

91. **Schwab, R. and Weksler, M. E.,** Cellular basis of immune senescence: impaired proliferation of T cell, in *Immunoregulation in Aging,* Facchini, A., Haaijman, J. J., and Labo, G., Eds., JH Pasmans Offsetdrukkerji BV, The Netherlands, 1986, 33.

92. **Segre, D., Miller, R. A., Abraham, G. N., et al.,** Aging and the immune system, *J. Gerontol.,* 44, 164, 1989.

93. **Shelton, E., Daves, S., and Hemmer, R.,** Quantitation of strain BALB-c mouse peritoneal cells, *Science,* 168, 1232, 1970.

94. **Simpson, R. J. A., Hoffman-Goetz, L., Thorne, R., et al.,** Exercise stress alters the percentage of splenic lymphocyte subsets in response to mitogen but not in response to interleukin-1, *Brain Behav. Immun.,* 3, 119, 1989.

95. **Solana, R., Villanueva, J. L., Pena, J., et al.,** Cell mediated immunity in aging, *Comp. Biochem. Physiol.,* 99A, 1, 1991.

96. **Tharp, G. D. and Preuss, T. L.,** Mitogenic response of T-lymphocytes to exercise training and stress, *J. Appl. Physiol.,* 70, 2535, 1991.

97. **Thoman, M. L.,** Lymphokines and aging of the immune system, in *Immunoregulation of Aging,* Facchini, A., Haaijman, J. J., and Labo, G., Eds., JH Pasmans Offsetdrukkerji BV, The Netherlands, 1986, 87.

98. **Thoman, M. L. and Weigle, W. O.,** Lymphokines and aging; interleukin-2 production and activity in aged animals, *J. Immunol.,* 127, 2101, 1981.

99. **Thoman, M. L. and Weigle, W. O.,** Reconstitution of *in vivo* cell-mediated lympholysis responses in aged mice with interleukin 2, *J. Immunol.,* 134, 949, 1985.

100. **Thoman, M. L. and Weigle, W. O.,** Partial restoration of Con A-induced proliferation, IL-2 receptor expression, and IL-2 synthesis in aged murine lymphocytes by phorbol myristate acetate and ionomycin, *Cell. Immunol.,* 114, 1, 1988.

101. **Thompson, J. S., Wekstein, D. R., Rhoades, J. L., et al.,** The immune status of healthy centenarians, *J. Am. Ger. Soc.,* 32, 274, 1984.

102. **Tomasi, T. B., Trudeau, F. B., Czerwinski, D., et al.,** Immune parameters in athletes before and after strenuous exercise, *J. Clin. Immunol.,* 2, 173, 1982.

103. **Tonnesen, E., Christensen, N. J., and Brinklov, M. M.,** Natural killer cell activity during cortisol and adrenaline infusion in healthy volunteers, *Eur. J. Clin. Invest.,* 10, 497, 1987.

104. **Umezawa, M., Hanada, K., Naiki, H., et al.,** Effects of dietary restriction on age-related immune dysfunction in the senescence accelerated mouse (SAM), *J. Nutr.,* 120, 1393, 1990.

105. **Utsuyama, M. and Hirokawa, K.,** Age-related changes of splenic T cells in mice. A flow cytometric analysis, *Mech. Ageing Dev.,* 40, 89, 1987.

106. **Utsuyama, M., Kasai, M., Kurashima, C., et al.,** Age influence on the thymic capacity to promote differentiation of T cells: induction of different composition of T cell subsets by aging thymus, *Mech. Ageing Dev.,* 58, 267, 1991.

107. **Vena, J. E., Graham, S., Zielezny, M., et al.,** Occupational exercise and risk of cancer, *Am. J. Clin. Nutr.,* 45, 318, 1987.

108. **Vie, H. and Miller, R. A.,** Decline, with age, in the proportion of mouse T cells that express IL-2 receptors after mitogen stimulation, *Mech. Ageing Dev.,* 33, 313, 1986.

109. **Weindruch, R. H., Kristei, J. A., Cheney, K. E., et al.,** Influence of controlled dietary restriction on immunologic function and aging, *Fed. Proc.,* 38, 2007, 1979.

110. **Weindruch, R., Devens, B. H., Raff, H. V., et al.,** Influence of dietary restriction and aging on natural killer cell activity in mice, *J. Immunol.,* 130, 993, 1983.

111. **Weksler, M. E., Innes, J. B., and Goldstein, A. L.,** Immunological studies of aging. IV. The contribution of thymic involution to the immune deficiencies of aging mice, and reversal with thymopoietin, *J. Exp. Med.,* 148, 996, 1978.

112. **Wu, W., Pahlavani, M., Cheung, H. T., et al.,** The effect of aging on the expression of interleukin 2 messenger ribonucleic acid, *Cell. Immunol.,* 100, 224, 1986.

113. **Zharhary, D. and Gershon, H.,** Allogeneic T cytotoxic reactivity of senescent mice: affinity for target cells and determination of cell number, *Cell. Immunol.,* 60, 470, 1981.

Chapter 11

PSYCHOLOGICAL EFFECTS OF EXERCISE FOR DISEASE RESISTANCE AND HEALTH PROMOTION

Rod K. Dishman

TABLE OF CONTENTS

I. INTRODUCTION

Exercise has been linked with mental health in the literatures of philosophy and medicine throughout recorded history,[1] and it was a popular adjunct to psychiatry earlier this century.[2] High costs of mental health care, coupled with a resurgence of psychosomatic medicine and preventive health care practices, have contributed to current interest in the psychological effects of exercise for disease resistance and health promotion. During the past 15 years, numerous reviews of the research literature have concluded that exercise and physical fitness are associated with reduced anxiety and depression. This also was the consensus of the Workshop on Exercise and Mental Health sponsored by the U.S. National Institute of Mental Health in 1984[3] and the International Conference on Exercise, Fitness and Health in 1988.[4] Another review has concluded that chronic exercise or physical fitness are accompanied by decreased reactivity to psychosocial stressors.[5]

Recent meta-analyses of nearly 250 studies concluded that the effects reported for depression and stress reactivity approximate one-half standard deviation,[6] while the effects for anxiety ranged from one-fourth to one-third of a standard deviation.[7] Although these effects are smaller than those seen for the influence of psychotherapy[8] and drug therapy[9] for reducing anxiety and depression, their magnitudes are comparable to population estimates of the relative risk of physical inactivity for increased incidence of coronary heart disease and all-cause mortality.[10]

The potential effectiveness of exercise as a preventive behavior for mental health is important because the lifetime prevalence rates for anxiety and depression disorders among Americans is estimated at 8 and 15%,[11] yet only 20 to 30% of those suffering will seek professional care.[12] Thus, exercise could be a salutary alternative for some individuals.

The effects reported in the descriptive epidemiology literature of anxiety and depression on coronary heart disease, arthritis, ulcers, asthma, and headaches are moderately strong and potentially causal.[13] Human[14] and animal[15] studies show that chronic anxiety and depression can be immunosuppressive, and there is accumulating evidence that cardiovascular reactivity to stressors is a risk factor for hypertension.[16] Thus, any impact of exercise or physical fitness on anxiety, depression, and stress reactivity might also exert a positive public health influence on some chronic diseases and immunity.

Despite these positive interpretations of the exercise literature, other reviews have concluded that the available evidence is not compelling. The U.S. Preventive Services Task Force of the U.S. Office of Disease Prevention and Health Promotion recently concluded that the quality of the available evidence was poor and stated that the relationship between exercise and the primary prevention of mental health problems was poorly understood.[17]

The purpose of this chapter is to characterize the quantity and quality of scientific evidence indicating that exercise or physical fitness is associated with reduced anxiety, depression, and physiological reactivity to nonexercise stressors. While there is sufficient evidence to conclude that some components of physical activity or physical fitness can be associated with positive outcomes on these variables, we do not yet know what forms or amounts of physical activity are most effective for whom or under what circumstances. In addition, potential psychological risks associated with overtraining or abusive exercise will be discussed. Also, while a number of reasonable hypotheses have been advanced for cognitive explanations for the reductions in anxiety and depression associated with exercise,[3,18] none have been experimentally verified. Most perplexing is the absence of supporting evidence for plausible biological mechanisms.

To provide some direction for enhancing both the internal and external validity of future research, the author will comment on selected measurement and design limitations of past studies and on some potential biologic mechanisms whereby the purported effects of exercise on anxiety, depression, and stress reactivity might be explained.

A large portion of the extant literature has serious design and methodology flaws. There are few randomized clinical trials and fewer population studies. Typically, anxiety and depression were not assessed by uniform measures or standard diagnostic criteria and exercise was not adequately quantified. The Diagnostic and Statistical Manual of Mental Disorders, 3rd Edition, Revised (DSM-III-R)[19] provides the most used standard for treatment and research on anxiety and depression. Although the etiology of the anxiety and depression disorders is not fully understood, refinements in diagnosis have led to the establishment of Research Diagnostic Criteria (RDC)[20] for the varieties of anxiety and depression. Only a handful of exercise studies have conformed to RDC definitions.[18,21,22]

There is also a lack of consensus over which psychosocial stressors are linked with specific patterns of cardiovascular, neuromuscular, hormonal, and immune responses and how the limbic system influences these responses. This lack of consensus has contributed to the current confusion surrounding the evidence linking exercise and physical activity with reactivity to non-exercise stressors. Lack of theory in this area has prevented clarification of the apparently contradictory findings in the exercise literature.[23]

The American College of Sports Medicine (ACSM) classifies exercise into three types: (1) cardiorespiratory of aerobic endurance, (2) muscular strength and endurance, and (3) flexibility. The majority of studies of exercise and depression have examined supervised programmatic exercise consistent with ACSM guidelines. Most have used aerobic exercise such as running, swimming, or bicycling. A few have investigated anaerobic exercise defined as weight training or vigorous sports. The author is unaware of studies using flexibility training as an intervention. Epidemiological definitions of exercise[24] measured by global estimates of energy expenditure or the frequency, intensity, and duration of free-living activity, regardless of type, must also be considered if the effectiveness of exercise as an effective health-promoting behavior is to be established.

II. EXERCISE AND DEPRESSION

A recent review by Martinsen[18] examined experimental studies of clinically depressed patients meeting RDC or DSM-III-R diagnostic categories of nonbipolar depression of mild to moderate severity who participated in aerobic forms of exercise. The conclusion was that aerobic exercise was as effective as group psychotherapy, individual psychotherapy, and meditative relaxation. Furthermore, exercise was more effective than no treatment or a placebo treatment.

A quantitative meta-analysis of exercise and depression[6] reported a mean effect size (ES) of $-0.53 \pm .85$, indicating that depression scores were decreased by about one-half of one standard deviation in exercise groups compared to leisure activity, psychotherapy, and nonexercising control groups. The meta-analysis indicated an effect for (1) all forms of depression reported including major and minor depressive disorders, primary and secondary types of depression, and self-rated depressive mood in nonpatients scoring in the normal range on questionnaires; (2) cardiorespiratory or aerobic endurance activities and muscular strength and endurance activities, as defined by ACSM; and (3) exercise programs ranging in length from less than 4 weeks to more than 24 weeks.

A number of issues cloud an interpretation of the meta-analysis. The finding that exercise combined with psychotherapy produced an effect ($+ .81 \pm .57$) that exceeds the effects of exercise alone ($.55 \pm 0.92$) or psychotherapy alone ($- .19 \pm .71$) is difficult to interpret because of the unusually low psychotherapy effect reported in exercise studies. Meta-analysis of the literature on psychotherapy and depression[8] has shown an independent effect size of 0.93 for psychotherapy compared to control conditions and an effect size approximating 0.20 for minimally effective or placebo interventions.[25] This suggests that the psychotherapy conditions contrasted in exercise studies have been ineffectively presented, poorly evaluated, or they involved individuals who were not depressed. In addition, the use of a true no-treatment control group in studies of depression is rare due to ethical concerns over withholding treatment. However, it is known that most episodes of moderate depression will remit spontaneously within several weeks or a few months, and this period falls within the duration of a number of prospective studies of exercise and depression. When all treatment groups respond with a reduction in depression symptoms within this period, it is difficult to discount that results are due to spontaneous remission or to nonspecific effects of the experimental or clinical setting rather than to specific therapeutic components of the interventions.

A dose-response relationship of exercise volume or increased fitness with decreased depression would present a more convincing case for an independent effect of physical activity on depression. Although many studies have followed ACSM guidelines for type, intensity, duration, and frequency known to increase fitness, several studies have shown no change in depression. Other studies show decreased depression with types and amounts of activity unlikely to influence fitness, while most studies have not assessed fitness with standardized measures. A recent study supports the efficacy of anaerobic exercise.[26] Aerobic and anaerobic training programs were compared, and both groups had similar improvements in depression that were not dependent on an improvement in VO_2 peak. This finding is consistent with North American population estimates showing a reduction in self-rated depression in both men and women when low energy expenditures were contrasted with inactivity,[27,28] but no further reduction in depression with increasing levels of energy expenditure.

Carefully controlled clinical trials addressing measurement and diagnostic errors, epidemiological issues of independence, time course, dose response, and population effectiveness will provide a greater understanding of the effects of exercise on depression. Also, biological plausibility must be established.

A. BIOLOGICAL PLAUSIBILITY?

The most widely studied biological hypotheses of affective disorders have involved the biogenic amines, norepinephrine (NE), dopamine (DA), and serotonin (5-HT). Other putative neurotransmitters have also been implicated in depression, e.g., acetylcholine and GABA, but the majority of exercise studies have examined NE and 5-HT.

The consensus view holds that monoaminergic neurons modulate a wide range of functions in the CNS. Noradrenergic neurons are implicated in hormonal release, cardiovascular function, sleep, and analgesic responses.[29,30] Serotonergic activity is associated with pain, fatigue, appetitive behavior, periodicity of sleep, and corticosteroid activity.[31] Both NE and 5-HT have been implicated in the regulation of emotion by virtue of their action in the limbic system and the frontal cortex. Noradrenergic cell bodies are most dense in the locus coeruleus (LC) region of the pons, and the LC is believed to be a major regulatory site for limbic dysfunction characteristic of both anxiety and depression.[30,32]

Evidence for involvement of central noradrenergic and serotonergic systems comes primarily from two sources. First, pharmacological studies have examined the actions and effects of antidepressant drugs which are known to raise the levels of amines in the synapse primarily by blocking their reuptake by the terminal nerve or by blocking their metabolism.

Second, clinical studies have examined monoaminergic systems in depressed patients by sampling metabolites of NE and 5-HT in cerebrospinal fluid (CSF) or urine. It is assumed that excretion of metabolites such as 3-methoxy-4-hydroxyphenylethylene glycol (MHPG) from NE and 5-hydroxy-indolacetic acid (5-HIAA) from 5-HT reflects the activity of noradrenergic and serotonergic systems. In general, the results of these studies demonstrate that in bipolar depression there are reduced levels of MHPG during depressive episodes and higher than normal levels during mania.[33,34] Reduced urinary MHPG has also been reported in schizoaffective depression and in subgroups suffering from unipolar depression.[33,35]

5-HIAA in urine has also been found to be below normal in depressed patients.[36] The same has been found to be true when examining 5-HIAA in CSF. However, sampling errors associated with diagnosis, tissue source (i.e., spinal fluid, plasma, urine), and circadian rhythms make this literature difficult to interpret.

It is biologically plausible that chronic exercise could affect monoamine systems in ways qualitatively similar to the effects of pharmacologic interventions. Baldessarini[37] has recently discussed consensus effects of antidepressants on NE and 5-HT systems. Chronic effects of tricyclic antidepressants include:[37]

1. Continuous blockade of reuptake
2. A temporary and reversible down-regulation of presynaptic and post-synaptic alpha-2 receptors
3. A normalization of firing rates and turnover which can lead to levels of monoamines that are above normal
4. Increased release of NE
5. A down-regulation of beta receptors
6. An increased affinity and sensitivity to alpha-1 agonists that may increase the number of alpha-1 receptors
7. A possible increase in the sensitivity to 5-HT receptors

B. EXERCISE STUDIES

Monoaminergic theories have been extended to exercise by describing changes in neurotransmitters such as NE and 5-HT with acute and chronic training in rats. They have also been investigated by observing changes in urinary MHPG in acute and chronic exercise in depressed and nondepressed humans.

In humans, changes in monoamines have been assessed by measuring MHPG in urine, plasma, or CSF; it has been assumed that increased MHPG would reflect increased central noradrenergic activity. Studies examining the effects of acute physical activity on MHPG have been summarized elsewhere.[38] Acute studies which measured urinary MHPG have found either increased MHPG excretion or no change. There are methodological problems with these studies. First, sample sizes were small and different types of depression were present in the same treatment group. Also, exercise levels were not quantified or very low levels of physical activity were used.

Studies of acute activity and MHPG in nondepressed subjects have typically quantified the exercise and some have relativized exercise intensity to work capacity. However, again the findings are mixed. Plasma MHPG typically has increased, but urinary MHPG has been unchanged. Other studies have found increases in glucuronide and sulfated subfractions of MHPG.[39,40] However, the continued debate over the central or peripheral origins of plasma and urinary MHPG and their meaning for NE metabolism in the brain hinder interpretations of the exercise studies for models of depression.[41] To determine the origin of the MHPG following exercise, a recent study[42] used ethanol to block the metabolism of MHPG to vanilmandelic acid in the liver. The findings were consistent with a central origin for MHPG sulfate, and showed similar excretion rates for MHPG subfractions in depressed patients and normal controls following high intensity exercise.

The author is unaware of chronic exercise studies that have examined MHPG responses. However, cross-sectional studies of nondepressed subjects have compared MHPG levels between fitness groups based on VO_2 peak and have found no differences.[43,44] An inverse relationship between VO_2 peak and self-rated depression has been reported,[45] and multivariate relationships among fitness and urinary NE metabolites with depression and anxiety have been reported for normal males following resting and occupational conditions.[23,46]

No clear conclusions can be drawn from these studies due to the absence of prospective controlled experiments, a lack of uniformity in diagnosis and quantification of exercise in the patient studies, the unclear relevance for depression of exercise studies with nonpatients, and the inherent limitations of peripheral metabolites of NE for understanding central noradrenergic activity.

A number of studies with rodents have examined brain NE, 5-HT, and 5-HIAA with acute and chronic training protocols.[47,48] Decreases in whole brain NE have been found with acute exercise. Conversely, chronic exercise studies have found elevation in brain NE levels. Acute and chronic exercise studies have found both increased and decreased concentrations and turnover of 5-HT and 5-HIAA that has differed by brain region.

It is not possible to determine from these studies how exercise affects noradrenergic and serotonergic activity because the lack of uniformity in their methods prevents direct comparisons of results. First, most studies have measured concentrations. Concentration of a neurotransmitter is not a direct indicator of neural activity. Turnover, estimated by the neurotransmitter and major metabolites, provides a better estimate of activity. Turnover can be measured directly by isotope methods, use of inhibitors, or indirectly through measurement of metabolites in CSF and plasma. All these methods make a number of assumptions which may lead to errors in the estimation of turnover.[32]

Most exercise studies have utilized other stressors in addition to exercise. Swim protocols can be confounded by fear and cold. Shock has commonly been used during treadmill exercise. It is possible that shock could differentially affect neurotransmitter systems. Also, very few studies have assessed fitness and the relationship between oxidative metabolism and neurotransmitter responses. Oxygen is a cofactor in the synthesis of both NE and 5-HT. At the present time, it is not known whether cardiorespiratory fitness induced by training or physical activity is necessary for changes in neurotransmitters to occur.

Studies also have not assessed the same brain regions. Neurotransmitter concentrations and turnover are likely to be different in specific brain regions because of specificity in neural activity and because monoaminergic neurons originate and terminate in different regions. Thus, it should be expected that turnover will vary from one brain region to another. Studies also are not comparable because different rat strains and genders were studied. Estrogen levels can differentially affect functioning of monoamine neurons.[49]

Exercise studies are needed to examine specific aspects of synthesis and metabolism of these neurotransmitters. Stone[50] compared running stress with injections of reserpine or methyltyrosine, all of which were later injected with radioactively labeled NE. Running stress did not adversely alter storage of NE, so it is likely that the NE depletion in the running condition was derived from newly synthesized NE and not from reuptake mechanisms. Chaouloff[48] has also conducted a series of studies which examine the effects of running on synthesis and metabolism of 5-HT in various brain regions. By injecting inhibitors into the synthetic pathways of control animals and examining increases in tryptophan, 5-HT, and 5-HIAA, he has reported that tryptophan is increased equally in hippocampus, midbrain, and striatum following running, but 5-HTP accumulation was increased in the midbrain, unchanged in the striatum, and decreased in the hippocampus. A follow-up study examined the effects of a tryptophan load on 5-HT and 5-HIAA levels and it was concluded from these studies that tryptophan utilization was affected differently in serotonergic nerve terminals, i.e., hippocampus and striatum but not in the cell bodies, i.e., midbrain.

Change in monoaminergic systems can also be assessed by studies of receptor-effector number and function. The author is unaware of studies that have examined changes in α or β receptors following exercise in depressed patients. However, it has been reported[51] that lymphocyte B-adrenoreceptor density is decreased with exercise training. Conversely, α_2-adrenergic receptors on platelets have been shown to increase following chronic exercise.[52] The mechanism of these changes in receptor density is unknown. Future studies also need to examine changes in receptor distribution because single neurotransmitters can have both inhibitory and excitatory effects. This can be done in animal models of exercise by labeling receptors with radioligands using autoradiography. It is also important to find plausible biological hypotheses explaining why monoamine systems might be stimulated by exercise. A number of candidates, including sensory afference from muscle and joint; metabolic influences on central neurotransmitters and motoric/limbic interactions are potentially plausible.[47]

Neurotransmitter systems not only influence each other, they also are linked to the hypothalamus-pituitary adrenal (HPA) axis. Growing evidence indicates a role for the HPA in anxiety and depression. More detail on the regulatory mechanisms of the HPA axis during stress is available elsewhere.[53,54,55]

C. THE HPA AXIS IN DEPRESSION AND ANXIETY

The symptomatology of typical Major Depression, including weight loss and early morning awakening, implicates the neuroendocrine system in the etiology and psychopathology of depression. Patients who are anxious and depressed typically show signs and symptoms of a disrupted HPA axis at rest and during challenge. These signs and symptoms include disturbances of mood, appetite, sleep, motivated behavior, and several indices of autonomic, endocrine, and immune status.[56] A common thread that binds these signs and symptoms is hypercortisolism, i.e., abnormally high secretion of cortisol. One of the major functions of cortisol is to maintain blood sugar levels during stress through the liberation and use of stored fat and glycogen and amino acids from muscle cells. In normal physiological concentrations, cortisol helps the body combat stress. However, in very high concentrations cortisol suppresses immune responses to infection and can inhibit healing. Collectively, the evidence[57] is consistent with the hypothesis that glucocorticoid regulation and the monaminergic systems reinforce one another's activity.

In melancholic depression, the glucocorticoids or the limbic monoaminergic system, or both, may fail to provide the appropriate regulation or restraint of the HPA axis. Sachar[58] has proposed that depletion of NE causes a loss of inhibition to the CRH neuron which then stimulates the secretion of ACTH; this may eventually lead to the hypercortisolism seen in depression.

Hypersecretion of cortisol can be explained by a disruption at any of several sites in the HPA axis.[59] These include but are not limited to: (1) hypersensitivity of the adrenal gland to ACTH, (2) hyposensitivity of the pituitary gland to cortisol, (3) hypersensitivity of the pituitary to CRF, (4) hypersecretion of CRF by the hypothalamus, and (5) resistance to neural feedback.

While the hypothalamus mediates HPA feedback, it appears subordinate to higher command. For example, deafferentation of the hypothalamus leads to resistance to dexamethasone suppression of ACTH. Sopolsky[60] argues that the hippocampus exerts an inhibitory central command on the hypothalamus and that damage or disruption of hippocampal activity can explain part of the hypercortisolism of depression. He has shown that sustained exposure to stressors also is associated with decreased receptor density in hippocampus. In addition to CRF, AVP, OT, catecholamines, and angiotensin stimulate ACTH directly or in synergy with CRF. The pattern of secretagogues appears stereotyped for different stressors.[53] Thus, it will be important to determine if exercise and depression share common patterns while examining the plausibility that either acute or chronic exercise might influence HPA regulation by influencing hippocampal activity or regulation.

1. Exercise Studies and the HPA Axis

In humans, post-exercise changes in the regulation of the HPA system and its interaction with the sympathetic nervous system have not been studied by methods directly relevant for understanding their effects on depression or anxiety. Acute effects during exercise regulate cardiovascular, thermoregulatory, fluid, electrolyte, and fuel needs of increased metabolism.[61] Aside from increases in NE and E that can range from 8- to 12-fold for intense prolonged exercise, several hormonal changes accompany exercise that may bear on HPA disruption in depression. Prolactin and growth hormone can increase two- to threefold during acute exercise, while increases in ACTH, Cortisol, and *B*-endorphin are similar in rate and magnitude during prolonged exercise at intensities approximating 80% VO_2 peak.[62] Some evidence from naltrexone blockade suggests that endogenous opioid peptides, including perhaps *B*-endorphin, inhibit secretion of growth hormone, cortisol, and catecholamines during acute exercise. Because all of these hormones have been implicated as potential secretagogues acting on the pituitary, hypothalamus, hippocampus, and locus coeruleus, research is needed to determine their patterns of release and action during exercise in relation to those observed with other stressors studied in HPA models of depression.

Due to the past unavailability of assay techniques sensitive to the small resting levels found in plasma, the effects of chronic exercise on tonic levels of monoamines and HPA hormones are poorly understood. Changes in response to ovine corticotropin releasing factor and synthetic corticosteroids such as dexamethasone may provide useful information regarding parallel regulatory responses of the HPA axis occurring with depression and with exercise. A recent study[63] reported a decreased resting ACTH and cortisol response to oCRH among highly trained runners compared with sedentary and moderately trained runners. This response was interpreted as consistent with sustained hypercortisolism in the highly trained group despite comparable increases in ACTH and cortisol during exercise that were proportional to relative exercise intensity for all groups. The cross-sectional design of this study precludes inferences about training status over other intrinsic HPA differences related to higher centers. Another recent cross-sectional comparison between highly trained endurance athletes and sedentary individuals showed no differences in plasma catecholamine responses to nonexertional stressors including a reaction-time shock avoidance task and the cold pressor test.[64,65]

D. ANXIETY AND DEPRESSION

Recent human evidence supports that the anxiety accompanying Major Depression is a principal clinical feature linked with HPA axis disruption measured by DST.[66] Weiss[67] has proposed that deficits in motivated behavior are the result of depleted NE in the locus coeruleus (LC) so that the normal inhibition of LC by its α-2 autoreceptors for NE is removed, leading to augmented release of NE from LC neurons projecting to other receptor fields in the limbic system and the spine.

It is believed that the LC fires in pulsatile bursts followed by a period of autoinhibition and α-2 autoinhibition modulates the response of LC neurons to excitatory stimuli. In addition to α-2 autoreceptor-mediated inhibition, it has been proposed that membrane changes in ion conductance lead to hyperpolarization of LC neurons due to a calcium-dependent influx of potassium.[68]

Gray[69] has argued that the LC-NE depletion model conceptualizes the role of the dorsal ascending noradrenergic bundle for the regulation of depression in a way similar to its established role in inhibiting behavior under conditions of threat that is characteristic of anxiety. Gray argues that the prevailing animal models of anxiety and neurotic depression share similar neurobiological pathways consistent with their shared clinical symptoms of agitation, hypervigilance, decreased motor activity under threat and HPA axis disruption.

A further parallel between depression and anxiety comes from the paradoxic phenomenon of "toughening up", in which chronic exposure (approximating two weeks) to the same uncontrollable stress that leads to a behavioral deficit (lasting 24 to 72 h) under acute exposure eliminates the behavioral deficit. The simple interpretation of this paradox is depletion or insufficient release of NE from LC following acute uncontrollable stress but increased synthesis of NE as an adaptive accommodation to chronic exposure. The similarity between the concept of "toughening up" with chronic monoamine or HPA adaptations to graduated exercise conditioning deserves study. It is plausible that acute episodes of both controlled and uncontrollable exercise stress could lead to increased metabolism and synthesis of monoamines and to an inoculation against central depletion and/or motivational deficits following acute uncontrollable stress.

III. EXERCISE AND ANXIETY

It is well established that subjective feelings of anxiety can be reduced 20 to 30 min following acute exercise, and the reduction may persist for one or more hours. However, the clinical significance and underlying mechanisms mediating the anxiolytic effect of exercise are unknown. A recent meta-analysis by Petruzzello et al.[7] concluded that exercise significantly reduced state anxiety with an overall effect size of one-fourth standard deviation, which held true regardless of which state anxiety measure was used. Chronic exercise was associated with a reduction in trait anxiety approximating one-third standard deviation. However, in experiments with adequate control conditions (e.g., quiet rest, reading), no difference in anxiety reduction was found between exercise and control conditions.[7] Thus, it is unknown if the relationship between exercise and anxiety reduction is causal, or if the anxiolytic effects can be attributed to some other factor common to exercise and the control conditions. This factor may be a distraction or "time-out" effect.[70] Distraction from sensory information can alter central neural processes, especially the ascending reticular system.[71]

Support for the "time-out" hypothesis of exercise and anxiety was first demonstrated by Bahrke and Morgan.[72] Subsequent research has shown exercise to have a similar anxiolytic affect as quiet rest,[73] taking a hot shower[73] and even eating a meal.[74]

A. BIOLOGICAL PLAUSIBILITY?

However, evidence indicates that some other mechanism mediates the anxiolytic effect of exercise. More reliable anxiety reduction is seen following aerobic exercise at an intensity of at least 60% $\dot{V}O_{2peak}$.[7,75] Some evidence also indicates that state anxiety reductions following exercise are more reliably seen in fit and/or trained individuals.[76,77,78] These differences could be due to an exercise training effect, a self-selection effect, a reappraisal of the physiological responses to exercise,[75] or to an expectancy influence. Taken collectively, available evidence suggests that the anxiolytic effect of acute exercise is due to some psychophysiological mechanism[7] and not simply the result of distraction or "time out" from environmental stressors.

The thermogenic hypothesis proposes that the anxiolytic effects of exercise may be due not to exercise per se, but to the environmentally independent increase in body core temperature that occurs during exercise.[38,79] This hypothesis has evolved from findings of similar reductions in subjective, electrocortical, cardiovascular, and neuromuscular indices of anxiety following exercise and passive heating. The hypothalamus plays a central role in autonomic nervous system regulation and thermal regulation. Afferent neurons convey temperature information to the hypothalamus which responds by initiating physiological adaptations including sweating and tachycardia. There are also close ties between the hypothalamus and limbic system structures. Thus, it is plausible that temperature activation of the hypothalamus during exercise, or perhaps deactivation following exercise, could influence hypothalamic input to the limbic system and to higher brain centers and thereby mediate, in part, the expression of and sensation of anxiety.[80]

Body core temperature (T_{core}) increases linearly as a function of relative exercise intensity,[81,82,83] and a modest elevation in relative exercise intensity (i.e., 10% increase) results in significant increases in T_{core}. Therefore, evidence of greater, or more reliable, anxiety reductions following vigorous vs. light exercise[7,84] suggests a thermally mediated influence of exercise intensity on anxiety reduction, but recent investigations from three different laboratories have found no support for the thermogenic hypothesis.[85,86,87]

Exercise studies have not adequately considered that anxiety is conceptually a multidimensional construct with cognitive, behavioral, and psychophysiological correlates.[32,69,88,89,90] Also, the signs and symptoms of anxiety can dissociate within individuals and across time and various conditions.[71,91,92]

The study of the anxiolytic effects of exercise requires a psychophysiological model. Blood pressure and brain electrocortical activity appear to be appropriate psychophysiological indices for testing anxiety reduction following acute exercise. Both variables have been associated with anxiety responses under nonexercise conditions.

B. BLOOD PRESSURE

Blood pressure typically increases during exposure to laboratory stressors, and decreases are associated with reductions in subjective assessment of anxiety.[93] The post-exercise hypotensive effect of acute exercise is well documented in humans.[94,95,96,97] Acute blood pressure reductions persist for 1 to 3 h following exercise and are observed following moderate exercise,[73,94] but they are greater following more vigorous exercise.[94] Significant acute blood pressure reductions have been found in normotensives as well as hypertensives[73] and in young as well as old individuals.[94] The mechanisms mediating the hypotensive effect of acute exercise are unknown.[98] Empirical evidence has failed to confirm the long-held assumption that decreased vascular resistance following exercise mediates the hypotensive response.[94,99] Recent evidence suggests that post-exercise hypotension is mediated by decreased sympathetic nervous system (SNS) activation following exercise. The decreased blood pressure following exercise reported by Hagberg et al. (1987) was attributed to a decreased cardiac output due to a 20% reduction in stroke volume. It was concluded that the reductions in stroke volume were due to a decreased myocardial contractility possibly mediated by a down regulation of myocardial β-adrenergic receptors as a result of acute elevation of plasma catecholamine concentration during exercise. This interpretation is supported by the work of Friedman et al.[100] in which decreased responsiveness to isoproterenol (an adrenergic agonist) in dogs persisted for 3 h following a 60-min treadmill run.

Other possible mediating factors influencing the hypotensive effect of exercise include peptides released from the atrium and ventricle of the heart, and endothelium relaxing factors.[98] Also, there is evidence that decreased SNS activity following exercise is due to endogenous opioid influences.[96,101] The degree to which these opioids are central in origin is unknown.

Also unknown is the extent to which decreases in anxiety and blood pressure following exercise are correlated or causally related. Few studies have concomitantly examined the effects of exercise on blood pressure and state anxiety or other psychophysiological indices of anxiety, but recent reports show that blood pressure and state anxiety responses can dissociate following acute exercise.[73,87] Much additional research is needed to establish the validity of blood pressure reduction as an index of reduced anxiety following exercise.

C. ELECTROENCEPHALOGRAPHY

Although there are a number of problems associated with attempting to infer psychological states from the electroencephalogram (EEG), it is generally agreed that subjective, behavioral, and psychophysiological correlates of relaxed wakefulness are associated with increased alpha brain activity (i.e., EEG in the 8 to 13 Hz frequency band) and decreased beta brain wave activity (i.e., EEG in the 14 to 40 Hz band) changes. Increases in alpha activity have been observed to follow acute aerobic exercise.[27,76,102-106] However, these studies are inconclusive because they have generally lacked control conditions or statistical analyses, and it is unclear whether standardized electroencephalographic recording techniques were employed. Also, with the exception of a study by Boutcher and Landers,[76] the studies did not measure concomitant changes in subjective feelings of anxiety. Many studies have only examined the alpha frequency band. Many factors unrelated to anxiety can affect the alpha rhythm (e.g., attention, blood sugar level, opening and closing the eyes). Blood pH changes due to exercise might also influence brain wave activity.[107] Also, perspiration could induce an artifact by decreasing electrode impedance and consequently increasing the strength of the recorded signal in all frequency bands. Limited psychological and physiological meaning can be ascribed to one frequency band without knowing what occurs in the other frequency bands.

Better controlled EEG studies have examined the acute effects of exercise on sleep and generally show increased slow-wave sleep (SWS) following exercise.[108,109,110] Slow-wave sleep is the deepest stage of sleep in which a deactivation of electrocortical activity and other markers of physiological arousal occur and is associated with a "well-rested" feeling upon wakening. Quasi-experimental studies of normal subjects have shown that acute exercise is followed by increased slow-wave sleep (SWS) during the evening of the exercise. High intensity (50 to 70% VO_2 max) exercise to exhaustion leads to increased SWS early in the sleep period concomitant with a decrease in rapid eye movement (REM) sleep. These effects have been seen most often when trained athletes are studied, and this has been attributed to greater energy expenditure during an exercise session by athletes when compared with non-athletes. A few acute studies of ultra endurance exercise show mixed results. Cross-sectional comparisons of fit and unfit subjects indicate that sleep differences are not dependent on daily exercise. Although this implies that a training effect is necessary for sleep effects, selection bias is an equally compelling explanation and convincing prospective studies of initially low fit persons have not been reported. Regional changes in brain blood flow and thermal effects have been proposed as plausible mechanisms for promoting sleep because of their established association with altered activity in both noradrenergic and serotonergic activity under resting conditions in rats. Porcine data indicate that during acute exercise, only blood flow to the cerebellum is increased following acute exercise.[111] Horne and Staff[110] found that vigorous exercise and passive heating conditions both resulted in significantly increased slow-wave sleep, while light exercise caused smaller, nonsignificant changes. Another study[109] found SWS increases to follow acute exercise, but when T_{core} was prevented from rising during exercise, no SWS changes were observed. The authors concluded that a high and sustained rate of body heating for 1 to 2 h might trigger a SWS response and that exercise might facilitate these effects. The author is unaware of prospective evidence that sleep is altered among patients with sleep disorders. No studies have been conducted with depressed or anxious patients to see if exercise may cause REM latency to lengthen or whether SWS may increase in depressed patients.

EEG activation techniques may prove to be more efficacious in establishing psychological significance of electrocortical activity. One such technique, photic stimulation (i.e., a flashing light stimulus), induces a phenomenon in which brain waves oscillate or "drive" at the same frequency, or at harmonics or subharmonics of the frequency of the light stimulus. There has been little research relating this phenomenon to anxiety levels, and the evidence is mixed. Only one exercise study was located that examined photic driving. Demeter and Nestianu[112] reported decreased photic driving following exercise. However, neither the exercise stimulus nor methods of photostimulation and recording were specified in this abstract report. No studies were located that have examined the effects of heating on photic driving.

It has been proposed that the effects of exercise on EEG may be due to sensory afference from baroreceptors.[113] Exercise may also reduce cortical arousal through inhibitory influence produced by prolonged and repetitive stimulation of the sensory afferents from muscle. Bonvallet and Bloch[114] have demonstrated in cats that an initial stimulation of the mesencephalic reticular activation system, or of afferent nerve fibers of anterior limbs, produces an initial cortical arousal.

In addition, recent evidence that photic driving decreases with increased adrenergic activity and decreases during cholinergically dominated states is of interest for exercise studies, because acute vigorous exercise can be accompanied by increases in both adrenergic and cholinergic activity. Drugs that induce an enhanced adrenergic state (e.g., noradrenalin, amphetamines, MAO inhibitors) have been shown to significantly reduce driving responses to photic stimulation.[115,116,117] Conversely, drugs which enhance cholinergic states by impairing central adrenergic mechanisms have been shown to enhance photically evoked brain-wave driving.[118] It has been proposed that ergotropic (e.g., exercise) and trophotropic behaviors are associated with decreased and increased driving, respectively.[119] However, the author is unaware of evidence supporting this hypothesis.

IV. AEROBIC FITNESS AND STRESS REACTIVITY

Resting heart rate (HR) and HR and catecholamine responses during standard submaximal aerobic exercise are decreased by aerobic exercise training. During the past decade, a small research literature has been interpreted as supportive that these adaptations to chronic exercise may generalize to nonexercise stressors. Thus, it has been proposed that increased aerobic fitness is accompanied not only by reduced physiological responses to a standard exercise stimulus but also by reduced physiological reactivity to nonexercise stressors.

A meta-analysis of 34 studies concluded that aerobically fit subjects had a stress response approximating one-half standard deviation less than that of unfit subjects.[5] The influence of a number of moderator variables, including published vs. unpublished study, type of exercise (acute/chronic), gender, statistical considerations (control/no control of initial values), study design (correlational/training program/control group/no control group), degrees of stress (high/low), source of results (during stress/post-stress recovery), and type of stress response measure was examined. It was concluded that the effect size was not statistically different for any of the moderating factors considered.

Although the statistical and design characteristics of the studies examined varied widely, effect sizes were statistically homogeneous for both controlled and uncontrolled studies. Despite this observation, there are a number of serious measurement and research design problems with the studies reviewed that preclude a consensus over their interpretation.

Relatively few of the studies included in the Crews and Landers meta-analysis objectively assessed fitness and/or activity status. In addition, most of the studies were cross-sectional and failed to assess additional variables that might confound the relationship between fitness and stress reactivity.

A. BIOLOGICAL PLAUSIBILITY?

None of the hypothesized mechanisms[5] for the presumed reduction in reactivity that accompanies aerobic fitness have been verified. Most have not been tested. Behavioral characteristics believed to be associated with exaggerated reactivity to stressors might confound the fitness/reactivity relationship. Enhanced parasympathetic and/or reduced sympathetic activation are believed to play an important role in fitness/related reductions of stress reactivity.[120,121] Alternatively, it has been reported that individuals characterized by the Type A behavior pattern (TABP) exhibit exaggerated cardiovascular reactivity to stressors.[122,123,124] In addition, there is evidence to suggest that individual differences in cardiovascular reactivity to stressors may be mediated primarily by differences in task-evoked β-adrenergic activity.[125,126] Thus, individuals exhibiting the Type A behavior pattern might also be characterized by exaggerated sympathetic activation in response to stressors. Exaggerated sympathetic activity might in turn be expected to oppose the influence of increased aerobic fitness. At least one study has reported such interactive effects of fitness and TABP on stress reactivity.[122]

Several studies have reported a smaller heart rate response to nonexercise stressors,[121,127,128] while others have reported no fitness-related reduction in the HR response to stressors but a more rapid HR recovery by fit individuals after stress.[129,130,131,132] Still other studies have reported no differences in the HR response patterns of fit and unfit groups.[120,122,133,134,135]

Fitness-related reductions in blood pressure reactivity to stressors have also been reported,[121,122,133,136,137] but negative results have also been reported.[135,138,139]

Heart rate and blood pressure have been the most commonly employed response measures in investigations of the relationship between aerobic fitness and stress reactivity. However, fitness-related reductions in other related stress responses have also been reported. Fit subjects were reported by van Doornen and de Geus[121] to exhibit a smaller stressor-induced decrement in cardiac pre-ejection period and a smaller increase in total peripheral resistance when compared to unfit subjects. Shulhan et al.[120] reported greater T-wave attenuation for low-fit vs. high-fit subjects in response to a difficult arithmetic task.

Brooke and Long[134] found that fit subjects showed more rapid plasma epinephrine (EPI) recovery after a rappelling task. However, they found no group differences in norepinephrine (NE) or cortisol recovery, and no group difference in response to the stressor for EPI, NE, or cortisol. Moreover, Hull and colleagues[133] reported no fitness-group differences in catecholamine responses to a battery of nonexertional stressors.

Much of the inconsistency can probably be explained by variation in the types of stressors employed in different studies. The various types of stressors employed include (1) cognitive performance tasks such as solving timed math problems, (2) passive tasks such as viewing films, (3) active physical tasks such as rappelling, and (4) passive physical tasks such as the cold pressor test.

The impact of aerobic fitness on physiological responses to stressors may be quite different for different types of stressors. Different types of stressors might be expected to elicit different degrees of sympathetic activation and require different degrees of physical effort. Cardiovascular response patterns to various stressors may show distinct differences in the degree to which cardiac or peripheral vasculature adjustments predominate. It is feasible that aerobic fitness level might interact differentially with these factors.

Another potential source of variability is a lack of standardization and objectivity of the methods for defining and assessing aerobic fitness and/or physical activity status.[140] Typically, determinations of aerobic fitness status were derived from estimates of $\dot{V}O_2$ max based on submaximal exercise HR measurements. Such estimates are subject to considerable error due to substantial individual variation in maximal HR. This source of error is compounded when HR is also used as a stress-response measure, as was the case in the majority of these studies. When HR defines both the independent and dependent variables, orthogonal tests of their association cannot be performed.[141]

V. PSYCHOLOGICAL MONITORING OF OVERTRAINING

While most evidence supports the potential for physical activity to exert positive mental health benefits, much less is known about risks for decreased mental health that may accompany intense and prolonged exercise. Irritability, apathy, lack of appetite, and sleep disturbances have been associated with overtraining among endurance athletes.[142-147] The work of Morgan and his students[145,146,148] indicates that mood disturbance may be an indicator of overtraining and staleness. In a series of cross-sectional and prospective studies with endurance athletes (runners, wrestlers, rowers, swimmers), Morgan and colleagues have repeatedly found that successful athletes (defined by Olympic and national team selection or consensus elite status) show profiles of mood states (POMS) that indicate positive mental health. At the outset of training or the team selection process, eventually successful athletes show less tension, depression, anger, fatigue, and confusion, but more vigor than do unsuccessful athletes or the average nonathlete of the same age.

Increasing mood disturbance shows a dose-response that accompanies increased training, and it correlates with decreased performance and increased muscle soreness among collegiate swimmers across the season. Conversely, as training volume decreases with tapering, mood disturbance lessens.

Studies of overtraining that combine assessments of psychological, neuroendocrine, and immune responses in order to establish dose-response relationships are needed. Stress emotions related to mood disturbance have been linked with immunocompetence and lymphocyte cytotoxicity.[149] In addition, evidence from psychoneuroimmunology suggests that stress hormones[150,151,152] may mediate psychological influences on immune responses. The relationship between psychological traits and states, stress hormones, and immune function has not been studied during exercise training,[153] but it is likely their interactions can explain important aspects of the etiology that underlies the clinical features of staleness.

Although daily cortisol levels may provide a practical marker of HPA disruption, the many sites for regulating the HPA axis may explain why studies have not always agreed over the autonomic and endocrine responses that accompany overtraining. Conflicting results can occur because of differences in the regulatory status of the HPA axis. Also, concentrations of HPA hormones under resting conditions may not be as sensitive or specific to overtraining as are hormone responses to challenge tests of the HPA axis.

A recent study[154] reported a decreased resting ACTH and cortisol response to CRF among highly trained runners compared with sedentary and moderately trained runners. This response was consistent with sustained hypercortisolism in the highly trained group. It occurred despite comparable increases for all groups in ACTH and cortisol during exercise. However, the cross-sectional design of the study prevents the conclusion that overtraining, rather than other intrinsic HPA differences, explained the results. Self-selection biases can cloud results in these types of studies. This is illustrated by another cross-sectional comparison between highly trained endurance athletes and sedentary individuals that found no differences in plasma DA and NE responses to nonexertional stressors including a reaction-time shock avoidance task and the cold pressor test.[155]

Uncontrolled prospective studies of overtraining also report mixed results. Increased salivary cortisol and mood disturbance have been reported after overtraining in female collegiate swimmers,[148] and these results are consistent with a hypercortisolism marker of staleness. However, another study of "stale" endurance athletes showed lower than expected plasma cortisol, ACTH, growth hormone, and prolactin response to insulin-induced hypoglycemia, and the responses returned to normal following 4 weeks of rest.[156] These results were interpreted as evidence for inhibition of the normal responsiveness by the hypothalamus as a result of overtraining. These two studies show that cortisol responses of stale athletes may differ between resting conditions and tests that challenge functions of the HPA axis. They also suggest that the response seen must be judged against a biologically appropriate index of normal HPA function. Related to hypercortisolism is the disruption of circadian rhythms[157,158] including sleep. The author is unaware of scientific studies of sleep during overtraining or sleep problems reported by stale athletes. Prospective studies of athletes undergoing systematic periods of overtraining and decreased training, contrasted with comparable athletes who do not overtrain or with a truly randomized control group, are necessary before the sensitivity, specificity, and predictive validity of staleness risk factors can be identified. Randomized experiments will also permit understanding of the physiological and psychological mechanisms responsible for staleness adaptations. Epidemiological studies with large representative samples are also needed to establish the prevalence and incidence of staleness, and its risk factors, among populations of athletes from sports where overtraining and staleness are believed to be problems.

Clinical parallels have also been drawn between excessively committed runners and patients diagnosed as suffering from anorexia nervosa. It is believed that the disciplined training and social milieu in sports that place a high premium on a lean body composition and dietary restriction may promote the development of eating problems or add to existing problems.

It remains unclear, however, if these circumstances reveal a common etiology, if they are each motivated by common goals or incentives, or rather, if each represent compulsions with similar surface behaviors, but with different origins, underlying processes, and medical outcomes. These are important questions to resolve because case studies have reported that running psychotherapy can aid the treatment of anorexia as exercise is an alternative to restrictive dieting among weight conscious females. It is clear that regular exercise can assist weight loss and weight management for many people. Although the link between exercise and body weight appears to offer healthful benefits for many, pathological extremes might be present as well. Case data have revealed instances where obsessions with weight loss might parallel excessive commitment to exercise and physical fitness.

Although concern over excessive exercise and risk for eating disorders appears to have some basis, results from other studies reveal that the issues are complex. Anorexics are commonly reported to augment food restriction by hyperactivity, but their aerobic fitness ($\dot{V}O_2$ peak) is well below average, while that of habitual runners and overtrained athletes is well above average. In addition, cross-sectional studies have no revealed a common psychopathology between obligatory (i.e., excessively committed) runners and anorexic patients.[159,160]

Scientific findings that are available do not yet permit clear conclusions. Previous studies lack generalizability and standardization of sampling and method. Small selected groups of athletes from different sport, regions, levels of competition, and socioeconomic backgrounds have been sampled. This makes it difficult to compare risks between types of sport when other influences on eating behaviors such as family history, personality, or socioeconomic status may differ between samples. Similarly, athletes' risk profiles have not been evaluated against those for nonathlete matched controls from the same academic, socioeconomic, or psychological background. Furthermore, standardized measures of eating attitudes and behaviors have not been uniformly used with athlete samples. Thus, it is difficult to compare study outcomes because different dependent measures have been used. Studies that have compared habitual exercisers from a community or population base with anorexic patients have not quantified the exercise behavior of either sample to verify the similarities or differences in physical activity assumed to exist between the two groups. This prevents conclusions that differences or similarities in eating behaviors or attitudes seen in athletes and anorexics are due to involvement in sport or exercise rather than due to attributes that existed prior to self-selection into the anorexic and exerciser groups. In any case, it is plausible that stress due to comorbid eating disorder and exercise abuse could contribute to immunosuppression; however, the author is unaware of any studies of these phenomena.

Morgan[161] described eight cases of "running addiction," when commitment to running exceeded prior commitments to work, family, social relations, and medical advice. Similar cases have been labeled as positive addiction, runner's gluttony, fitness fanaticism, athlete's neurosis, obligatory running, and exercise abuse.[159] However, little is understood about the origins, diagnostic validity, or the mental health impact of abusive exercise. For most people, the benefits of exercise exceed the risks of exercise abuse; sedentariness represents a more prevalent public health problem.

Because endurance exercise continues to be promoted as a health behavior, it is important to accurately identify overall risks, and individuals at risk, for mental health disorders that might accompany an exercise training regimen. In two recent controlled experimental studies of risks,[162,163] we have not observed the negative health consequences we expected based on earlier cross-sectional studies. Healthy inactive women showed no pathological signs of eating disorders or mental health problems following a 6-month overtraining period during which weekly running mileage was increased from less than 10 to more than 60 miles per week. We have also observed increased muscular strength and cardiorespiratory endurance following 12 weeks of training in males diagnosed as seropositive for the HIV-1 human immunodeficiency virus and symptomatic for AIDS or AIDS related complex. The increased fitness occurred with no change in T-lymphocyte phenotypes or in clinical diagnosis of health status. In both studies, overtraining was gradual according to the guidelines of the American College of Sports Medicine. Thus, our results show that the amount of physical activity that will increase risk for mental health problems or immune suppression is unknown and may vary widely from person to person.

VI. SUMMARY

There are a sufficient number of studies that show consistent results to conclude that acute and chronic physical activity can improve mood in normal individuals and that chronic exercise is accompanied by reduced symptoms or minor and major unipolar depression and generalized anxiety in symptomatic patients. Nearly all of these studies have sampled young and middle-aged white males and females. Collectively, a few population-based studies also suggest that physical activity reduces risk for depression in the population. However, there are not enough population studies available to determine if the effects seen in clinical settings generalize to the population. It is not yet clear that chronic activity or physical fitness reduce reactivity to nonexercise stressors or whether the risks of overtraining or abusive exercise are prevalent enough to represent a public health concern. The author is unaware of studies that directly show decreased morbidity or risk for morbidity and mortality that accompany physical activity are mediated by changes in anxiety, depression, or stress reactivity. The roles of these variables as potential mediators or moderators of the relationship between physical activity and immunity are also unestablished and have received very little research attention.

For all the areas of research reviewed, epidemiological criteria for causality, including independence of the effect observed, persistence of the effect over time, a dose-response relationship, and biological plausibility, have not been satisfied by the available evidence from physical activity studies. Also, the studies reviewed have been atheoretical, conducted without consideration of broader based theoretical models of human emotion[88,164] and mental health disorders.[29,30,32,65] There is sufficient evidence to warrant accelerated research on the psychological effects of exercise for disease resistance and health promotion. However, if advances in our scientific and applied knowledge are to be made, future research should also study ethnic and minority groups, gender comparisons, children and older adults, and individuals of varying health status. Studies must begin to experimentally examine cognitive and neurobiological mechanisms, using human and animal comparative models when appropriate, and apply epidemiological traditions within broader theories of emotion and disease.

ACKNOWLEDGMENTS

Thanks go to my doctoral students, Andrea L. Dunn, Ralph E. Graham, and Shawn D. Youngstedt, for their scholarly contributions to the preparation of this chapter.

REFERENCES

1. **Burton, R.,** *The Anatomy of Melancholy,* Henry Cripps, Oxford, 1632.
2. **Campbell, D. D. and Davis, J. E.,** Report of research and experimentation in exercise and recreational therapy, *Am. J. Psychiatry,* 96, 925, 1939.
3. **Morgan, W. P. and Goldston, S. E.,** Eds., *Exercise and Mental Health,* Washington Hemisphere Publishing, Washington, D.C., 1987.
4. **Bouchard, C., Shephard, R. J., Stephens, T., Sutton, J. R., and McPherson, B. D.,** *Exercise, Fitness, and Health: a Consensus of Current Knowledge,* Human Kinetics, Champaign, IL, 1990.
5. **Crews, D. J. and Landers, D. M.,** A meta-analytic review of aerobic fitness and reactivity to psychosocial stressors, *Med. Sci. Sports Exercise,* 19(Suppl.), S114, 1987.
6. **North, T. C., McCullagh, P., and Vu Tran, Z.,** Effect of exercise on depression, *Exercise Sport Sci. Rev.,* 18, 379, 1990.
7. **Petruzzello, S. J., Landers, D. M., Hatfield, B. D., Kubitz, K. A., and Salazar, W.,** A meta-analysis on the anxiety reducing effects of acute and chronic exercise: outcomes and mechanisms, *Sports Med.,* 11, 142, 1991.
8. **Smith, M. L., Glass, G. V., and Miller, T. E.,** *The Benefits of Psychotherapy,* Johns Hopkins University Press, Baltimore, MD, 1980.
9. **Regier, D. A., Hirschfield, R. M. A., Goodwin, F. K., Burke, J. D., Lazar, J. B., and Judd, L. L.,** The NIMH depression awareness, recognition, and treatment program: structure, aims, and scientific basis, *Am. J. Psychiatry,* 145, 1351, 1988.
10. **Powell, K. E., Thompson, P. D., Caspersen, C. J., and Kendrick, J.,** Physical activity and the incidence of coronary heart disease, *Annu. Rev. Public Health,* 8, 253, 1987.
11. **Tonind, L. N., Helzer, J. E., Weissman, M. M., Orvaschel, H., Gruenberg, E., Burke, J. D., and Regier, D. A.,** Lifetime prevalence of specific psychiatric disorders in three sites, *Arch. Gen. Psychiatry,* 41, 949, 1984.
12. **Shapiro, S., Skinner, E. A., Kessler, L. G., et al.,** Utilization of health and mental services, *Arch. Gen. Psychiatry,* 41, 971, 1984.
13. **Friedman, H. S. and Booth-Kewley, S.,** The "disease-prone personality". A meta-analytic view of the construct, *Am. Psychol.,* 42, 539, 1987.
14. **Kiecolt-Glaser, J. K. and Glaser, R.,** Psychosocial moderators of immune function, *Ann. Behav. Med.,* 9, 16, 1987.
15. **Shavit, Y. and Martin, F. C.,** Opiates, stress, and immunity: animal studies, *Ann. Behav. Med.,* 91, 11, 1987.
16. **Menkes, M. S., Matthews, K. A., Krantz, D. S., Lundberg, U., Mead, L. A., Qagish, B., Liang, K., Thomas, C. B., and Pearson, T. A.,** Cardiovascular reactivity to the cold pressor test as a predictor of hypertension, *Hypertension,* 14, 524, 1989.
17. **Harris, S. S., Caspersen, C. J., DeFriese, G. H., and Estes, Jr., E. H.,** Physical activity counseling for healthy adults as a primary preventive intervention in the clinical setting, *JAMA,* 261, 3590, 1989.
18. **Martinsen, E. W.,** The role of aerobic exercise in the treatment of depression, *Stress Med.,* 3, 93, 1987.
19. American Psychiatric Association, Diagnostic and Statistical Manual of Mental Disorders, 3rd ed., Revised, (DSM-III-R), American Psychiatric Association, Washington, D.C., 1987.
20. **Spitzer, R. L., Endicott, J., and Robins, E.,** Research diagnostic criteria rationale and reliability, *Arch. Gen. Psychiatry,* 35, 773, 1978.
21. **Greist, J. H., Klein, M. H., Eischens, R. R., Faris, J. W., Guirman, A. S., and Morgan, W. P.,** Running through your mind, *J. Psychosom. Res.,* 22, 259, 1978.
22. **Klein, M. H., Greist, J. H., Gurman, R. A., et al.,** A comparative outcome study of group psychotherapy vs. exercise treatments for depression, *Int. J. Ment. Health,* 13, 148, 1985.

23. **Sothmann, M. S.**, Catecholamines, behavioral stress, and exercise — introduction to the symposium, *Med. Sci. Sports Exercise,* 23, 836, 1991.
24. **Caspersen, C. J., Powell, K. E., and Christenson, G. M.**, Physical activity, exercise, and physical fitness: definitions and distinctions for health-related rsearch, *Public Health Rep.,* 100, 126, 1985.
25. **Dush, D. M.**, The placebo in psychosocial outcome evaluations, *Eval. Health Prof.,* 9, 421, 1986.
26. **Martinsen, E. W., Hoffart, A., and Solberg, O.**, Comparing aerobic with nonaerobic forms of exercise in the treatment of clinical depression: a randomized trial, *Compr. Psychiatry,* 30, 324, 1989.
27. **Farmer, M. E., Locke, B. Z., Moscicki, E. K., Dannenberg, A. L., Larson, D. B., and Radloff, L. S.**, Physical activity and depressive symptoms: the NHANES I epidemiologic follow-up study, *Am. J. Epidem.,* 128, 1340, 1988.
28. **Stephens, T.**, Physical activity and mental health in the United States and Canada: evidence from four population surveys, *Prev. Med.,* 17, 35, 1988.
29. **Post, R. M. and Ballenger, J. C., Eds.**, *Neurobiology of Mood Disorders,* Williams and Wilkins, Baltimore, MD, 1984.
30. **Koob, G. F., Ehlers, C. L., and Kupfer, D. J., Eds.**, *Animal Models of Depression,* Birkhauser, Boston, 1989.
31. **Cooper, J. R., Bloom, F. E., and Roth, R. H.**, *The Biochemical Basis of Neuropharmacology,* 5th ed., Oxford University Press, New York, 1986.
32. **Burrows, G. D., Roth, M., and Noyes, Jr., R., Eds.**, *Handbook of Anxiety,* Elsevier, Amsterdam, 1990.
33. **Beckmann, H. and Goodwin, F. K.**, Urinary MHPG in subgroups of depressed patients and controls, *Neuropsychobiology,* 6, 91, 1980.
34. **Schildkraut, J. J.**, The catecholamine hypothesis of affective disorders: a review of supporting evidence, *Am. J. Psychiatry,* 122, 509, 1965.
35. **Schildkraut, J. J., Orsulak, P. J., Schatzberg, A. F., and Rosenbaum, A. H.**, Relationship between psychiatric diagnostic groups of depressive disorders and MHPG, in *MHPG: Basic Mechanism and Psychopathology,* Maas, J. W., Ed., Academic Press, New York, 1983, 129.
36. **Coppen, A.**, Depressed states and indolealkylamines, in *Advances in Pharmacology,* Vol. 6, Academic Press, New York, 1968, 283.
37. **Baldessarini, R. J.**, Current status of antidepressants: clinical pharmacology and therapy, *J. Clin. Psychiatry,* 50, 117, 1989.
38. **Morgan, W. P. and O'Connor, P. J.**, Exercise and mental health, in *Exercise Adherence: Its Impact on Public Health,* Dishman, R. K., Ed., Human Kinetics, Champaign, IL, 1988, 91.
39. **Peyrin, L.**, Urinary MHPG sulfate as a marker of central norepinephrine metabolism: a commentary, *J. Neural. Transm.,* 80, 51, 1990.
40. **Tang, S. W., Stancer, H. C., Takahashi, S., Shephard, R. J., and Warsh, J. J.**, Controlled exercise elevates plasma but not urinary MHPG and VMA, *Psychiatr. Res.,* 4, 13, 1981.
41. **Maas, J. W. and Leckman, J. F.**, Relationships between central nervous system noradrenergic function and plasma and urinary MHPG and other norepinephrine metabolites, in *MHPG: Basic Mechanisms and Psychopathology,* Maas, J. W., Ed., Academic Press, New York, 1983, 33.
42. **Filser, J. G., Spira, J., and Fischer, M., et al.**, The evaluation of 4-hydroxy-3-methoxyphenyglycol sulfate as a possible marker of central norepinephrine turnover: studies in health volunteers and depressed patients, *J. Psychiatr. Res.,* 22, 171, 1988.
43. **Sothmann, M. S. and Ismail, H. H.**, Relationships between urinary catecholamine metabolites, particularly MHPF, and selected personality and physical fitness characteristics in normal subjects, *Psychosom. Med.,* 46, 523, 1984.

44. **Sothmann, M. S., Ismail, A. H., and Chodepko-Zajiko, W.,** Influence of catecholamine activity on the hierarchical relationships among physical fitness condition and selected personality characteristics, *J. Clin. Psychol.,* 40, 1308, 1984.
45. **Lobstein, D. D., Mosbacher, B. J., and Ismail, A. H.,** Depression as a powerful discriminator between physically active and sedentary middle-aged men, *J. Psychosom. Res.,* 27, 69, 1983.
46. **Sothmann, M. S. and Ismail, A. H.,** Factor analytic derivation of the MHPG/NM ration. Implications for studying the link between physical fitness and depression, *Biol. Psychiatry,* 20, 570, 1985.
47. **Dunn, A. L. and Dishman, R. K.,** Exercise and the neurobiology of depression, *Exercise Sport Sci. Rev.,* 19, 41, 1991.
48. **Chauloff, F.,** Physical exercise and brain monoamines: a review, *Acta Physiol. Cand.,* 137, 1, 1989.
49. **Fuxe, K., Cintra, A., and Agnati, L. F., et al.,** Studies on the cellular localization and distribution of glucocorticoid receptor and estrogen receptor immunoreactivity in the central nervous system of the rat and their relationship to the monoaminergic and peptidergic neurons of the brain, *J. Steroid Biochem.,* 27, 159, 1987.
50. **Stone, E. A.,** Accumulation and metabolism of NE in rat hypothalamus after exhaustive stress, *J. Neurochem.,* 21, 589, 1973.
51. **Butler, J., O'Brien, M., O'Malley, K., and Kelly, J. G.,** Relationship of B-adrenoceptor density to fitness in athletes, *Nature,* 298, 60, 1982.
52. **Lockette, W., McCurdy, R., Smith, S., and Carretero, O.,** Endurance training and alpha 2-adrenergic receptors on platelets, *Med. Sci. Sports Exercise,* 19, 7, 1987.
53. **Antoni, F. A.,** Hypothalamic control of adrenocorticotropin secretion: advances since the discovery of 41-residue corticotropin releasing factor, *Endocrine. Rev.,* 7, 351, 1986.
54. **Axelrod, J. and Resine, T. D.,** Stress hormones: their interaction and regulation, *Science,* 224, 452, 1984.
55. **Jones, M. T. and Gillham, B.,** Factors involved in the regulation of adrenocorticotropic hormone/B-lipotropic hormone, *Physiol. Rev.,* 68, 743, 1988.
56. **Gold, P. W., Goodwin, F. K., and Chrousos, G. P.,** Clinical and biochemical manifestations of depression, relation to the neurobiology of stress, I, *N. Engl. J. Med.* 319, 348, 1988.
57. **Gold, P. W., Goodwin, F. K., and Chrousos, G. P.,** Clinical and biochemical manifestations of depression, relation to the neurobiology of stress. II, *N. Eng. J. Med.,* 319, 413, 1988.
58. **Sachar, E. J., Asnis, G., Halbreich, U., Nathan, R. S., and Halpern, F.,** Recent studies in the neuroendocrinology of major depressive disorders, *Psychiatr. Clin. North. Am.,* 3, 3113, 1980.
59. **Sapolsky, R. M., Krey, L. C., and McEwen, B. S.,** Stress down-regulates corticosterone receptors in a site-specific manner in the brain, *Endocrinology,* 114, 287, 1984.
60. **Sapolsky, R. M. and Plotsky, P. M.,** Hypercortisolism and its possible neutral bases, *Biol. Psychiatry,* 27, 937, 1990.
61. **Galbo, H., Kjaer, M., and Mikines, M., et al.,** Discussion: hormonal adaptation to physical activity, in *Exercise, Fitness and Health: A Consensus of Current Knowledge,* Bouchard, C., Shepard, R. J., Stephens, T., Sutton, J. R., and McPherson, B. D., Eds., Human Kinetics Publisher, Champaign, IL, 1990, 259.
62. **Sutton, J. R., Farrell, P. A., and Harber, V. J.,** Hormonal adaptations to physical activity, in *Exercise, Fitness and Health: A Consensus of Current Knowledge,* Bouchard, C., Shepard, R. J., Stephens, T., Sutton, J. R., and McPherson, B. D., Ed., Human Kinetics Publishers, Champaign, IL, 1990, 17.
63. **Luger, A., Deuster, P. A., and Kyle, S. B., et al.,** Acute hypothalamic-pituitary-adrenal responses to the stress of treadmill exercise: physiological adaptations to physical training, *N. Engl. J. Med.,* 316, 1309, 1987.

64. **Claytor, R. P., Cox, R. H., Howley, E. T., Lawler, K. A. and Lawler, J. E.,** Aerobic power and cardiovascular response to stress, *J. Appl. Physiol.,* 65, 1416, 1988.

65. **Willner, P.,** *Depression: A Psychobiological Synthesis,* John Wiley & Sons, New York, 1985.

66. **Meador-Woodruff, J. H., Greden, J. F., Grunhaus, L., and Haskett, R. F.,** Severity of depression and hypothalamic-pituitary-adrenal axis dysregulation: identification of contributing factors, *Acta Psychiatr. Scand.,* 81, 364, 1990.

67. **Weiss, J. M., Glazer, H. I., and Pohorecky, L. A.,** Coping behavior and neurochemical changes: an alternative explanation for the "learned helplessness" experiments, in *Animal Models in Human Psychobiology,* Serban, G. and King, A., Eds., Plenum Press, New York, 1976, 141.

68. **Adrade, R. and Aghajanian, G. K.,** Locus coeruleus activity in vitro: intrinsic regulation by a calcium-dependent potassium conductance but not alpha-2 adrenoreceptors, *J. Neurosci.,* 4, 161, 1984.

69. **Gray, J. A.,** Issues in the neuropsychology of anxiety, in *Anxiety and the Anxiety Disorders,* Tuma, A. H. and Masser, J. D., Eds., Lawrence Erlbaum Associates, Hillsdale, New Jersey, 1985, 5.

70. **Morgan, W. P.,** Physical activity and mental health, in *Exercise and Health,* Eckert, H. M. and Montoye, H. J., Eds., Human Kinetics, Champaign, IL, 1984, 132.

71. **Teichner, W. H.,** Interaction of behavioral and physiological stress reactions, *Psychol. Rev.,* 75, 271, 1968.

72. **Bahrke, M. S. and Morgan, W. P.,** Anxiety reduction following exercise and mediation, *Cog. Ther. Res.,* 2, 323, 1978.

73. **Raglin, R. S. and Morgan, W. P.,** Influence of acute execise and distraction on state anxiety and blood pressure, *Med. Sci. Sports Exercise,* 19, 456, 1987.

74. **Wilson, V. E., Berger, B. C., and Byrd, E. L.,** Effects of running and an exercise class on anxiety, *Percept. Mot. Skills,* 53, 4772, 1981.

75. **Dishman, R. K.,** Mental health, in *Physical Activity and Well Being,* Seefeldt, V., Ed., AAHPERD, Reston, VA, 1986.

76. **Boutcher, S. H. and Landers, D. M,** The effects of vigorous exercise on anxiety, heart rate and Alpha activity of runners and nonrunners, *Psychophysiology,* 23, 696, 1988.

77. **Dishman, R. K., Farquhar, R., and Cureton, K. J.,** Subjective and physiological responses during preferred exertion levels in physically active and inactive men, submitted for publication.

78. **Roth, D. L.,** Acute emotional and psychophysiological effects of aerobic exercise, *Psychophysiology,* 26, 593, 1989.

79. **Morgan, W. P.,** Affective beneficence of vigorous physical activity, *Med. Sci. Sports Exercise,* 17, 94, 1985.

80. **Reeves, D. L., Levinson, D. M., Justesen, D. R., and Lubin, B.,** Endogenous hyperthermia in normal human subjects. II. Experimental study of emotional states, *International J. Psychosom.,* 32, 18, 1985.

81. **Davies, J. R., Brotherhood, J. B., and Zeiderford, E.,** Temperature regulation during severe exercise with some observations on effect of skin wetting, *J. Appl. Physiol.,* 41, 772, 1976.

82. **Gilsolfi, C. V. and Weger, C. B.,** Temperature regulation during exercise: old concepts, new ideas, *Exercise Sports Sci. Rev.,* 12, 339, 1984.

83. **Sawka, M. N. and Weger, C. B.,** Physiological responses to acute exercise-heat stress, in *Human Performance Physiology and Environmental Medicine at Terrestrial Extremes,* Pandolf, K. B., Sawka, M. N., and Gonzalez, R. R., Eds., Benchmark Press, Indianapolis, 1988, 97.

84. **Farrell, P. A., Gustafson, A. B., Morgan, W. P., and Pert, C. B.,** Enkephalins, catecholamines and psychological mood alterations: effects of prolonged exercise, *Med. Sci. Sports Exercise,* 19, 347, 1987.

85. **Koltyn, K. F. and Morgan, W. P.,** Psychobiological responses to paced scuba exercise, *Med. Sci. Sports Exercise,* 23(Suppl), S41, 1991.

86. **Petruzzello, S. J., Landers, D. M., and Salazar, W.,** Exercise and anxiety reduction: examination of the thermogenic hypothesis, *Med. Sci. Sports Exercise,* 23(Suppl), S41, 1991.

87. **Youngstedt, S. D., Dishman, R. K., Cureton, K., Peacock, L., Wells, W., Fluech, D., and Hinson, B.,** Does body temperature mediate anxiolytic effects of acute exercise? *Med. Sci. Sports Exercise,* 23(Suppl.), S41, 1991.

88. **Lang, P. J.,** The cognitive psychophysiology of emotion: fear and anxiety, in *Anxiety and Anxiety Disorders,* Tuma, A. H. and Maser, J., Eds., Lawrence Erlbaum Associates Publishers, Hillsdale, New Jersey, 1985.

89. **Spielberger, C. D.,** The measurement of state and trait anxiety: conceptual and methodological issues in research, in *Anxiety: Current Trends in Theory and Research,* Vol. 1, Spielberger, C. D., Ed., Academic Press, New York, 1975.

90. **Tuma, A. H. and Maser, J. D.,** *Anxiety and the Anxiety Disorders,* Lawrence Erlbaum Associates, Hillsdale, New Jersey, 1985.

91. **Andreassi, J. L.,** *Psychophysiology,* Oxford Press, New York, 1980.

92. **Lacey, J. I. and Lacey, B. C.,** Verification and extension of the principle of atonomic response sterotypy, *Am. J. Psychol.,* 71, 50, 1958.

93. **Lader, M. H.,** *The Psychophysiology of Mental Illness,* Routledge & Kegan Paul, Boston, 1975.

94. **Hagberg, J. M., Montain, S. J., and Martin, W. H.,** Blood pressure and hemodynamic responses after exercise in older hypertensives, *J. Appl. Physiol.,* 63, 270, 1987.

95. **Kaufman, F. L., Hughson, R. L., and Schaman, J. P.,** Effect of exercise on recovery blood pressure in normotensive and hypertensive subjects, *Med. Sci. Sports Exercise,* 19, 17, 1987.

96. **Hoffmann, P. and Thoren, P.,** Long-lasting cardiovascular depression induced by acupuncture-like stimulation of the sciatic nerve in unanesthetized rats. Effects of arousal and type of hypertension, *Acta Physiol. Scand.,* 135, 275, 1986.

97. **Shyu, B. C. and Thoren, P.,** Circulatory events following spontaneous muscle exercise in normotensive and hypertensive rats, *Acta Physiol. Scand.,* 128, 515, 1986.

98. **Tipton, C. M.,** Exercise, training and hypertension: an update, *Exercise Sports Sci. Rev.,* 19, 447, 1991.

99. **Overton, J. M., Joyner, M. J., and Tipton, C. M.,** Reduction in blood pressure after acute exercise by hypertensive rats, *J. Appl. Physiol.,* 64, 748, 1988.

100. **Friedman, D. B., Ordway, G. A., and Williams, R. S.,** Exercie-induced functional desensitization of canine cardiac b-adrenergic receptors, *J. Appl. Physiol.,* 62, 1721, 1987.

101. **Boone, J. B., Levine, M., Flynn, M. G., Pizza, F. X., Kubitz, G. R., and Andres, F. F.,** Opiod receptor modulation of post exercise hypotension, *Med. Sci. Sports Exercise,* 22(Abstr.), S106, 1990.

102. **Daugherty, P. L., Fernhall, B., and McCanne, T. R.,** The effects of three exercise intensities on the alpha brain wave activity, *Med. Sci. Sports Exercise,* 19, S23, 1987.

103. **Kamp, A. and Troost, J.,** EEG signs of cerebrovascular disorder, using physical exercise as a provocative method, *Electroencephal. Clin. Neurophysiol.,* 45, 295, 1978.

104. **Pineda, A. and Adkisson, M. A.,** Electroencephalographic studies in physical fatigue, Texas Reports, *Biol. Med.,* 19, 332, 1987.

105. **Severtson, B. M. A.,** Effects of meditation and aerobic exercise on EEG patterns, *J. Neurosci. Nursing,* 18, 206, 1986.

106. **Wiese, J., Singh, M., and Yuedall, L.,** Occipital and parietal alpha power before, during and after exercise, *Med. Sci. Sports Exercise,* 15, 117, 1983.

107. **Remond, A., Ed.,** *Handbook of Electroencephalography and Clinical Neurophysiology,* Elsevier, Amsterdam, 1976.

108. **Horne, J. A.,** The effects of exercise on sleep: a critical review, *Bio. Psychol.,* 3, 241, 1981.
109. **Horne, J. A. and Moore, V. J.,** Sleep effects of exercise with and without additional body cooling, *Electroencephal. Clin. Neurophysiol.,* 60, 33, 1985.
110. **Horne, J. A. and Staff, L. H. E.,** Exercise and sleep: body heating effects, *Sleep,* 6, 36, 1983.
111. **Norton, K. I., Delp, M. T., Jones, M. T., Duan, C., Dengel, D. R., and Armstrong, R. B.,** Distribution of blood flow during exercise following blood volume expansion in swine, *J. Appl. Physiol.,* in press.
112. **Demeter, A. and Nestianu, V.,** The dynamics of photic driving under conditions of effort in athletes, *Electroencephal. Clin. Neurophysiol.,* 18, 635, 1965.
113. **Koriath, J. J., Lindholm, E., and Landers, D. M.,** Cardiac-related cortical activity during variations in mean heart rate, *Int. J. Psychophysiol.,* 5, 289, 1987.
114. **Bonvallet, M. and Bloch, V.,** Bulbar control of cortical arousal, *Science,* 133, 1133, 1961.
115. **Floru, R., Costin, A. Nestianu, V., and Sterescu-Volanschi, M.,** Research concerning the effect of noradrenaline upon the electric activity of the central nervous system and upon the evoked rhythm of intermittent photic stimulation in cats with chronic electrodes, *Electroencephal. Clin. Neurophysiol.,* 14, 561, 1962.
116. **Shetty, T.,** Photic responses in hyperkinesis of childhood, *Science,* 174, 1356, 1971.
117. **Vogel, W., Broverman, D. M., Klaiber, E. L., and Kobayashi, Y.,** EEG driving responses as a function of monoamine oxidase, *Electroencephal. Clin. Neurophysiol.,* 10, 325, 1958.
118. **Jorgensen, R. S. and Wulff, M. H.,** The effect of orally administered chlorpromazine on the electroencephalogram of man, *Electroencephal. Clin. Neurophysiol.,* 10, 325, 1958.
119. **Vogel, W., Broverman, D. M., Klaiber, E. L., and Kun, K. J.,** EEG response as a function of cognitive style, *Electroencephal. Clin. Neurophysiol.,* 27, 186, 1969.
120. **Shulhan, D., Scher, H., and Furedy, J. J.,** Phasic cardiac reactivity to psychological stress as a function of aerobic fitness level, *Psychophysiology,* 23, 562, 1986.
121. **van Doornen, L. J. P. and deGeus, E. J. C.,** Aerobic fitness and the cardiovascular response to stress, *Psychophysiology,* 26, 17, 1989.
122. **Lake, B. W., Suarez, E. C., Schneiderman, N., and Tocci, N.,** The type A behavior pattern, physical fitness, and psychophysiological reactivity, *Health Psychol.,* 4, 169, 1985.
123. **Jamieson, J. L. and Lavoie, N. F.,** Type A behavior, aerobic power, and cardiovascular recovery from a psychosocial stressor, *Health Psychol.,* 6, 361, 1987.
124. **Harbin, T. J.,** The relationship between the Type A behavior pattern and physiological responsivity: a quantitative review, *Psychophysiology,* 26, 110, 1989.
125. **Obrist, P. A.,** *Cardiovascular Psychophysiology: A Perspective,* Plenum Press, New York, 1981.
126. **Light, K. C.,** Cardiovascular responses to effortful active coping: implications for the role of stress in hypertension development, *Psychophysiology,* 18, 216, 1981.
127. **Holmes, D. S. and Roth, D. L.,** Association of aerobic fitness with pulse rate and subjective responses to psychological stress, *Psychophysiology,* 22, 525, 1985.
128. **Holmes, D. S. and Cappo, B. M.,** Prophylactic effect of aerobic fitness on cardiovascular arousal among individuals with a family history of hypertension, *J. Psychosom. Res.,* 5, 601, 1987.
129. **Cox, J. P., Evans, J. F., and Jamieson, J. L.,** Aerobic power and tonic heart rate response to psychosocial stressors, *Pers. Soc. Psychol. Bull.,* 5, 160, 1979.
130. **Hollander, B. J. and Seraganian, P.,** Aerobic fitness and psychophysiological reactivity, *Can. J. Behav. Sci.,* 16, 257, 1984.

131. **Sinyor, D., Schwarts, S. G., Peronnet, F., Brisson, G., and Seraganian, P.,** Aerobic fitness level and reactivity to psychosocial stress: physiological, biochemical, and subjective measures, *Psychosom. Med.,* 45, 205, 1983.

132. **Sinyor, D., Golden, M., Steiner, Y., and Seraganian, P.,** Experimental manipulation of aerobic fitness and the response to psychosocial stress: heart rate and self-report measures, *Psychosom. Med.,* 48, 324, 1986.

133. **Hull, E. M., Young, S. H., and Ziegler, M. G.,** Aerobic fitness affects cardiovascular and catecholamine responses to stressors, *Psychophysiology,* 21, 353, 1984.

134. **Brooke, S. T. and Long, B. C.,** Efficiency of coping with a real-life stressor: a multimodal comparison of aerobic fitness, *Psychophysiology,* 24, 173, 1987.

135. **Claytor, R. L., Cox, R. H., Howley, E. T., Lawler, K. A., and Lawler, J. E.,** Aerobic power and cardiovascular responses to stress, *J. Appl. Physiol.,* 65, 1416, 1988.

136. **Cantor, J. R., Zillmann, D., and Day, K. D.,** Relationship between cardiorespiratory fitness and physiological responses to films, *Percep. Mot. Skills,* 46, 1123, 1978.

137. **Sherwood, A., Light, K. C., and Blumenthal, J. A.,** Effects of aerobic exercise training on hemodynamic responses during psychosocial stress in normotensive and borderline hypertensive Type A men: a preliminary report, *Psychosom. Med.,* 51, 123, 1989.

138. **Holmes, D. S. and Roth, D. L.,** Effects of aerobic exercise training and relaxation training on cardiovascular activity during psychological stress, *J. Psychosom. Res.,* 32, 469, 1988.

139. **Gurley, K. R., Peacock, L. J., and Hill, D. W.,** The effect of a training program and induced cognitive stress on heart rate, blood pressure, and skin conductance, *J. Sports Med.,* 27, 318, 1987.

140. **Blumenthal, J. A.,** Response to Abbott and Peters, *Psychosom. Med.,* 51, 219, 1989.

141. **Dishman, R. K. and Landy, F. J.,** Psychological factors and prolonged exercise, in *Perspective in Exercise Science and Sports Medicine: Prolonged Exercise,* Lamb, D. R. and Murray, R., Eds., Benchmark Press, Indianapolis, IN, 1988.

142. **Kereszty, A.,** Overtraining, in *Encyclopedia of Sports Science and Medicine,* Larson, L. A. and Hermann, D. E., Eds., Macmillan, New York, 1971, 218.

143. **Mellerowicz, H. and Barron, D. K.,** Overtraining, in *Encyclopedia of Sports Science and Medicine,* Larson, L. A. and Hermann, D. E., Eds., Macmillan, New York, 1971, 1310.

144. **Wolf, J. G.,** Staleness, in *Encyclopedia of Sport Sciences and Medicine,* Larson, L. A., Ed., Macmillan, New York, 1971, 1048.

145. **Morgan, W. P., et al.,** Psychological monitoring of overtraining and staleness, *Br. J. Sports Med.,* 21, 107, 1987.

146. **Morgan, W. P., et al.,** Mood disturbance following increased training in swimmers, *Med. Sci. Sports Exercise,* 20, 408, 1988.

147. **Ryan, A. J., et al.,** Overtraining in athletes: a round table, *Phys. Sportsmed.,* 11, 92, 1983.

148. **O'Connor, P. J., et al.,** Mood state and salivary cortisol levels following overtraining in female swimmers, *Psychoneuroendocrinology,* 14, 303, 1989.

149. **Eskola, J., et al.,** Effect of sport stress on lymphocyte transformation and antibody formation, *Clin. Exp. Immun.,* 32, 339, 1978.

150. **Bateman, A., et al.,** The immune-hypothalamic-pituitary-adrenal axis, *Endocrine. Rev.,* 10, 92, 1989.

151. **Rabin, B. S., Cunnick, J. E., and Oysle, D. T.,** Stress-induced alteration of immune function, *Prog. Neuroendocrin. Immunol.,* 3, 116, 1990.

152. **Shavit, Y. and Martin, F. C.,** Opiates, stress, and immunity: animal studies, *Ann. Behav. Med.,* 91, 11, 198.

153. **Keast, D., Cameron, K., and Morton, A. R.,** Exercise and the immune response, *Sports Med.,* 5, 248, 1988.

154. **Luger, A., et al.,** Acute hypothalamic-pituitary-adrenal responses to the stress of treadmill exercise: physiologic adaptations to physical training, *N. Eng. J. Med.,* 316, 1309, 1987.

155. **Claytor, R. P., et al.,** Aerobic power and cardiovascular response to stress, *J. Appl. Physiol.,* 65, 1416, 1988.
156. **Barron, J. L., et al.,** Hypothalamic dysfunction in overtrained athletes, *J. Clin. Endocrin. Metabl.,* 60, 803, 1985.
157. **Krieger, D. T.,** Rhythms in CRFT, ACTH, and corticosteroids, in *Endocrine Rhythms,* Krieger, D. T., Ed., Raven Press, New York, 1979, 123.
158. **Meltzer, H. Y. and Lowy, M. T.,** Neuroendocrinine function in psychiatric disorders and behavior, in *American Handbook of Psychiatry,* Vol. 8, 2nd ed., Berger, P. A. and Brodie, H. K. H., Basic Books, New York, 1986, 111.
159. **Dishman, R. K.,** Medical psychology in exercise and sport, *Med. Clin. N. Am.,* 69, 123, 1985.
160. **Blumenthal, J. A., Rose, S., and Chang, J. L.,** Anorexia nervosa and exercise, *Sports Med.,* 2, 237, 1985.
161. **Morgan, W. P.,** Negative addition in runners, *Phys. Sportsmed.,* 7, 57, 1979.
162. **Dishman, R. K., et al.,** Psychological and behavioral effects of overtraining in healthy women: no evidence of health risk, submitted for publication.
163. **Rigsby, L., Dishman, R. K., Jackson, A. W., Maclean, G. S., and Raven, P. B.,** Effects of exercise training on men seropositive for the human immunodeficiency virus-1, *Med. Sci. Sports Exercise,* 24(1), 6, 1992.
164. **Lazarus, R. S.,** *Emotion and Adaptation,* Oxford University Press, Oxford, 1991.

INDEX

A

Accessory cell/T-cell interaction, age-associated deterioration of, 161–162
Acetylcholine, in depression, 183
Acquired immune deficiency syndrome
associated opportunistic infections and cancers of, 140
exercise by patients with, 139–143
with overtraining, 198–199
sports and, 141–142
Acquired immunity, types of, 73
ACTH, see Adrenocorticotrophic hormone
Activity limitations, all types, 67–68
Acute-phase proteins, 132
Acute-phase response, 131–132
Adhesins, response of to exercise training, 107
Adrenalin, see also Epinephrine
exercise-induced, 99
varied levels of with exercise, 107
Adrenergic activity, 193
Adrenocorticotrophic hormone
cortisol release and, 108
exercise-induced, 99
immunomodulatory properties of, 99
increase in with exercise, 188
Aerobic energy system, 94
Aerobic exercise
in AIDS patients, 142
alpha activity and, 191–192
in asthmatics, 98
beneficial effects of on disease prevention and rehabilitation, 160
cardio-protective effect of, 34
energy expenditure and, 18
functional capacity of cancer survivors and, 64
Aerobic fitness, stress reactivity and, 193–195
Aerobic threshold intensity, determination of, 28
Affective disorders, biological hypotheses of, 183–184
Aging
cell-mediated immunity and, 161–165
decline in immune function and, 160–172

AIDS, see Acquired immune deficiency syndrome
AIDS-related complex (ARC), 140, 198–199
Aldosterone, exercise-modified levels of, 108
α-2 autoinhibition, 188–189
Alpha-adrenergic antagonists, for exercise-induced asthma, 97
α_2-adrenergic receptors, increased density of on platelets with exercise, 186
Alpha brain activity, 191–192
American Cancer Society, exercise guidelines of, 68
American College of Sports Medicine (ACSM), 67, 181–183
Anaerobic energy system, 94
Anaphylatoxins, functions of, 151
Angina, as initial presentation of CHD in women, 12
Animal studies
of exercise effects on immunosenescence, 168–171
on long-term training and humoral immunity, 95–96
of lung tumors and exercise, 43–44
of physical activity and cancer link, 38, 41, 44, 52
Anorexia nervosa, among runners, 197
Anti-asialo GM_1, 46
Anti-cholinergics, for exercise-induced asthma, 97
Antidiuretic hormone, exercise-modified levels of, 108
Antigen presenting cell (APC), interleukin-1 production by, 100
Antigen processing, 91
Antineoplastic agents, effects of, 66
Anxiety
electroencephalographic study of, 191–193
HPA axis in, 186–189
prevalence of, 180
reasons for reduction of with exercise, 181
subjective feelings of, 192
Apolipoproteins, effect of physical activity on peripheral metabolism of, 30, 33